DIGESTIVE SYSTEM DISEASES AND DISORDERS

Also Available from
Bloomsbury Academic

The Geography of Disease: How Location and Culture Influence Health in Today's World
Jing Luo

Treatments for Anxiety: Fact versus Fiction
Myrna Chandler Goldstein and Mark A. Goldstein, MD

Prescription for Inequality: Exploring the Social Determinants of Health of At-Risk Groups
Jillian M. Duquaine-Watson

DIGESTIVE SYSTEM DISEASES AND DISORDERS

UNDERSTANDING SYMPTOMS AND TREATMENTS

Myrna Chandler Goldstein and Mark A. Goldstein, MD

BLOOMSBURY ACADEMIC
NEW YORK • LONDON • OXFORD • NEW DELHI • SYDNEY

BLOOMSBURY ACADEMIC
Bloomsbury Publishing Inc.1359 Broadway, 12th FloorNew York, NY 10018USA
Bloomsbury Publishing Plc, 50 Bedford Square, London, WC1B 3DP, UK

BLOOMSBURY, BLOOMSBURY ACADEMIC and the Diana logo are trademarks of Bloomsbury Publishing Plc

First published in the United States of America 2026

A catalog record for this book is available from the Library of Congress.

ISBN: HB: 979-8-7651-2197-9
ePDF: 979-8-7651-2199-3
eBook: 979-8-7651-2198-6

Typeset by Deanta Global Publishing Services, Chennai, India
Printed and bound in the United States of America

For product safety related questions contact productsafety@bloomsbury.com.

To find out more about our authors and books visit www.bloomsbury.com and sign up for our newsletters.

We would like to dedicate this book to our parents
Craig and Sarah Chandler
and
Samuel and Jeanne Goldstein
May their memory be a blessing

CONTENTS

ACKNOWLEDGMENTS

We would like to thank our editor, Maxine Taylor, who has edited most of our books. Tirelessly dedicated, Maxine had repeatedly offered excellent suggestions and advice.

PREFACE

When we initially proposed writing a book on gastrointestinal health, we submitted a list of potential entries to our editor, Maxine Taylor. It contained approximately fifty entries. After we actually began researching and writing the book, it soon became evident that the entries that would be included had to meet two main criteria. Obviously, they had to interest the widest number of people. But, they also had to have a reasonable amount of peer-reviewed published research. In the end, we were able to include thirty entries. A few entries were eliminated because they were rare illnesses that had very little published research. Others could not be included simply because of a lack of adequate space. Still, we hope that the majority of readers agree with the selections that we made.

Each of the entries in this book has a similar format. They all begin with an overall introduction to the medical problem. What is it? Is there a known cause? If so, the cause is explained. What are the subcategories? The introduction section ends with a little historical perspective. The next section addresses the symptoms, risks, and potential complications of the medical problem. Symptoms may include signs such as nausea, vomiting, constipation, fever, dizziness, weight loss, bloating, headache, pain, gas, anemia, abdominal distension, rashes, heartburn, and diarrhea. That is followed by risks, such as age, gender, and rural or urban residence. And, risks are followed by complications, such as dehydration and malnutrition. The next section addresses the prevalence. How common is this disorder? That section is followed by one on diagnosis and treatment. How do medical providers determine exactly what is wrong? What tests do they order? And, how will the medical problem be treated? The main body of each entry includes the presentation of a number of different relevant research studies. These address various approaches. Some are clearly more traditional, and others are complementary. Finally, every entry ends with the endnotes and a listing of further references.

It is our hope that each of the entries presents a comprehensive introduction to the medical problems discussed. At the very least, the entries should provide those newly diagnosed with a gastrointestinal problem the fundamental tools they require to continue their search to obtain the best medical care available.

Myrna Chandler Goldstein
Mark A. Goldstein, MD

INTRODUCTION

Even as a young girl, I remember my parents, grandparents, and other relatives distressing over various gastrointestinal problems. In fact, almost every one of my biological relatives had at least one gastrointestinal problem. Most seemed to have several. And, these problems were a frequent topic of discussion. Just about everyone had heartburn. In our family, calcium carbonate tablets or Tums® was eaten like candy. Men often carried them in their jackets and women had them in their purses. Another common malady was nausea. Of course, all too often, the nausea would trigger bouts of vomiting. For the nausea and vomiting, the treatment was bismuth subsalicylate or Pepto-Bismol®. Then, there was flatulence, usually called bloating. Even at a young age, I was quite aware that the adults in the room believed that certain foods had the potential to cause bloating. They would comment that they had to avoid this food or that food, such as fatty meats or cheesecake. And, while it was less frequently discussed, especially in mixed company, I was acutely aware that the adults suffered profoundly from their repeated bouts of constipation. These bouts often required the relief that only enemas could provide. In those days before disposable enemas were readily available, at least in the world in which I lived, those dreaded enemas were considered frightful medical interventions and greatly feared by me and my young friends. At the same time, we were very much aware of how much they were part of the daily lives of the older generations. Every relative and family friend I knew had a large rubber blue or red bag hanging from a hook on the top of the bathroom door and an elongated tube that ended with a slightly curved plastic white nozzle.

And, although it has been decades since I have seen an enema bag in a bathroom, it is still evident that people today continue to suffer from a host of different gastrointestinal concerns. Every day, in the United States and throughout the world, millions of people are forced to deal with gastrointestinal problems. Some, such as gastritis and dyspepsia, tend to be mild; with these, minor changes in lifestyle factors may be sufficient to quell the discomfort. Others, such as food poisoning and gastroenteritis, are quite debilitating, but fortunately usually last for relatively short periods of time. Still others, such as esophageal, liver, and stomach cancer, are potentially life-threatening. However, most of the gastrointestinal complaints seem to be chronic conditions that require adherence to a specialized diet and/or medications. Thus, people with celiac disease must permanently remove gluten—found in wheat, barley, rye, and sometimes oats, from their diets. And, that is not as easy as it may initially appear to be. Since people with celiac disease must eliminate even the tiniest amounts of gluten from their diets, they must also avoid the cross-contamination of gluten-containing products into their foods, something that may easily occur in a restaurant or group setting. Thus, if a utensil from a gluten-containing food is transferred to a gluten-free food, the gluten-free food may no longer be consumed by the person with celiac disease. People with celiac disease must also be vigilant about everything orally consumed, including medications and supplements. If they are careless, they may easily cause permanent damage to their bodies, which time may be unable to remedy. Though the consequences are not as serious, people with lactose intolerance also face daily challenges, especially if they are not careful label readers. Milk and other dairy products are found in a host of different items. Obviously, they are in milk and many creamers, cheeses, and yogurts. But, they may also be in cakes, breads, muffins, prepared soups, prepared foods, canned foods, desserts, frozen foods, breakfast foods, snacks, luncheon meats, as well as medications and supplements. Fortunately, people with lactose intolerance have the option of taking a lactase supplement before consuming the lactose-containing product. And, while people with lactose intolerance may be forced to deal with the discomforts of gas, their symptoms tend to pass over time.

If you are reading this book, there is a good chance that you or someone you care for has been dealing with gastrointestinal issues, probably for an extended period of time. In all likelihood, you have already searched the internet for answers to your many questions. And, there is a good chance your searching has triggered more questions rather than offered solutions. We hope that this book will finally provide you with the answers you need and desperately want and that it will serve as a guide to the restoration of your health and well-being.

ORGANS AND FUNCTIONS OF THE DIGESTIVE SYSTEM

Before beginning a discussion of the diseases and conditions that can affect the digestive system, it is important to understand the roles and functions of the various components of this system that are so integral to the maintenance of the human body. What are the specific organs and what exactly do they do?

Of course, the digestive system begins with the mouth, which is the home to the tongue, teeth, and gums. When food enters the mouth, it is chewed into smaller amounts by the teeth, which are anchored in the gums. The tongue, which secretes lingual lipase, also plays an integral role in the process. At the same time, the salivary glands secrete mucins and salivary amylase. Thus, begins the process of digestion.

From the mouth, it takes only a few seconds for the food to be propelled into the esophagus, which is about 10–13 inches in length in adults and about ¾ inch in width. Within a few more seconds, the esophagus moves the food along into the stomach, which is about the size of a fist but is greatly expandable. The stomach has a variety of functions. While in the stomach, food is mixed with stomach enzymes, such as pepsin, lipase, amylase, urease, as well as hydrochloric acid. This breaks down the food into smaller, more digestible amounts. Hydrochloric acid, in particular, destroys most of the microorganisms ingested with food, breaks down the plant cell walls, and denatures protein. The stomach also secretes an intrinsic factor that plays a role in the absorption of vitamin B12. The amount of time that food remains in the stomach varies according to the type of food. Simple carbohydrates like sugars and fruits remain in the stomach for thirty minutes to an hour; proteins and complex carbohydrates stay for one to two hours, and fats and complex carbohydrates remain for two to four hours. Eventually, food is expelled from the stomach into the small intestine, which is about twenty to 23 feet long and 1 inch wide.

The small intestine produces lipase for fat digestion, peptidase for protein breakdown, and sucrase, maltase, and lactase for the breakdown of sugar. It also absorbs electrolytes and water. It mixes the digesting food and propels it into the large intestine. Food stays in the small intestine for two to six hours. Meanwhile, several other organs make products that are absorbed into the small intestine. For example, the pancreas, which is a 6-inch, flat, elongated organ that lies behind the stomach and in front of the spine, produces the enzymes pancreatic trypsin for protein digestion, pancreatic amylase for carbohydrate digestion, and pancreatic lipase for fat digestion. The liver, which is a large organ about the size of a football and weighing about 3 pounds, is located in the upper right abdomen, produces bile salts that help to emulsify fat, enabling them to be digested by the body. Located under the liver, the gallbladder is a thin-walled, pear-shaped organ that is 2.7 to 3.9 inches long and up to 2 inches wide. The gallbladder stores the bile produced by the liver and contains bile salts. Bile empties into the duodenum of the small intestine. The appendix, which is located in the lower right abdomen where the small and large intestines connect, is a small worm-shaped pouch that is 3 or 4 inches long and ¼ inch wide. It is a reservoir for beneficial bacteria that restore the gut biome, and it may play a role in maintaining immunity. The digesting food passes from the small intestine into the large intestine, which is about 6 feet long and varies from 2 to about 3½ inches wide. The microbiome of the large intestine helps to break down undigested food, and it absorbs fluids and electrolytes. Undigested food is passed into the lower section of the large intestine, known as the rectum, and finally to the anus, where it is expelled from the body. This functioning of the entire digestive system generally takes between ten and fifty-nine hours, but times vary from person to person.

THE FUNCTIONS OF THE GASTROINTESTINAL SYMPTOM

Of course, the primary function of the gastrointestinal system is the breaking down of food into smaller amounts and the absorption of the nutrients of these foods into the body. It is well known that bacteria help with this crucial function. But, the gastrointestinal system is also the site of a good deal of the body's immune system and, because of the connection to the brain ("the gut-brain axis"), a source of mental health and overall well-being.

Immunity and the Gut

The microbiome is a complex system involved in the growth and proliferation of immune cells that help to support the intestine. The human gut microbiome is composed of more than 1,500 types of microorganisms, including bacteria, fungi, viruses, and protozoa that fight infectious diseases. The microorganisms in the microbiome produce metabolites that interact with human cells and may influence the immune response. It has been shown that disorders that cause changes in the microbiome may lead to imbalances in human immune regulation. For example, inflammatory bowel diseases, such as ulcerative colitis and Crohn's disease, are associated with an imbalance of the microorganisms found in the microbiome. Other diseases associated with these changes include rheumatoid arthritis, lupus, and psoriasis. In addition, through physical barriers such as mucous and cells, the gut protects us from infections. The microbiome may produce antiviral proteins that help to eliminate viral infections.

Gut-Brain Axis

Also known as the gut-brain connection, the gut-brain axis describes the interrelationship between the gastrointestinal system and the brain and the entire body. Communicating with different organs, the microbiome helps to regulate brain and body activity. For example, the central nervous system and the gut communicate through hormones, chemicals, and other routes. If the gut microbiome is altered, this may lead to symptoms such as migraine headaches. Other symptoms and responses include signaling for hunger, satiety, food cravings, sensitivities, intolerances, gut motility, digestion, mood, behavior, stress levels, pain sensitivity, cognitive function, and immunity.

UNDERSTANDING COMMON GASTROINTESTINAL SYMPTOMS

In all probability, you have reached for this book because you are dealing with at least one ongoing common gastrointestinal symptom. And there are a number of different possibilities. These include abdominal pain, belching, bloating, flatulence, constipation and defecation problems, diarrhea, fecal incontinence, and nausea and vomiting. These symptoms may be benign and of little concern, especially when they occur only briefly and occasionally, or they may be a sign of a more serious underlying medical condition. And, while you may have your own personal definition for each of these symptoms, they actually all have a precise medical definition.

ABDOMINAL PAIN

Abdominal pain, or stomach pain, is pain that is felt anywhere between the chest and the groin. At some point, just about everyone has felt abdominal pain. It is probably one of the most frequent gastrointestinal problems. Yet, the seriousness of the precipitating condition is not necessarily related to the degree of pain. People may feel strong pain with benign conditions, and there may be essentially no pain with a life-threatening medical problem. Thus, gas, which is benign, may be quite painful, while early colorectal or esophageal cancer may cause no pain or even mild discomfort. Most people tend to ignore benign abdominal pain. However, if it persists over time, it should definitely be discussed with a medical provider, who may well recommend a few imaging tests, such as a CT scan, to check for any abnormalities.

BELCHING, BLOATING, AND FLATULENCE

A normal process, belching is caused by swallowed air that accumulates in the stomach. The air may either be sent back up (belched) or passed into the intestines where it may be released as rectal gas. Bloating is the feeling of fullness in the upper abdomen. It is caused by food accumulating in the stomach and/or gas. Flatulence is the passage of rectal gas. It is caused by swallowing air and the action of colon bacteria on undigested carbohydrates. Everyone has experienced rectal gas. For some, it is an occasional discomfort; for others, it is a daily occurrence. Sometimes, persistent gas is a symptom of a food intolerance. It may be useful to keep a food diary to see if there is any correlation between the consumption of certain foods or food groups and gas. For example, people with a dairy intolerance often have gas when they consume dairy products. And, people with the autoimmune disease known as celiac disease may well have excess gas when they consume foods with gluten. (See the entry on celiac disease.)

CONSTIPATION AND DEFECATION PROBLEMS

A very common gastrointestinal complaint, it has been estimated that there are at least 2.5 million physician visits every year for constipation. That figure is probably a serious underestimate. Many people with constipation are too uncomfortable or embarrassed to mention it to their medical providers. It is known that people spend hundreds of millions of dollars every year for laxatives and other constipation-relieving medications. In contrast to the prevailing misconception, constipation is not the number of bowel movements a person passes in a single day. Rather, it refers to the incomplete emptying of the bowels, straining to have a bowel movement, or the elimination of hard stools. So, a person may actually have several bowel movements and, if the evacuation is incomplete, may still feel constipated. Constipation most often occurs when stool moves slowly through the digestive tract. This may be caused by decreases in water consumption, changes in the diet, reductions in physical activity, a sluggish gut, and/or certain medications. When stool moves slowly through the digestive track, too much water is absorbed, and it becomes hard and dry. Of course, constipation may be caused by a bowel obstruction. But, fortunately, that is a far less frequent cause. An occasional bout of constipation should generally be of no concern. It may well be caused by eating too many constipation-causing foods, such as white rice and bananas, and too little fluid. Chronic constipation may be a symptom of an underlying problem and should be discussed with a medical provider.

DIARRHEA

Diarrhea, which may be acute, persistent, or chronic, is the presence of loose, watery stools that occur three or more times on the same day. Acute diarrhea is more common than persistent or chronic diarrhea, and diarrhea may result in the malabsorption of nutrients or dehydration. The causes of diarrhea include infections, food allergies or intolerances, celiac disease, digestive tract problems, and the side effects of certain medications. An occasional bout of diarrhea is most likely no reason for concern and may well be caused by a virus or dietary changes. However, persistent diarrhea should be investigated further by a medical provider.

FECAL INCONTINENCE

Also known as accidental bowel leakage, fecal incontinence is the uncontrolled passage of solid or liquid stool from the anus. It is the inability to control stool from leaking from the anus. While most people are aware of this loss of control, in some instances, people are unaware of the leakage. Fecal incontinence may range from the occasional leakage of tiny or small amounts of stool to the complete loss of control. Among the causes of fecal incontinence are digestive tract disorders, chronic diseases, diarrhea, constipation, and muscle or nerve damage, which may be associated with aging or giving birth. While an occasional bout of fecal incontinence is probably more of a psychological than physical concern, repeated or persistent fecal incontinence should always be discussed with a medical provider and investigated further. Medications, biofeedback, and/or sessions with a specially trained physical therapist may be useful.

NAUSEA AND VOMITING

Nausea is an uncomfortable feeling in the back of the throat or an uneasiness in the stomach. It frequently appears with dizziness and lightheadedness, as well as problems with swallowing and a feeling that one needs to vomit. But, nausea does not always lead to vomiting or the forcible emptying of the contents of the stomach. For some, nausea is an occasional problem; for others, it is a daily concern. It may also be a symptom of a medical problem, such as a gastroenteritis flu, or a medical condition, such as pregnancy. As with other symptoms, an occasional bout of nausea or vomiting is probably of little or no concern. Still, persistent nausea and vomiting should always be discussed with a medical provider who will order tests, such as an upper endoscopy. During this procedure, a thin tube is inserted into the throat, esophagus, and stomach. A medical provider is able to determine if the condition is functional or without a biological basis or is actually caused by a medical condition, such as gastroparesis, that needs to be addressed. (See entry on gastroparesis.)

APPENDICITIS

INTRODUCTION

Appendicitis is the inflammation of the appendix, a finger-shaped pouch located in the cecum at the intersection of the small and large intestines, on the lower right side of the abdomen. The appendix actually has a purpose, as it plays a role in the immune system.

Most likely, appendicitis is caused by an obstruction in the lining of the appendiceal lumen. A frequent source of this blockage is stool, but in adults, it can also be due to cancer or fibrosis. The blockage may, in turn, cause distention, tissue destruction, and infection. An infection can lead to the appendix becoming inflamed, swollen, and filled with pus. If not treated quickly, within a few days, the appendix may burst open and spread pus throughout the abdomen, a true medical emergency.

There are two types of appendicitis—acute and chronic. In the vast majority of cases, appendicitis is acute. The condition begins suddenly and worsens quickly. On the other hand, chronic appendicitis is considered a rare medical problem. It occurs when something periodically irritates the appendix, but the condition mostly remains stable. Chronic appendicitis may continue for an indefinite period of time, or it may worsen, become acute, and require treatment.

The first successful appendectomy was performed in 1735 by Charles Amyand, MD, at St. George's Hospital in London. The patient was an eleven-year-old boy whose appendix had become perforated. It is important to note that this operation was performed many decades before the availability of general anesthesia.[1]

SYMPTOMS, RISKS, AND COMPLICATIONS

Appendicitis causes pain around the umbilicus, which then moves to the lower right section of the abdomen. As the inflammation worsens, this pain increases markedly. The pain worsens when coughing, moving, taking deep breaths, sneezing, walking, or making jarring movements. Other symptoms include nausea and vomiting, upset stomach, loss of appetite, fever and chills, constipation or diarrhea, intense need to urinate, bloating, and gas. However, children, the elderly, and pregnant women are less likely to have these common symptoms.

Although anyone may develop appendicitis, it most often occurs in people between the ages of ten and thirty. Men have a slightly higher risk than women. Having a family history of appendicitis does appear to increase the risk.

Appendicitis has the potential to cause serious complications, such as a ruptured appendix, which may spread the infection throughout the abdomen, a condition called peritonitis. Because peritonitis may be life-threatening, it requires immediate surgery to remove the appendix. Intravenous antibiotics are an integral part of the treatment. In addition, when an appendix bursts, a pocket of infection, called an abscess, may develop. Normally, this requires a surgeon to place a tube through the abdominal wall into the abscess, enabling it to drain. This tube remains in place for about two weeks; antibiotics are prescribed. And, the appendix is surgically removed. Often, appendicitis complications may be treated during surgery, but these may require open abdominal surgery. Recovery from a laparoscopic appendectomy should be fairly quick; recovery from an open abdominal procedure takes longer.

PREVALENCE

Acute appendicitis is considered a common medical problem. In children, it occurs most often during the teenage years, but younger children may also be affected. In the United States, about 5 percent of the population will have an attack of acute appendicitis. It is the leading cause of abdominal pain that results in emergency abdominal surgery. Although far less is known about chronic appendicitis, it has been estimated that chronic appendicitis affects about 1 percent of the US population. Worldwide, an appendectomy, or the surgical removal of the appendix, is one of the most frequently performed surgical procedures.

DIAGNOSIS AND TREATMENTS OPTIONS

Healthcare providers diagnose appendicitis from the symptoms described by the patient and a physical examination. If necessary, a few tests may be ordered. These include a blood test that may show signs of inflammation, such as a high white blood cell count and a high C-reactive protein count. Generally, the imaging test used is the computerized tomography or CT scan, which provides X-ray images of the abdomen and a swollen appendix. When a CT is not available or the patient is concerned about radiation to the area, an abdominal ultrasound, which shows images of the abdomen, may be used. In addition, for pregnant women and those concerned about radiation, a magnetic resonance imaging or MRI scan, which uses a giant magnet to show images of the abdomen, may be used instead of a CT scan.

Treatment of appendicitis almost always includes antibiotics. Very frequently, surgery is performed to remove the appendix. Often, surgery will be combined with antibiotics. In certain cases, antibiotics alone may be sufficient, and surgery may not be needed or may be postponed. However, because appendicitis may reoccur, as it does in about 40 percent of the cases, healthcare providers tend to recommend surgery. Once the appendix is removed, there is no chance for another attack of appendicitis. The appendix never regrows. Following surgery, patients are given medication for pain relief.

RESEARCH FINDINGS

There May Be an Association between Some Aspects of Dietary Intake and Childhood Appendicitis

In a study published in the *International Journal of Food Sciences and Nutrition*, researchers from Greece examined the association between the intake of fiber and childhood appendicitis. The cohort consisted of 203 consecutive cases of children who had an appendectomy—121 boys and 82 girls with a mean age of nine years—and 1,922 healthy controls—1,011 boys and 911 girls with a mean age of eight years. All of the cases of appendicitis were histologically confirmed. Data for the cases and controls were collected during the same time period. On the second postoperative day, a researcher interviewed parents and children about their usual diet during the previous twelve months. Questions were asked about food frequency and quantity of seventy-two simple food items and food groups, and inquiries were made about abdominal pain and chronic constipation. Other questions addressed body weight, height, socioeconomic data, the child's and family's medical history, and appendectomy surgery in other family members. The researchers learned that the children with appendicitis consistently ate diets that were lower in fiber, and they had more recurrent abdominal pain and chronic constipation than the controls. Thirteen percent of the children who had an appendectomy and 5 percent of the controls had fewer than three bowel movements per week. A positive family history of appendectomy was found in 6.4 percent of the cases and 1.5 percent of the controls. At the same time, there was no statistical correlation between acute appendicitis and energy, protein, carbohydrate, and fat intake. The researchers concluded that a low-fiber intake could play a role in the pathophysiology of appendicitis. "This study gives evidence that low-fiber intake could play an important role in the pathogenesis of appendicitis."[2]

In a hospital-based, case-control study published in the *American Journal of Public Health*, researchers from Seattle, Washington, evaluated the association between fiber intake in children and the risk of appendicitis. The cohort consisted of 135 children who had appendicitis and 256 comparison children. The children and their parents were residents of Washington State, and all of the children were white. The comparison children were chosen from the orthopedic service and short stay unit of the same hospital. They were matched to the children with appendicitis by age, sex, and admission date. Telephone interviews were conducted with a parent of each of the children about the child's intake of whole grain breads and cereals, fruits, vegetables, legumes, nuts, and seeds. Monthly total fiber and whole grain bread and cereal intake scores were calculated. The researchers found that the children with higher intakes of fiber had lower rates of appendicitis, "but the effect was modest and reasonably consistent with chance departure from no actual trend." The researchers noted that age might affect the data. Thus, the higher intake of bran for children between the ages of seven and eighteen was associated with lower rates of appendicitis. But, this association did not exist for children six years and younger. Still, these results could also have been caused by chance alone. In addition, since the information on the diet was obtained from a parent, the researchers wondered if it was not entirely accurate, especially for the older children who may be eating at least some of their food away from home. Still, the researchers concluded "that a liberal intake of whole grain breads and cereals may decrease the risk of appendicitis during childhood."[3]

In a trial published in the *Journal of Epidemiology and Community Health*, researchers from the UK studied the association between diets and appendicitis. The cohort consisted of fifty-three adolescents—thirty-four males and nineteen females—who had appendicitis followed by emergency surgery and two sets of age- and sex-matched controls, who had not had appendicitis. The teens were between the ages of thirteen and fifteen. One set of the controls included classmates of the students; the other was a random sample of all schoolchildren in the city. With the help of the parents, diets were measured with a seven-day weighed food record. The heights and weights of each teen were determined. The researchers learned that the adolescents with appendicitis weighed less and were shorter in height; they had lower intakes of energy, protein, fat, carbohydrate, fiber, and water. The differences in weight and water intake were statistically significant. Low water intake was identified as a risk factor for appendicitis, and it was independent of other risk factors. But, fiber intake had no independent effect on appendicitis.[4]

Certain Environmental Factors Appear to Increase the Risk of Acute Appendicitis

In an observational study published in the journal *Heliyon*, researchers from Belgium and the Netherlands examined environmental factors that may play a role in acute appendicitis. The cohort consisted of 374 patients who had cases of acute appendicitis and 513 healthy controls, who were mostly university students. Patients and controls completed questionnaires with questions about demographics, lifestyle characteristics, such as diet and smoking, and environmental exposures. Compared to the controls, the patients were more likely to be male and a few years older, 32.8 versus 28.3 years. Patients tended to live with family or communities and in rural areas, while the controls were more often single and living in urban areas, such as student housing. A notable 55.8 percent of the patients had a family history of acute appendicitis; only 6.7 percent of the controls had such a family history. Patients were breastfed significantly less than controls, 69.1 percent versus 85.3 percent, and those who were, were breastfed for shorter periods of time. Patients consumed significantly less fruit and fiber-rich vegetables, more sugar-containing drinks, had less education, used more antibiotics and probiotics, and were more often smokers. The researchers determined that the family history was the most important risk factor for appendicitis. Patients with more complicated cases of appendicitis tended to be male. They were older, 37.3 versus 30.8 years, and they more often lived in rural areas, 50.6 versus 35.7 percent. These patients tended to have contact with farm animals during their youth, and they waited longer before going to the hospital, 5.3 versus 2.6 days. The researchers concluded that "lifestyle and environment may affect the risk of developing acute appendicitis, and to a lesser extent the severity of the disease. It may be beneficial to take these factors into account in future research into the etiology of acute appendicitis."[5]

Appendicitis May Be a Complication of a Colonoscopy

In a study published in *JAMA Surgery*, researchers from North Dakota compared the risk of developing appendicitis during the first week after a colonoscopy to the risk of developing appendicitis during the following fifty-one weeks. Their cohort consisted of 392,485 veterans from the US Department of Veterans Affairs Administration who had a colonoscopy during a five-year period of time. Using this data, the researchers compared the incidence rate ratio for appendicitis or appendectomy during the first week after a colonoscopy to the incidence rate during the remaining weeks. They learned that the incidence rates occurred more often during that first week than the remaining fifty-one weeks. By contrast, this increase was not seen in the same cohort after a bronchoscopy, knee replacement procedure, cataract surgery, or knee arthroscopy. According to the researchers, their findings "suggest that undergoing a colonoscopy predisposes patients to appendicitis within one week." Still, "the mechanism of this effect awaits elucidation."[6]

A Child's Age May Affect the Management and Outcome of Pediatric Appendicitis

In a retrospective review published in the *Journal of Pediatric Surgery*, researchers from California examined the association between the age of children diagnosed with appendicitis and the management and outcome of the illness. The cohort consisted of 5,894 patients, with a median age of 10.3 years, who were treated for appendicitis over a ten-year period of time. Sixty-one percent were boys. Study outcomes included thirty-day postoperative morbidity, the use of laparoscopy, and the length of hospitalization. Postoperative morbidity included rates of wound infection, postoperative abscess drainage, and readmission. Patients were categorized into three age groups—young (five years or younger), middle (six to nine years), and older (ten years or older). No one was over the age of fourteen years. The researchers learned that the perforation rate was highest for the patients who were young and lowest for those who were older, 51 percent versus 27 percent. The perforation rate for the group of middle children was 32 percent. The need for postoperative abscess drainage was greatest in the older children, but the readmission rate and length of hospitalization were highest in the young children. Laparoscopic appendectomy was used the least often in the young children, who most frequently had nonoperative management. Wound infection rates were similar in all three groups. As might be expected, perforated appendicitis significantly increased the risk of wound infection, postoperative abscess drainage, readmission, and length of hospitalization. The researchers concluded that their findings may be useful, "as little data exist regarding outcomes of pediatric appendicitis based on age."[7]

There Seems to Be an Association between Socioeconomic Status and Appendiceal Perforation in Childhood Appendicitis

In a study published in the *Journal of Pediatrics*, researchers from Houston, Texas, evaluated the association of socioeconomic status and appendiceal perforation in childhood appendicitis. The cohort consisted of 1,501 patients under the age of eighteen years who had an appendectomy for acute appendicitis over a four-year period of time. Five hundred and ten of these patients, or 34 percent, had perforated appendicitis. The researchers learned that there was an association between rates of perforated appendicitis and lower household income, lower percentage of adults with a college education, and a higher percentage of adults with less than a twelfth-grade education. Children younger than ten years and those without insurance or on public insurance also had an increased risk. In fact, younger age and public insurance were stronger predictors of appendiceal perforation than socioeconomic status.[8]

Certain Factors Appear to Increase the Risk of a Complicated Case of Appendicitis

In a multicenter, case-control study published in the journal *Surgery in Practice and Science*, researchers from eastern Ethiopia wanted to determine what factors increased the risk for a complicated case of appendicitis. The cohort consisted of 402 patients; there were 134 complicated cases of appendicitis and 268 cases of simple appendicitis. The vast majority, 278 patients, were between the ages of eleven and thirty years; 246 were from urban areas, and the remainder were from rural areas. Patients with complicated cases of appendicitis tended to have visited other primary healthcare centers and private clinics that did not have surgical experts and facilities. In addition, patients with complicated cases had a history of constipation, and they waited longer before coming for treatment. Those who waited thirty-six to seventy-two hours before coming to the hospital had a 3.2 increased odds of complicated appendicitis, and those who waited more than seventy-two hours had an 8.5 increased odds of a complicated case. "The longer time interval between intervention and onset of pain, the more likelihood of ending up with complicated appendicitis."[9]

People with Disabilities Are More Likely to Have Complicated Cases of Appendicitis

In a study published in the journal *Frontiers in Public Health*, researchers from South Korea and Boston, Massachusetts compared the rates of complicated appendicitis between people with different levels of disability and people without disability. The cohort consisted of 310,833 men and 300,174 women without a disability and 21,990 men and 14,071 women with a disability. Patients with a disability and appendicitis were slightly older than those without a disability, and those with a disability had a lower economic status. The proportion of patients with medical aid was higher in the disabled group, but the people with a disability were more than twice as likely to have a complicated case of appendicitis than those without a disability. "Accessing medical facilities is more difficult for disabled than non-disabled due to physical and transportation problems; this leads to late diagnosis or treatment of appendicitis, which in turn increases the likelihood of complicated appendicitis developing." In addition, people with disabilities may also have a harder time dealing with the financial costs associated with medical care. And, these problems may be particularly challenging for those with severe disabilities or mental disabilities.[10]

Both Surgery and Antibiotics Seem to Be Useful for Many Adults with Appendicitis

In a nonblinded, randomized trial published in the *New England Journal of Medicine*, researchers based in Seattle, Washington, compared the treatment of appendicitis with a ten-day course of antibiotics to treatment with surgery. The cohort consisted of 1,552 adults with appendicitis from twenty-five different medical locations in the United States; 414 of these patients had an appendicolith or a small, hard deposit in the appendix. The patients were assigned to one of two groups: 776 received antibiotics and 776 had an appendectomy. The two groups of patients had similar demographic characteristics.

Patients in the antibiotics group received an intravenous formulation for at least twenty-four hours, followed by oral antibiotics, for an overall ten-day course of therapy. In the patients assigned to the appendectomy group, both laparoscopic and conventional surgical approaches were allowed. The usual preoperative and postoperative care were followed. Adherence to the treatment was 90 percent in the antibiotics group and more than 99 percent in the appendectomy group. Complications were more common in the antibiotics group than in the appendectomy group. After thirty days and again after ninety days, both groups had similar outcomes. While some of the patients in the antibiotics group eventually required trips to the emergency department and/or an appendectomy, many recovered completely, and they and their caregivers missed less time from work and required less hospitalization. The researchers noted that their findings were consistent with the "noninferiority" of the antibiotics, at least in the short term.[11]

The Nonoperative Management of Appendicitis in High-Risk Patients Has an Advantage but Also Potential Problems

In a retrospective cohort study published in the journal *Surgery*, researchers from several locations in the United States but based in Dallas, Texas, wanted to learn if patients with preexisting medical problems would be at a higher risk for complications if the condition was managed medically instead of surgically. The cohort consisted of 21,242 high-risk patients with a median age of sixty-eight years. They were 42 percent female, 68 percent white, and 59 percent had four or more comorbidities. Thirty-one percent of the patients were managed medically, and 69 percent were managed with surgery. Compared with the operative group, nonoperative management was associated with a 9 percent absolute decrease in morbidity. The primary reason for the difference in morbidity was a higher incidence of gastrointestinal complications. However, the nonoperative management was associated with a 2 percent increase in mortality, higher patient costs, and a greater likelihood of discharge to a skilled facility. As a result, the researchers commented that "nonoperative management is not a panacea for avoiding risks in patients who might not be the ideal surgical candidates. . . . Surgeons should exercise caution when considering nonoperative management in these vulnerable patients."[12]

Seven Years after an Attack of Uncomplicated Acute Appendicitis, Patients Were More Satisfied with Some Treatments than Others

In a randomized clinical trial published in *JAMA Surgery*, researchers from several different locations in Finland compared the long-term levels of satisfaction of patients who were treated for uncomplicated acute appendicitis with antibiotics or an appendectomy. The initial cohort consisted of 530 patients; there were 257 in the antibiotics group and 273 in the appendectomy group. The antibiotics group had a median age of thirty-three years, and the appendectomy group had a median age of thirty-five years. After seven years, 423 patients were available for a telephone interview; 206 patients had taken antibiotics and 217 had an appendectomy. Patients who had an appendectomy were more satisfied with their treatment than patients taking antibiotics. That may have been because eighty-one patients taking antibiotics had to have a subsequent appendectomy. However, those patients who had a successful experience with antibiotics had the same levels of satisfaction as the patients who had an appendectomy. "Patients with appendectomy or with successful antibiotic therapy were more satisfied than antibiotic group patients who later underwent appendectomy."[13]

For Children with Acute, Uncomplicated Appendicitis, Surgery Seems to Be a Better Option than Antibiotics

In a multicenter, parallel group, open-label, randomized trial published in the journal *Lancet*, researchers from many locations and countries but based in Kansas City, Missouri, compared the surgical and nonsurgical treatments of acute uncomplicated appendicitis in children aged five to sixteen years. Between January 20, 2016, and December 3, 2021, 936 patients were enrolled and assigned to either an appendectomy or antibiotics; there were 459 in the appendectomy group and 477 in the antibiotics group. At the twelve-month follow-up, primary outcome data were available for 846 (90 percent) of the patients. While treatment failure occurred in 153 (34 percent) of the 452 patients in the antibiotic group, treatment failure occurred in only twenty-eight (7 percent) of the 394 patients in the appendectomy group. There were no deaths or serious adverse events in either group.

During the initial hospitalization, the median length of stay for the appendectomy group was one to zero days compared to one to twenty-five days for the antibiotic group. Patients in the antibiotic group also spent more total time in the hospital during the twelve-month follow-up period, with a median of one to six days compared to zero to one day for the appendectomy group. On the other hand, the patients in the antibiotic group returned to school and activities sooner than the appendectomy patients, and, unlike the appendectomy patients, they tended not to require pain medication. Seventy-three percent of the families in both groups were satisfied with their treatment. Families in the antibiotic group were satisfied that they avoided surgery, and those in the appendectomy group were satisfied that the surgery was effective and the appendicitis could not recur. According to the researchers, their findings determined that "antibiotic treatment for uncomplicated appendicitis in children was inferior to appendectomy."[14]

Acute Appendicitis May Be Caused by a Slowed Colon Transit Time and a Trapped Foreign Object in the Appendix

In a case report published in the *Middle East Journal of Digestive Diseases*, researchers from Iran described the case of a patient who appeared to develop appendicitis as a complication of constipation caused by slowed transit time and a trapped foreign object. The patient was a forty-five-year old male who was referred to a colorectal research clinic in southern Iran. He had been dealing with chronic constipation for many years. To evaluate colon motility, the researchers ordered a colon transit time study, and the man was diagnosed with "colon inertia." He was treated with "medical management." One month later, the man arrived at the hospital's emergency department with abdominal pain. Soon, he was evaluated and admitted to the hospital's surgery department to rule out appendicitis. After further testing, he was found to have appendicitis caused by the foreign body ingestion of radio-opaque markers, and an appendectomy was performed. The researchers commented that "the position of the appendix and its wide orifice can be a threatening factor for trapping the markers."[15]

There May Be an Association between Gastroesophageal Reflux Disease and Appendicitis and Appendectomy

In a population-based, case-control study published in *Scientific Reports*, researchers from Taiwan investigated the association between gastroesophageal reflux disease (GERD) and appendicitis. Using administrative claims data from the Taiwan Longitudinal Health Insurance Database, the cohort consisted of 7,113 patients with appendicitis and 28,452 matched patients without appendicitis. The two groups of patients had a mean age of 41.3 years. While the groups were matched for gender, age, and index year, there were significant differences in monthly income and geographic regions. The researchers determined that 359 (5.05 percent) of the patients with appendicitis had GERD and 728 (2.56 percent) of those without had GERD. In all of the age groups, appendicitis was associated with prior GERD; patients with appendicitis were 2.05 times more likely to be diagnosed with prior GERD than those without appendicitis. Yet, "the actual mechanisms of the association between GERD and appendicitis still remain unclear." Nevertheless, the researchers concluded that "physicians should notice the association between GERD and appendicitis and be alert in suspecting appendicitis for abdominal pain in patients with a medical history of GERD."[16]

In a study published in the journal *Medicine*, researchers from Korea examined the association between GERD and the risk of an appendectomy. Using data from the Korean National Health Insurance Service—National Sample Cohort, the cohort consisted of 13,484 patients who had an appendectomy; they were matched to 53,936 controls for age, sex, income, region of residence, and histories of hypertension, diabetes, and dyslipidemia. The appendectomy group had higher rates of ischemic heart disease, cerebral stroke, and depression. When the researchers determined the numbers of people in each group who had GERD, they found that 11.4 percent of those in the appendectomy group had GERD, while the number in the control group was 8.2 percent. And, these results were observed for all age groups and in both males and females.[17]

REFERENCES AND FURTHER READING

Adamidis, D., E. Roma-Giannikou, K. Karamolegou et al. "Fiber Intake and Childhood Appendicitis." *International Journal of Food Sciences and Nutrition* 51 (2000): 153–157.

Basson, Marc D., Daniel Persinger, and William P. Newman. "Association of Colonoscopy with Risk of Appendicitis." *JAMA Surgery* 153, no. 1 (January 1, 2018): 90–91.

Bayissa, Badhaasaa Beyene, Pufa Miressa, Adnan Abulkadir, and Gelana Fekadu. "Predictors of Complicated Appendicitis Among Patients Presented to Public Referral Hospitals in Harari, Eastern Ethiopia: A Case-Control Study." *Surgery in Practice and Science* 9 (2022): 100072.

Brender, Jean D., Noel S. Weiss, Thomas D. Koepsell, and Edgar K. Marcuse. "Fiber Intake and Childhood Appendicitis." *American Journal of Public Health* 75, no. 4 (1985): 399–400.

Flum, D. R., G. H. Davidson, S. E. Monsell et al. "A Randomized Trial Comparing Antibiotics with Appendectomy for Appendicitis." *New England Journal of Medicine* 383, no. 20 (November 12, 2020): 1907–1919.

Ghahramani, Leila, Reza Roshanravan, Shahin Khodaei et al. "Acute Appendicitis as Complication of Colon Transit Time Study: A Case Report." *Middle East Journal of Digestive Diseases* 7, no. 3 (July 2015): 185–188.

Kao, Li-Ting, Ming-Chieh Tsai, Herng-Ching, and Cha-Ze Lee. "Association Between Gastroesophageal Reflux Disease and Appendicitis: A Population-Based Case-Control Study." *Scientific Reports* 6, no. 1 (March 2016): 22430.

Kim, So Young, Hyung-Jong Kim, Hyun Lim et al. "Increased Risk of Appendectomy in Patients with Gastroesophageal Reflux Disease." *Medicine* 97, no. 52 (2018): e13700.

Lee, Steven L., Rebecca Stark, Arezou Yaghoubian et al. "Does Age Affect the Outcomes and Management of Pediatric Appendicitis?" *Journal of Pediatric Surgery* 46 (2011): 2342–2345.

Lunardi, Nicole, Melissa Thornton, Ben L. Zarzaur et al. "Potential Risks of Nonoperative Management of Appendicitis in High-Risk Patients." *Surgery* 176, no. 6 (December 2024): 1568–1575.

Nelson, M., J. Morris, D. J. P. Barker, and S. Simmonds. "A Case-Control Study of Acute Appendicitis and Diet in Children." *Journal of Epidemiology and Community Health* 41 (1986): 316–318.

Peeters, Toon, Bert Houben, Peter Cools et al. "An Observational Study on Lifestyle and Environmental Risk Factors in Patients with Acute Appendicitis." *Heliyon* 9 (2023): e15131.

Putnam, Luke R., KuoJen Tsao, Hoang T. Nguyen et al. "The Impact of Socioeconomic Status on Appendiceal Perforation in Pediatric Appendicitis." *Journal of Pediatrics* 170 (March 2016): 156–160.e1.

St. Peter, Shawn D., Janelle R. Noel-MacDonnell, Nigel J. Hall et al. "Appendectomy versus Antibiotics for Acute Uncomplicated Appendicitis in Children: An Open-Label, International, Multicentre, Randomised, Non-Inferiority Trial." *Lancet* 405, no. 10474 (January 2025): 233–240.

Sippola, Suvi, Jussi Haijanen, Lauri Viinikainen et al. "Quality of Life and Patient Satisfaction at Seven-Year Follow-Up of Antibiotics Therapy vs Appendectomy for Uncomplicated Acute Appendicitis." *JAMA Surgery* 155, no. 4 (February 19, 2020): 283–289.

Yeob, K. E., S. Y. Kim, J. E. Park, and J. H. Park. "Complicated Appendicitis Among Adults with and Without Disabilities: A Cross-Sectional Nationwide Study in South Korea." *Frontiers in Public Health* 10 (2022): 813608.

BARRETT'S ESOPHAGUS

INTRODUCTION

With Barrett's esophagus, there is a change in the cellular structure of the lining of the lower end of the esophagus, the flexible tube that carries food from the mouth to the stomach. If something irritates the lining of the esophagus for a long period of time, it may damage the tissues and reprogram the cells. These changes alter the structure and appearance of the esophageal lining. Instead of looking like the lining of the esophagus, which should be white, it looks more similar to the lining of the intestines, which is a salmon-pink color. This is termed "internal metaphsia." Barrett's esophagus tends to occur in people with chronic, untreated gastrointestinal reflux disease (GERD). But, not everyone fits this profile. While it is a risk factor for cancer, treating the underlying condition may help prevent Barrett's esophagus from progressing to esophageal cancer.

There are two main types of Barrett's esophagus. In short-segment Barrett's esophagus, the affected area is less than 3-centimeter long; in long-segment Barrett's esophagus, the affected area is longer than 3 centimeter. There are also different stages of Barrett's esophagus. With non-dysplastic (abnormal cell) metaplasia, there is no dysplasia and a low risk of cancer; with metaplasia with low-grade dysplasia, there is some dysplasia and cancer risk. With metaplasia with high-grade dysplasia, there is significant dysplasia and cancer risk, and with carcinoma, the dysplasia has progressed to cancer.

According to an article in the journal *American Family Physician*, Barrett's esophagus was first referenced in 1950 by Norman Barrett, a thoracic surgeon. It was then that he described a case of chronic peptic ulcer in the lower esophagus that was covered by the epithelium.[1]

SYMPTOMS, RISKS, AND COMPLICATIONS

While Barrett's esophagus does not cause specific symptoms, and many do not experience any related symptoms, people with this medical problem often have the more notable symptoms associated with GERD. These include heartburn, indigestion, chest pain, sore throat, blood in the vomit or stool, difficulty swallowing foods, especially solid foods, and nocturnal regurgitation.

Some people are at an increased risk for Barrett's esophagus. These include people assigned male at birth, people who are older than fifty or fifty-five years, people who have GERD, especially for longer periods of time, such as five or ten years, and those who smoke. People who have higher levels of abdominal fat and non-Hispanic whites have a higher risk, and family history may also play a role.

The most serious and significant complication associated with Barrett's esophagus is the fact that the esophageal cells may become precancerous or even develop into esophageal cancer, which often has a poor prognosis. (See entry on esophageal cancer.) That is why it is so important that people with Barrett's esophagus undergo periodic upper endoscopy screenings. Effectively treating GERD and Barrett's esophagus may prevent this potentially life-threatening complication. Additionally, people with Barrett's esophagus have an increased risk of some other medical problems. These include esophageal stricture or the narrowing of the esophagus, primarily due to scarring, and peptic ulcers or open scores caused by stomach acid or enzymes.

PREVALENCE

About thirty million people in the United States have GERD. About 5 percent of the people with chronic GERD develop Barrett's esophagus. The condition is more common in men than in women and is seen more often in Caucasian Americans than in African Americans. The average age at diagnosis is fifty-five years.

DIAGNOSIS AND TREATMENT OPTIONS

While medical providers may initially suspect Barrett's esophagus from a medical history, it is usually diagnosed during an upper endoscopy, also known as an esophagogastroduodenoscopy. During this procedure, under anesthesia, a thin tube is inserted from the throat into the esophagus, stomach, and the first part of the small intestine. A gastroenterologist views the esophageal lining and takes cell samples to biopsy. A chromoendoscopy may be used to stain and identify potentially abnormal cells. During the upper endoscopy, the gastroenterologist applies stain to the esophagus with a liquid called Lugol's solution. The dye stains only the normal cells; unstained areas, which may be easily seen due to color differences, may be cancerous. A few centers in the United States employ endoscopic confocal microscopy (endomicroscopy), which uses a powerful microscope to help diagnose the condition. These microscopes use high-resolution images to identify abnormalities.

Barrett's esophagus is a complication of GERD. So, the treatment is similar to the treatment for GERD. The goal is to heal the esophageal lining and to prevent the condition from spreading. Treatment generally begins with diet and lifestyle changes and acid-blocking medication, such as antacids and proton pump inhibitors. Omeprazole, lansoprazole, pantoprazole, rabeprazole, esomeprazole, and dexlansoprazole are examples of proton pump inhibitors. Other medications include histamine 2 blockers, promotility agents, and baclofen. To check on the progression of the disease, periodic endoscopy exams will be advised. If precancerous cells are detected, they will be removed; this stops their progression into cancer. Generally, Barrett's esophagus without dysplasia may require an upper endoscopy every few years. People with Barrett's esophagus after dysplasia usually have an upper endoscopy every year.

There are a number of endoscopic procedures used to treat dysplasia. In general, they will be carried out by gastroenterologists and/or surgeons. With ablation therapy, very high or low temperatures are used to eliminate affected tissue. A medical provider may freeze or burn off the layer of intestinal metaplasia with cold gas (cryotherapy), a thermal balloon, a laser, or radiofrequency. If these initial procedures are not effective, a medical provider may surgically remove the affected localized area. If this too is not effective or if high-grade dysplasia or carcinoma is present, a medical provider may remove the affected portion of the esophagus, then rebuild the area with pieces of the gastrointestinal tract. This is known as an esophagectomy. Once the affected area is removed, Barrett's esophagus is considered cured. But, it may return. In addition, a layer of metaplasia may be hidden under a layer of new, normal tissue.

RESEARCH FINDINGS

Higher Intakes of Some Antioxidants and Fruits and Vegetables May Lower the Risk of Barrett's Esophagus

In a case-control study published in the *American Journal of Gastroenterology*, researchers from the San Francisco (Bay) area of California evaluated the association between the intake of antioxidants, fruits and vegetables, and the risk of Barrett's esophagus. The cohort consisted of 296 people with Barrett's esophagus, 308 with gastroesophageal reflux disease, and 309 controls. Nutrient intake was measured using a validated 110-item food frequency questionnaire. The antioxidant results were stratified by dietary versus total intake of antioxidants. Among the long-term supplement users, 83 percent used a multivitamin at least once per week, approximately 50 percent took vitamin C and/or vitamin E, 7 percent took beta-carotene, and none used selenium. The researchers learned that the dietary intakes of vitamin C, vitamin E, and beta-carotene were inversely associated with the risk of Barrett's esophagus. For example, the subjects in the fourth quartile of dietary intake of vitamin C had a 50 percent lower risk of Barrett's esophagus than those in the first quartile. On the other hand, there was no association between total intake (dietary plus supplement) of vitamin C and the risk of Barrett's esophagus. In addition, there was a strong inverse association between the consumption of fruits and vegetables and the risk of Barrett's esophagus. When compared to those in the lowest category, people with the highest intakes of fruits and vegetables (median intake of 8.3 servings per day) had a 73 percent lower risk of developing Barrett's esophagus. Each additional serving per day of fruits and vegetables was associated with a 14 percent reduction in risk. When fruits and vegetables were analyzed separately, the consumption of vegetables had a slightly stronger effect than fruits. The researchers noted that they demonstrated that antioxidant intake lowered the risk of Barrett's esophagus, and this benefit appeared to be derived primarily from dietary sources, rather than supplements. The consumption of fruits and vegetables also lowered the risk. The researchers concluded that future avenues of research "could include an intervention study to evaluate whether changes in diet can modify the risk of esophageal adenocarcinoma."[2]

In a similar trial published in the *American Journal of Clinical Nutrition*, researchers from Washington State and Bethesda, Maryland, also examined the association between fruit and vegetable intake and the risk of Barrett's esophagus. They compared the fruit and vegetable intake of 170 patients with newly diagnosed Barrett's esophagus to that of 182 controls from the general population. Both groups were matched according to age and sex. The participants were men and women between the ages of twenty and eighty years who were residents of western Washington State. The vast majority of the participants were non-Hispanic whites, and most reported having some college-level education. Fruit and vegetable intake was estimated using a food frequency questionnaire. The researchers learned that the participants who ate more fruits and vegetables appeared to have lower rates of Barrett's esophagus than those who ate fewer fruits and vegetables. In fact, the researchers found that those in the second and third tertiles of vegetable and fruit intake had a lower risk than those in the first tertile. The researchers concluded that their findings confirmed the limited number of published studies that support the belief that a diet with higher levels of fruits and vegetables may help prevent GERD, Barrett's esophagus, and esophageal cancer. More studies on the "relations between fruit and vegetables intake (as well as other dietary patterns) and occurrence of BE [Barrett's esophagus] are needed."[3]

Higher Fiber Intake Seems to Lower the Risk of Barrett's Esophagus

In a systematic review and meta-analysis published in the journal *Critical Reviews in Food Science and Nutrition*, researchers from China and Boston, Massachusetts, examined the association between fiber intake and the risk of Barrett's esophagus. The researchers identified fifteen studies with 16,885 subjects that met their criteria; seven were population-based case-control studies and eight were hospital-based case-control studies. Sample sizes ranged from 143 to 4,740. Overall, the studies found that dietary fiber intake was associated with a decreased risk of Barrett's esophagus and esophageal cancer. Four of the studies evaluated the dose-response relationship between dietary fiber intake and the risk of Barrett's esophagus and esophageal cancer. They found that a 10-gram-per-day increase in the intake of dietary fiber decreased the risk of Barrett's esophagus and esophageal cancer by 31 percent. The researchers concluded that "well-designed large prospective studies for dietary fiber supplementation are warranted to confirm this association and to better establish the potential dose-response relationship, which may play an important role for the prevention of esophageal cancer in the future."[4]

There Appear to Be Certain Factors That Increase the Risk That a Person with GERD Will Develop Barrett's Esophagus

In a trial published in the journal *Acta Informatica Medica*, researchers from the Republic of Kosovo wanted to learn which factors fostered the development of Barrett's esophagus in people with GERD. The cohort consisted of forty-two patients with diagnosed Barrett's esophagus; there were twenty-five males and seventeen females with a mean age of 52.8 years. The researchers examined factors such as age, sex, obesity, alcohol consumption, smoking, duration of symptoms, prevalence of short- and long-segment Barrett's esophagus, and the presence of a hiatal hernia. The researchers learned that obesity was present in twenty-four of the patients, and twenty-seven of the patients were smokers. Symptom duration was approximately 9.4 years. Sixty-four percent of the patients had hiatal hernias. Twelve percent of the patients had H. pylori. The researchers determined that there were several factors that increased the risk that people with GERD would develop Barrett's esophagus. The most important of these were male sex, middle age, smoking, and alcohol consumption. The number of males was significantly higher than females, and the most represented age group was fifty to fifty-nine years. Sixty-four percent of the patients smoked and 45 percent drank alcohol. Other important factors include obesity and having a hiatal hernia. In contrast, the prevalence of H. pylori in these patients was very low, "which suggests the possibility of protective role of this microorganism."[5]

While They May Increase the Risk of GERD and Esophageal Cancer, Higher Intakes of Fat and Meats May Not Increase the Risk of Barrett's Esophagus

In a case-control trial published in the *International Journal of Cancer*, researchers from Belfast, Ireland, assessed the association between the intake of dietary fat and meat and the risk of GERD, Barrett's esophagus, and esophageal adenocarcinoma. Using a food frequency questionnaire, dietary information was collected from 219 patients with GERD, 220 patients with Barrett's esophagus, 224 patients with esophageal cancer, and 256 frequency-matched controls. The patients with GERD were younger and more likely to be male and have H. pylori. Patients with Barrett's esophagus had a higher intake of energy; they were more likely to have less education and to work in manual jobs. Meanwhile, the patients with esophageal cancer had higher body mass indexes (BMIs), higher energy intake, were more likely to smoke and were less educated. They were more likely to hold manual occupations, consume less alcohol, and were less likely to have H. pylori. The researchers found that patients in the highest quartile of total fat intake had a higher risk of GERD; patients in the highest quartile of saturated fat and monounsaturated fat intake had a higher risk for GERD and esophageal cancer; patients in the highest quartile of fresh red meat intake had a higher risk of esophageal cancer; patients in the highest category of processed meat intake had a higher risk of GERD. But there were no consistent associations between Barrett's esophagus and any fat or meat intakes. The researchers commented that "further studies, investigating the association between dietary fat intakes and food sources of fat are needed to confirm these results."[6]

Tobacco Smoking Increases the Risk of High-Grade Dysplasia and Cancer among People with Barrett's Esophagus

In a study published in the journal *Gastroenterology*, researchers from Northern Ireland analyzed data from 3,167 patients with Barrett's esophagus with specialized intestinal metaplasia (cells that have changed). Data on clinical, demographic, and lifestyle factors related to their diagnosis of Barrett's esophagus were collected from hospital notes. The researchers used the Northern Ireland Cancer Registry to identify which of these patients later developed esophageal adenocarcinoma, adenocarcinomas of the gastric cardia, or esophageal high-grade dysplasia. During a total of 23,692 person-years of follow-up and a mean follow-up period of 7.5 years, 117 of these patients progressed to develop a type of gastric cancer or high-grade dysplasia. The mean interval from Barrett's esophagus diagnosis to cancer or high-grade dysplasia diagnosis was 4.5 years. Those patients with Barrett's esophagus who developed the types of gastric cancers or high-grade dysplasia were twice as likely to be smokers. They also tended to be seventy years or older and male and to have had indefinite or low-grade dysplasia at their diagnosis. Even past smokers had an increased risk. In fact, tobacco smoking was the strongest risk factor for progression. While acknowledging that their findings need to be supported by other studies, the researchers concluded "that tobacco smoking be discouraged and smoking cessation strategies considered in BE [Barrett's esophagus] patients in order to reduce future cancer risk."[7]

Obesity, Especially Abdominal Obesity, Seems to Be Associated with the Risk of Barrett's Esophagus

In a retrospective case-control study published in the *American Journal of Gastroenterology*, researchers from Houston, Texas, evaluated the association between overweight/obesity and Barrett's esophagus. The cohort consisted of thirty-six people with Barrett's esophagus and ninety-three controls; they all had an endoscopy and an abdominal CT scan at a single large VA medical center. From the results of the CT scan, the researchers calculated surface and subcutaneous adipose tissue or degrees of abdominal obesity. There were no significant differences between cases and controls in age, gender, or race; they had a mean age of sixty-three years; 98 percent were men, and 71 percent were Caucasian. There were no significant differences in the proportions of patients with GERD symptoms, abdominal pain, anemia, nausea, dysphagia, varices, diarrhea, or follow-up of abnormal imaging. The researchers determined that the subjects with Barrett's esophagus had significantly higher BMIs than the controls and their visceral adipose tissue was about 1.5 times higher. In fact, the researchers found that higher BMI was significantly associated with Barrett's esophagus. There was an 11 percent increase in risk for each unit increase in BMI. Further, the surface area of visceral adipose tissue was 59 percent larger in those with Barrett's esophagus. Subjects with the higher tertile of visceral adipose tissue surface area comprised 55.6 percent of the cases compared to 24.7 percent of the controls. Subjects with the highest tertile of visceral adipose tissue surface area were 3.2 times more likely to have Barrett's esophagus than those in the lowest tertile. On the other hand, there were no significant differences between the cases and controls in subcutaneous adipose tissue, and the surface area of the subcutaneous adipose tissue was not significantly associated with Barrett's esophagus. The researchers commented that obesity, especially abdominal obesity, and a higher BMI increase the risk of Barrett's esophagus. "Larger studies utilizing prospective enrollment of patients are required to further examine this issue."[8]

Physical Activity May or May Not Increase the Risk of Barrett's Esophagus

In a case-control trial published in the journal *Diseases of the Esophagus*, researchers based in Houston, Texas, examined the role that physical activity may play in the risk of Barrett's esophagus. The cohort consisted of 307 people with Barrett's esophagus and 1,724 controls. The study participants completed a short form of the International Physical Activity Questionnaire, which measured physical activity during the previous seven days. The researchers determined that most of the participants (73.6 percent) were in the lowest category of physical activity; 14.4 percent had moderate levels of physical activity, and 12 percent had high levels. The researchers determined that, when compared to the controls, the participants with Barrett's esophagus were "slightly" more likely to be in the high category of physical activity. The researchers commented that there have been studies that have found that physical activity triggers or worsens GERD and, therefore, at least hypothetically, increases the risk of Barrett's esophagus. The researchers emphasized the need for more studies on the association between Barrett's esophagus and physical activity. Nevertheless, they concluded that "recent amount and intensity of physical activity are not associated with a reduction in the risk of BE."[9]

In another study, published in the *European Journal of Gastroenterology & Hepatology*, researchers from the UK also reviewed the association between physical activity and Barrett's esophagus. For their study, the researchers used the European Prospective Investigation of Cancer-Norfolk, which recruited 30,445 men and women between 1993 and 1997. The subjects, who were all between the ages of thirty-nine and seventy-nine years, were followed until 2015. They were identified from thirty-five general practices across the county of Norfolk. Using a baseline questionnaire, occupational and recreational levels of physical activity were measured. During the mean follow-up of 17.6 years, 203 participants developed Barrett's esophagus; they had a mean age of 70.6 years and the majority (70.9 percent) were men. When compared to the controls, the people who developed Barrett's esophagus were more likely to be male and older at the time of recruitment. They were also more likely to have previously smoked, to be overweight, and to drink more alcohol. The researchers observed an inverse association between standing occupations and the risk of Barrett's esophagus. At the same time, while heavy manual occupations were positively associated with disease risk, statistical significance was not reached. No associations were found between recreational activity and the risk of Barrett's esophagus. The researchers concluded that "although differing levels of recreational exercise were not associated with disease risk, occupational physical activity may be either protective (as in standing occupations) or possibly hazardous (as in heavy metal occupations)."[10]

People with Barrett's Esophagus May Benefit from Taking Aspirin and the Proton Pump Inhibitor Esomeprazole

In the AspECT trial published in the journal *Lancet*, researchers based in the UK wanted to learn if patients with Barrett's esophagus would benefit from aspirin combined with the proton pump inhibitor esomeprazole. (Proton pump inhibitors reduce acid reflux, which is believed to be one of the primary causes of Barrett's esophagus.) The cohort consisted of 2,557 people with Barrett's esophagus that was at least 1 centimeter in length; they were from eighty-four centers in the UK and one in Canada. The patients, who were recruited by gastroenterologists and gastroenterological surgeons, were divided into four groups—high-dose esomeprazole (n = 704), high-dose esomeprazole with low-dose aspirin (n = 577), low-dose esomeprazole (n = 705), or low-dose esomeprazole and low-dose aspirin (n =

571). (High-dose esomeprazole was defined as 40 mg twice daily; low-dose esomeprazole was defined as 20 mg twice daily. Patients who were assigned aspirin took 300 mg per day in the UK and 325 mg per day in Canada.) Follow-ups were held once per year, and patients had endoscopies on alternate years. Patients were monitored for a median of 8.9 years. The primary "endpoint" was time of death from any cause, diagnosis of esophageal cancer, or diagnosis of high-grade dysplasia. The researchers determined that compared to the low-dose esomeprazole, high-dose esomeprazole had a statistically significant benefit on whatever the cause of the "endpoint." Still, the most effective treatment was high-dose esomeprazole with low-dose aspirin. Only twenty-eight patients (1 percent) reported study-related serious adverse events. The researchers noted that it appears that the administration of esomeprazole and aspirin for at least nine years would improve survival rates of Barrett's esophagus. The researchers commented that their findings have important implications for clinical practice. At present, guidelines recommend treating GERD and Barrett's esophagus with low doses of proton pump inhibitors. But, they found that higher doses were more effective than the lower ones for treating Barrett's esophagus, "in terms of delaying death, cancer, and dysplasia." And, the combination of a high dose of a proton pump inhibitor and aspirin was most useful. "Our results suggest that a review of the existing guidelines is warranted."[11]

But, Aspirin Alone May Help Lower the Risk of Barrett's Esophagus in Women

In a study published in the journal *Clinical and Translational Gastroenterology*, researchers from Boston, Massachusetts, St. Louis, Missouri, and New Haven, Connecticut evaluated the use of aspirin to reduce the risk of Barrett's esophagus in women. They used data from 121,700 women enrolled in the Nurses' Health Study, a large prospective cohort study. Almost all of the participants were Caucasian, and they had a mean age of sixty-six years. Forty-eight percent reported regular aspirin use. During eighteen years of follow-up, there were 667 cases of Barrett's esophagus among the 27,881 women who had an upper endoscopy. The researchers determined that regular aspirin users had a 15 percent lower risk of Barrett's esophagus, which was statistically significant. And, the risk declined with increasing doses and longer durations of aspirin use. Aspirin appeared to "influence both the initiation and progression of BE." In contrast, the regular use of any other NSAIDs was not associated with the risk of Barrett's esophagus. The researchers concluded that their findings may provide further "insight into the earliest mechanisms of BE pathogenesis." And, according to these researchers, there is the possibility that aspirin may prevent esophageal adenocarcinoma "by influencing the initiation as well as progression of esophageal neoplasia, and provide the rationale for future trials for high-risk patients."[12]

And, Proton Pump Inhibitors May Not Reduce the Risk of Esophageal Adenocarcinoma in People with Barrett's Esophagus

In a systematic review and meta-analysis published in the online journal *PLoS ONE*, researchers from China and Baltimore, Maryland, wanted to learn if the use of proton pump inhibitors in people with Barrett's esophagus would reduce the risk of the development of high-grade dysplasia or esophageal adenocarcinoma. The researchers identified nine observational studies (five cohort studies and four case-control studies) that had 5,712 patients with Barrett's esophagus. These studies were conducted in the United States, the Netherlands, Australia, the UK, and Denmark. Sample sizes ranged from 77 to 1,437. At the time of diagnosis, the mean age of the patients with Barrett's esophagus ranged from fifty-eight to sixty-five years, and about 73 percent of those with this illness were men. The researchers deemed that the quality of their studies was moderate to high. In addition to the use of proton pump inhibitors, some of the patients also used NSAIDs, aspirin, and statins. The researchers determined that the use of proton pump inhibitors seemed to have no association with the risk of high-grade dysplasia or esophageal adenocarcinoma, and they offered no protection from either medical problem. So, clinicians who tell their patients that proton pump inhibitors may offer protection "should be aware that such an effect, if [it] exists, has not been proven with statistical significance."[13]

People with Metabolic Syndrome Appear to Have an Increased Risk for Barrett's Esophagus

In a systematic review and meta-analysis published in the journal *BMC Gastroenterology*, researchers from Iran evaluated the association between metabolic syndrome and Barrett's esophagus. They identified fourteen prospective and retrospective studies that met their criteria; the total sample size was 108,416. The researchers found that metabolic syndrome significantly increased the risk of Barrett's syndrome. Other risk factors included GERD, age, male gender, smoking, longer Barrett's esophagus segments, and low-grade dysplasia. The researchers concluded that "the results of this study can help health practitioners by identifying a treatable risk factor for the most important risk factor for esophageal carcinoma (ie, BE)." Moreover, future research should attempt to determine if treatment for metabolic syndrome reduces the risk of Barrett's esophagus.[14]

Alcohol Consumption May or May Not Be Associated with the Risk of Barrett's Esophagus

In a systematic review and meta-analysis published in the journal *Scientific Reports*, researchers from China examined the association between alcohol consumption and the risk of Barrett's esophagus. Their analysis included twenty cohort studies with 42,925 participants and 3,775 cases of Barrett's esophagus. A total of 41,593 subjects were from Western countries and 1,332 subjects were from Asia. The researchers found a positive association between higher alcohol consumption and incidence of Barrett's esophagus in the studies from Asia but not in the Western countries. Women who consumed more alcohol were less likely to suffer from Barrett's esophagus. But, no statistically significant findings could be noted from the studies on men. When they used a dose-response analysis, the researchers did not find an association between an increase in alcohol consumption of 10 g per day and the risk of developing Barrett's esophagus. However, there was a statistically significant inversion between an increase in alcohol consumption of 10 g per day and the risk of Barrett's esophagus in women. After pooling all of the data from the highest and lowest comparisons, the researchers commented that alcohol consumption was not associated with an increased incidence of Barrett's esophagus. The researchers concluded that "further large prospective cohort studies, with careful control of confounding factors, are needed to reach a more definitive conclusion as to whether the consumption of alcohol can lead to BE."[15]

Despite the Prevailing Beliefs, People with Barrett's Esophagus Are Actually at a Relatively Low Risk for Progression to Cancer

In a systematic review and meta-analysis published in the journal *Clinical Gastroenterology and Hepatology*, researchers from the Netherlands wanted to determine the actual risk that people with Barrett's esophagus have of developing and dying from esophageal adenocarcinoma. The researchers located fifty-one studies that met their criteria. Twenty of these studies were from the UK, sixteen from the United States, thirteen from European countries, and two from Australia. The overall mean age of the people with Barrett's esophagus was sixty-one years, and the overall proportion of males was 64 percent. Fifty studies reported on the incidence of esophageal adenocarcinoma; these studies included 14,109 patients who were followed for 61,804 person-years. During this follow-up, there were 344 incident cases of esophageal adenocarcinoma. According to the researchers, a random effects model produced a pooled estimate for esophageal adenocarcinoma incidence in Barrett's esophagus of 6.3 per 1,000 person-years. Nineteen studies reported on esophageal adenocarcinoma-related mortality in Barrett's esophagus patients. These studies included 7,930 patients followed for 33,022 person-years. There were eighty-eight deaths from esophageal adenocarcinoma and 1,271 deaths from other causes. The pooled incidence of fatal esophageal adenocarcinoma was 3.0 per 1,000 person-years. The researchers concluded that patients with Barrett's esophagus "are at low risk of malignant progression and predominantly die due to causes other than EAC [esophageal adenocarcinoma]." According to the researchers, "this undermines the cost-effectiveness of BE surveillance and supports the search for valid risk stratification tools to identify the minority of patients that are likely to benefit from surveillance."[16]

REFERENCES AND FURTHER READING

Coleman, Helen G., Shivaram Bhat, Brian T. Johnston et al. "Tobacco Smoking Increases the Risk of High-Grade Dysplasia and Cancer Among Patients with Barrett's Esophagus." *Gastroenterology* 142 (2012): 233–240.

El-Serag, Hashem B., Peter Kvapil, Joan Hacken-Bitar, and Jennifer R. Kramer. "Abdominal Obesity and the Risk of Barrett's Esophagus." *American Journal of Gastroenterology* 100 (2005): 2151–2156.

Gashi, Zaim, Ljube Ivkovski, Ragip Shabani et al. "What Are Protective Factors for Developing of Barrett's Esophagus in Patients with GERD – Our Experience." *Acta Informatica Medica* 19, no. 3 (September 2011): 146–148.

Hilal, J., H. B. El-Serag, D. Ramsey et al. "Physical Activity and the Risk of Barrett's Esophagus." *Diseases of the Esophagus* 29 (2016): 248–254.

Hu, Q., T. T. Sun, J. Hong et al. "Proton Pump Inhibitors Do Not Reduce the Risk of Esophageal Adenocarcinoma in Patients with Barrett's Esophagus: A Systematic Review and Meta-Analysis." *PLoS One* 12, no. 1 (2017): e0169691.

Jankowski, J. A. Z., J. de Caestecker, S. B. Love et al. "Esomeprazole and Aspirin in Barrett's Oesophagus (AspECT): A Randomized Factorial Trial." *Lancet* 392 (2018): 400–408.

Jovani, M. Y. Cao, D, Feskanich et al. "Aspirin Use Is Associated with Lower Risk of Barrett's Esophagus in Women." *Clinical and Translational Gastroenterology* 8, no. 12 (December 2017): e131

Karimian, M., M. Salamati, and M. Azami. "The Relationship Between Metabolic Syndrome and Increased Risk of Barrett's Esophagus: An Updated Systematic Review and Meta-Analysis." *BMC Gastroenterology* 20 (2020): 138.

Kubo, Ai, T. R. Levin, Gladys Block et al. "Dietary Antioxidants, Fruits and Vegetables, and the Risk of Barrett's Esophagus." *American Journal of Gastroenterology* 103, no. 7 (July 2008): 1614–1624.

Lam, Stephen, Leo Alexandre, Robert Luben, and Andrew Hart. "The Association Between Physical Activity and the Risk of Symptomatic Barrett's Oesophagus: A UK Prospective Cohort Study." *European Journal of Gastroenterology & Hepatology* 30 (2018): 71–75.

O'Doherty, Mark G., Marie M. Cantwell, Liam J. Murray et al. "Dietary Fat and Meat Intakes and Risk of Reflux Esophagitis, Barrett's Esophagus and Esophageal Adenocarcinoma." *International Journal of Cancer* 129, no. 6 (September 15, 2011): 1493–1502.

Ren, Lin-Lin, Ting-Ting Yan, Zhen-Hua Wang et al. "Alcohol Consumption and the Risk of Barrett's Esophagus: A Comprehensive Meta-Analysis." *Scientific Reports* 5 (2015): 16048.

Shalauta, Mark a., and Richard Saad. "Barrett's Esophagus." *American Family Physician* 69, no. 9 (May 1, 2004): 2113–2118.

Sikkema, M., P. J. F. De Jonge, E. W. Steyerberg, and E. J. Kuipers. "Risk of Esophageal Adenocarcinoma and Mortality in Patients with Barrett's Esophagus: A Systematic Review and Meta-Analysis." *Clinical Gastroenterology and Hepatology* 8 (2010): 235–244.

Sun, Lingli, Zhizhong Zhang, Jian Xu et al. "Dietary Fiber Intake Reduces Risk for Barrett's Esophagus and Esophageal Cancer." *Critical Reviews in Food Science and Nutrition* 57, no. 13 (2017): 2749–2757.

Thompson, Olivia M., Shirley A. A. Beresford, Elizabeth A. Kirk, and Thomas I. Vaughan. "Vegetable and Fruit Intakes and Risk of Barrett's Esophagus in Men and Women." *American Journal of Clinical Nutrition* 89 (2009): 890–896.

CANCER, COLORECTAL

INTRODUCTION

Colorectal cancer is a type of cancer that begins either in the large colon or rectum, which comprise the lower section of the digestive system. The colon is a muscular tube, about 5 feet long, that absorbs water from the remaining food matter. The colon has four main parts—ascending colon, transverse colon, descending colon, and sigmoid colon. The rectum is the last 6 inches of the colon. It is the storage place for feces before they leave the body through the anus.

The vast majority of the cancers that form in the colon or rectum are adenocarcinomas. The tumors start in the gland cells that release or secrete the fluids that help move along the stool. Other types of cancers that may begin in the colon or rectum are gastrointestinal stromal tumors, lymphomas, carcinoids, and sarcomas.

At first, most colorectal cancers are polyps or fleshy clumps of tissue that form on the inner lining of the colon or rectum. Small polyps are rarely cancerous. But, as they grow, polyps may develop into adenomatous polyps or adenomas that may become cancerous.

Colorectal cancer has probably always existed. Historically, it has been traced to an ancient Egyptian mummy. However, it was an American pathologist, Aldred Warthin, MD/PhD, who first documented the genetic basis for this disease. In 1895, he suspected the presence of a hereditary form of colorectal cancer in a family he called Family G. For years, Dr. Warthin, who is often said to be the father of cancer genetics, studied this family, and he published his first report on Family G in 1913.[1]

SYMPTOMS, RISKS, AND COMPLICATIONS

People with colorectal cancer often have no symptoms. By the time symptoms begin to appear, the cancer may well have spread beyond the colon and rectum. Still, there are several symptoms associated with the disease. These include a change in bowel habits that lasts more than a few days or the feeling that the bowel is not emptying after a bowel movement; bright red or very dark blood in the stool, fatigue, pain, aches, or cramps in the abdomen; thin stools, slimy stools, stools with mucous; and bloating, flatulence, fullness, unexplained weight loss, and vomiting. If the cancer has spread beyond the colon, one may have symptoms related to the area where the cancer has spread. For example, if the cancer has spread to the liver, a person may have jaundice.

Personal and familial genetics play an important role in increasing the risk of colorectal cancer. Thus, people who have a family member with a history of colonic polyps may be at increased risk for colorectal cancer. But, there are several other proven risks. Older people have a greater risk than younger people; this is especially true for people over the age of fifty years. Black individuals and Ashkenazi Jews have a higher risk, as do males. Certain illnesses increase the risk, such as ulcerative colitis, Crohn's disease, Lynch syndrome, familial adenomatous polyposis (FAP), obesity, and type 2 diabetes. People who eat a lot of red or processed meats, have a low-fiber diet and/or high-fat diet, smoke cigarettes, are inactive, and drink excessive amounts of alcohol have a higher risk. And, finally, people who have had a cholecystectomy (gallbladder removal) are at higher risk for right-side colon cancer.

There are several complications associated with colorectal cancer. These include bowel obstructions that cause a blockage of the bowel or rectum, cancer that returns after treatment, cancer that spreads to other organs, such as the liver, lungs, or brain, and the development of a second primary colorectal cancer.

PREVALENCE

Colorectal cancer is the third most prevalent cancer in the world and the second most fatal cancer. In the United States, colorectal cancer is a leading cause of cancer deaths. This is particularly unfortunate, because an early diagnosis often results in a complete cure. The American Cancer Society estimated that in 2024 there were about 106,590 new cases of colon cancer in the United States; there were 54,210 in men and 52,380 in women. During the same year, there were 46,220 new cases of rectal cancer; there were 27,330 in men and 18,890 in women. Combining these figures, there were about 152,810 cases of colorectal cancer. Approximately, 53,010 died from colorectal cancer.[2] The lifetime risk for colorectal cancer in people of average risk is about 4 percent.

DIAGNOSIS AND TREATMENT OPTIONS

The best way to diagnose colorectal cancer is with a colonoscopy or the insertion of a flexible tube into the rectum and colon. But, there are other tests available. These include a flexible sigmoidoscopy or the viewing of the lower one-third of the colon with a flexible tube. However, this does not allow the viewing of the ascending or transverse colon and could miss cancers in those locations. There is also a CT colonography, also known as a virtual colonoscopy, which takes pictures of the digestive system with a CT scan. And, there are stool-based screening tests that may look for blood or DNA mutations.

For most people, screening should begin at age forty-five. People with a family history of colorectal cancer or with a digestive illness such as ulcerative colitis or Crohn's disease may wish to begin earlier, around age forty. Screening should continue at least until the age of seventy-five years.

Once diagnosed, colorectal cancer will be staged. In stage 0 (in situ), there is only cancer on the innermost layer of the lining of the intestine; in stage 1 colorectal cancer, there is cancer in the inner layers of the colon or rectum; in stage 2 cancer, the cancer has spread through the muscular wall of the colon; in stage 3 cancer, the cancer has spread to the lymph nodes; and in stage 4, the cancer had spread to other organs, such as the liver or lungs.

Usually, the first treatment for colorectal cancer is surgery, endoscopic surgery, or cryosurgery—the use of an extremely cold liquid or instrument. That may or may not be followed by radiation therapy, chemotherapy, targeted therapy, and/or ablation and embolization. All of these are designed to kill the cancer cells directly. Another type of therapy, immunotherapy, enhances the immune system of the body, enabling it to fight the cancer.

RESEARCH FINDINGS

Several Factors Appear to Play a Role in the Etiology of Colorectal Cancer

In a prospective cohort study published in the journal *Nutrients*, researchers from China and the UK evaluated factors associated with increasing the risk of colorectal cancer. The researchers examined lifestyle factors and the consumption of 139 foods and nutrients in a cohort of 118,210 UK subjects. During a mean follow-up of 12.8 years, there were 1,466 incident cases of colorectal cancer. The mean age of the colorectal patients was 55.87 years, and almost 44.6 percent of the study population was male. Compared to the general population, people with colorectal cancer were more likely to be male and white, older and less educated, have less physical activity, and a higher BMI. Further, they were more likely to have a family history of colorectal cancer, a personal history of smoking, and a higher prevalence of diabetes. While alcohol and white bread were associated with an increased risk for colorectal cancer, dietary fiber, calcium, magnesium, phosphorus, and manganese were associated with a lower risk. The researchers commented that their findings "provide evidence and suggestions for dietary prevention of CRC [colorectal cancer]."[3]

Several Factors Place People at Increased Risk for Early-Onset Colorectal Cancer

In a systematic review and meta-analysis published in the journal *Clinical Gastroenterology and Hepatology*, researchers from Canada reviewed the non-genetic risk factors that placed people at increased risk for early-onset colorectal cancer, defined as before the age of fifty years. The researchers located twenty studies that met their criteria and examined at least one risk factor for early-onset colorectal cancer; fourteen of these studies were included in the meta-analysis. The twenty studies had a total of 47,692 cases of early-onset colorectal cancer. Thirteen of the studies were conducted in North America, three in Europe, three in Asia, and one in Australia. Ten of the studies were case-control, eight were cohort, and two were cross-sectional. While six of the studies were believed to be of high quality, the majority were considered to be of moderate quality. Ten studies examined the association of demographic factors with the development of early-onset colorectal cancer; nine studies reviewed the relationship between preexisting comorbidities and early-onset colorectal cancer. And, nine studies discussed the association between lifestyle or occupational factors and early-onset colorectal cancer. The researchers learned that early-onset colorectal cancer was significantly associated with the male sex, Caucasian ethnicity, colorectal cancer history in a first-degree relative, hyperlipidemia, obesity, and alcohol consumption. While many believe that smoking plays a role, the results were not statistically significant. With the exception of alcohol consumption, there was a good deal of heterogeneity between the studies. Other less studied potential risk factors included ulcerative colitis, chronic kidney disease, hypertension, diet-related factors, sedentary behavior, and occupational exposure to organic dusts. The researchers concluded that "high-quality studies conducted on generalizable populations and that comprehensively examine risk factors for EoCRC [early-onset colorectal cancer] are required to inform primary and secondary prevention initiatives for EoCRC."[4]

Researchers Have Found That Certain Foods Tend to Be Directly Associated with Colorectal Cancer and Other Foods Have an Inverse Association

In a study also published in *Clinical Gastroenterology and Hepatology*, researchers from many different countries but based in Greece wanted to learn which foods and nutrients contribute to colorectal cancer and which foods and nutrients help fight this illness. To conduct their study, the researchers used data from the European Prospective Investigation into Cancer and Nutrition, which is a large European multicenter prospective cohort that had 521,324 participants, who were primarily between the ages of 35 and 70 years. After excluding certain people, the researchers had a cohort of 386,792 participants, in which 71 percent were female. During a mean follow-up of 14.1 years, there were a total of 5,069 (56.8 percent women) cases of colorectal cancer. The researchers assessed the intake of sixty-three foods and twenty-nine nutrients during the previous twelve months, and they determined that there were many foods and nutrients that were positively or negatively associated with colorectal health.

Thus, increased intakes of alcohol, liquor, spirits, wine, beer/cider, soft drinks, and pork were associated with a higher risk of colorectal cancer. Conversely, higher intakes of milk, cheese, calcium, phosphorous, magnesium, potassium, riboflavin, vitamin B6, beta-carotene, fruits, fibers, nonwhite bread, banana, and total protein were associated with a lower risk of colorectal cancer. The researchers concluded that their findings "confirm a positive association for alcohol and an inverse association for dairy products and calcium with CRC risk, and also suggest a lower risk at higher dietary intakes of phosphorous, magnesium, potassium, riboflavin, beta carotenes, and total protein."[5]

Dietary Fiber May or May Not Be Useful for the Prevention of Colorectal Cancer

In a systematic review published in the *Journal of Healthcare Engineering*, researchers from Hunan, China evaluated studies on the relationship between dietary fiber and the risk of colorectal cancer in East Asian countries. The researchers located nine studies that met their criteria. Five were case-control studies and four were prospective cohorts. The five case-control studies and one prospective study found that fiber had a significant protective effect against colorectal cancer. Interestingly, one of these studies even found that a high intake of cereal fiber was related to a low risk of colorectal cancer. Meanwhile, three of the prospective cohorts suggested that fiber had no protective effects. One of these studies determined that colorectal cancer was more a function of being elderly, postmenopausal, or having less education than the dietary consumption of fiber, such as fruits and vegetables. Since the researchers were unable to find consistent findings on the protective effects of fiber against colorectal cancer, they noted that they were unable to "substantiate the preventive effect of dietary fiber intake on colorectal cancers." They underscored the need for more studies among East Asian populations.[6]

Consumption of Red Meat and Processed Meats Increases the Risk of Colorectal Cancer

In a systematic review and meta-analysis published in the online journal *PLoS One*, researchers from the UK and the Netherlands examined the association between the consumption of red and processed meat and colorectal cancer. Twenty-four prospective studies—two case-control, three nested case-control, and nineteen cohort studies—were included in the highest versus the lowest meta-analyses. There were thirteen cohorts of men and women, three male cohorts, and eight female cohorts. Twelve studies were from North America, including a multiethnic cohort, and a European study had results from ten European countries. There were two studies each from Finland, the Netherlands, and Japan, and one study each from Australia, Canada, Sweden, China, and a Singaporean study with Chinese participants. The researchers determined that red and processed meats were associated with an increased risk of colorectal cancer. In fact, in a linear response model, they found that the risk of colorectal cancer increased 14 percent for every 100 g/day increase of total red and processed meat. At the same time, in nonlinear models, colorectal cancer appeared to increase almost linearly with increasing intake of red and processed meats up to approximately 140 g/day. Above that level, the risk was "less pronounced." The researchers concluded that "high intake of red and processed meat is associated with significant increased risk of colorectal, colon, and rectal cancers." Moreover, "the overall evidence of prospective studies supports limiting red and processed meat consumption as one of the dietary recommendations for the prevention of colorectal cancer."[7]

Flexible Sigmoidoscopy Screening Reduces the Incidence and Mortality from Colorectal Cancer

In a systematic review and meta-analysis published in the *World Journal of Gastroenterology*, researchers from Houston, Texas, and Canada compared the incidence and mortality of colorectal cancer in a group of people who had flexible sigmoidoscopy screening to a group who did not have this screening. The researchers located four randomized controlled trials with a total of 165,659 people in the screened groups and 249,707 in the control groups. The trials were conducted in the United States, the UK, Italy, and Norway. The trials had different follow-up times. The age range of the US study was fifty-five to seventy-four years, and the age range in the other three studies was fifty-five to sixty-four years. There tended to be about equal numbers of males and females. These four trials had 5,865 cases of colorectal cancer. The researchers learned that flexible sigmoidoscopy screening significantly reduced the incidence and mortality from colorectal cancer, with similar reductions in men and women. In addition, the meta-analysis indicated that there was a significant decrease in the incidence of distal colorectal cancer and proximal colorectal cancer between the flexible sigmoidoscopy groups and the controls, as well as mortality from distal colorectal cancer. However, there was no reduction in mortality from proximal colorectal cancer. The researchers concluded that "the pooled results from this meta-analysis confirms that screening FS [flexible sigmoidoscopy] reduces the overall incidence of and mortality from CRC [colorectal cancer]." Furthermore, "it reduces the incidence and mortality from distal CRC, incidence of proximal CRC, and decreases the likelihood of subsequent diagnosis of advanced CRC."[8]

People with Obesity Who Have Bariatric Surgery May or May Not Lower Their Risk of Colorectal Cancer

In a systematic review and meta-analysis published in the journal *Nutrients*, researchers from France and Italy wanted to determine if people with obesity who have bariatric surgery reduce their risk of colorectal cancer. They located eighteen studies that met their criteria. A meta-analysis was performed on 12,517,893 patients. Half of these studies were conducted in the United States. The researchers noted that people with morbid obesity who had bariatric surgery experienced a 54 percent reduction in the risk of developing colorectal cancer during the follow-up period. The researchers concluded that "bariatric surgery reduces the incidence of colorectal cancer in individuals independently from gender and surgical procedure."[9]

On the other hand, in a retrospective study published in the journal *Annals of Surgery*, researchers from the UK and Sweden also evaluated the association between bariatric surgery and the risk of colorectal cancer. They used data obtained from a nationwide retrospective register-based cohort study that was conducted in Sweden. There were a total of 15,095 patients with obesity that had bariatric surgery and 62,016 patients with obesity that did not have bariatric surgery. During a median of ten years and 146,810 person-years of follow-up in the obesity surgery group, there were seventy new cases of colorectal cancer. In the no surgery group, during a median follow-up of seven years and 411,041 person-years of follow-up, there were 373 colorectal cases. The majority of patients in both groups were female. The patients in the surgery group had a mean age of thirty-nine years, while the patients in the non-surgery group had a mean age of forty-nine years. Diabetes, hypertension, and cardiovascular disorders were more common in the non-surgery group. The researchers found that the patients in the surgery group had an increased risk of colorectal cancer, and the risk tended to increase over time. No such pattern was observed in the non-surgery group. In fact, the researchers concluded that their data "suggested that increased colorectal cancer risk may be a long-term consequence of such surgery."[10]

Consumption of Ultra-Processed Foods Increases the Risk of Colorectal Cancer

In a matched case-control study published in the journal *Nutrition and Cancer*, researchers from Lubbock, Texas, and Iran evaluated the relationship between the consumption of ultra-processed food and the incidence of colorectal cancer. The cohort consisted of seventy-one colorectal cancer patients and 142 control patients; the study was conducted at four hospitals in Tehran, Iran. At the time of diagnosis, all of the patients were between the ages of forty and seventy-five years. The control patients were recruited from the same hospitals and within the same time periods. They had other medical problems, including fractures and sprains, osteoarticular disorders, disk disorders, acute surgical conditions, traumas and injuries, skin diseases, and other illnesses. The patients with colorectal cancer and the controls had similar demographic characteristics. Dietary intakes were assessed using a 125-item semi-quantitative food frequency questionnaire based on foods that Iranians commonly consume. The researchers learned that when compared to those with the lowest intake of ultra-processed foods, the subjects with the highest intake of ultra-processed foods were more likely to have colorectal cancer. This association remained even after "adjustment for BMI, income, smoking, type of job, educational level, and physical activity."[11]

Cigarette Smoking Appears to Increase the Risk of Colorectal Cancer

In a study published in *Clinical Gastroenterology and Hepatology*, researchers from many countries but based in the Netherlands examined the association between cigarette smoking and colorectal cancer. They used data obtained from the European Prospective Investigation into Cancer and Nutrition Study; their cohort had 465,879 participants. During an 8.7-year follow-up period, 2,741 participants developed colorectal cancer; there were 1,058 men and 1,683 women. There were 1,791 cases of colon cancer and 950 cases of rectal cancer. At baseline, detailed information about cigarette smoking was collected in a questionnaire. This included information about smoking status at recruitment, age when smoking began, time since quitting, duration of smoking, type of smoking, and number of cigarettes smoked per day. The researchers determined that smokers had a higher risk of colon cancer, but apparently not rectal cancer. Only when smoking had ended for a minimum of twenty years were the rates of colon cancer between ex-smokers and non-smokers the same. The researchers noted that "smoking cessation pays off."[12]

Vitamin D May Well Play a Role in the Prevention of Colorectal Cancer

In a systematic review and meta-analysis of case-control and prospective cohort studies published in the journal *Cancers*, researchers from Spain and the UK assessed the role that vitamin D may play in the prevention of colorectal cancer. The researchers located thirty-one original studies that they included in a quantitative meta-analysis; these studies had a total of 47,540 cases and 70,567 controls in case-control studies and a total of 14,676 colorectal cancer incident subjects (out of 808,130 subjects) in prospective cohort studies, from sixteen countries around the world. The follow-up of the prospective cohort studies ranged from five to sixteen years. Eighty-one percent of the case-control studies were considered good; the remainder were fair. Seventy-five percent of the prospective studies were rated scores of eight out of nine. When analyzing the case-control studies, the researchers found that dietary intake of vitamin D was significantly associated with a lower risk of colon cancer, rectal cancer, and colorectal cancer. Vitamin D supplementation reduced levels of colon cancer, and total intake of vitamin D was associated with reductions in colorectal cancers. In their analyses of prospective studies, the researchers observed an association between total and supplemental vitamin D intake and reductions of colorectal cancer risk. The researchers concluded that their findings "support the idea that both dietary and supplemental intake of vitamin D are associated with a reduced risk of CRC [colorectal cancer], which suggests a significant influence on vitamin D on the prevention of CRC."[13]

There Seems to Be an Association between Vitamin B6 and the Risk of Colorectal Cancer

In a prospective case-control study published in the *American Journal of Clinical Nutrition*, researchers from Sweden and Norway investigated the association between vitamin B6 status and colorectal cancer. The cohort consisted of 613 people with colorectal cancer and 1,190 matched controls, who were all part of the Northern Sweden Health and Disease Study (n = 114,679). Participants were followed from 1985 to 2009, with a median follow-up from baseline to colorectal cancer diagnosis of 8.2 years. The median age at diagnosis was 65.2 years. Baseline data for BMI, physical activity, and alcohol intake were comparable for cases and controls. The researchers determined that the subjects with the lowest levels of markers for vitamin B6 had the highest risk for colorectal cancer. Similarly, the subjects with low functional vitamin B6 status had high rates of colorectal cancer. Yet, from their analyses, the researchers concluded that vitamin B6 appeared to play a role in "tumor progression rather than [tumor] initiation."[14] While vitamin B6 deficiency seemed to support the growth of colorectal cancer, it did not appear to trigger their growth.

Other B Vitamins May Also Play a Role in Colorectal Cancer Prevention

In a case-control study published in the *British Journal of Nutrition*, researchers from China wanted to learn if other B vitamins as well as the amino acid methionine could help lower the risk of colorectal cancer. They recruited 2,502 patients with colorectal cancer (1425 men and 1077 women) and 2,538 age and sex-matched controls. Among the cases, 1,565 were diagnosed with colon cancer and 937 were diagnosed with rectal cancer. Compared to the control subjects, the patients with colorectal cancer were more likely to be married, live in a rural area, have less education and lower income, have lower BMI, work as a farmer, and have fewer household and leisure activities. They were more likely to be smokers, regular consumers of alcohol, and to have a family history of cancer. And, their intake of vitamins B2, B6, B9 (folate), and B12 was significantly lower. (No significant difference was observed for methionine intake.) When the researchers stratified their analyses by sex, they found that intakes of vitamins B2, B6, and folate were inversely associated with colorectal cancer in both men and women. On the other hand, vitamin B12 was associated with decreased rates of colorectal cancer only in women. The researchers concluded that "the present study indicated that higher intake of folate, vitamin B2, vitamin B6, and vitamin B12 was inversely associated with the risk of colorectal cancer in a Chinese population."[15]

Vitamin C and Vitamin E Supplementation Do Not Appear to Impact Colorectal Cancer Mortality

In a study published in the journal *Cancer Epidemiology, Biomarkers & Prevention*, researchers from Atlanta, Georgia, used data from the American Cancer Society's Cancer

Prevention Study II to determine if vitamin C and E supplementation would impact the mortality of people diagnosed with colorectal cancer. The data consisted of 711,891 men and women in the United States who completed a four-page self-administered questionnaire that included information on demographic characteristics and various behavioral, environmental, occupational, and dietary factors; at baseline, none of the subjects had been diagnosed with cancer. At enrollment, the median age for men was fifty-seven years and for women was fifty-six years. No one was younger than thirty years. During the fourteen years of follow-up, there were 4,404 deaths from colorectal cancer. Of these deaths, 2,468 occurred in men and 1,936 occurred in women. After the researchers adjusted for multiple colorectal cancer risk factors, they observed that the regular and/or long-term use of vitamins C and E were not associated with colorectal cancer mortality. The researchers concluded that their findings "do not support a substantial effect of even relatively long-term use of vitamin C or vitamin E supplementation on risk of colorectal cancer mortality." At the same time, the researchers noted that their findings "cannot rule out effects on populations with poor nutrition or effects that are modest or limited to specific subgroups."[16]

Electroacupuncture Appears to Be Useful for Postoperative Ileus

In a multicenter, randomized, sham-controlled trial published in *AMA Surgery*, researchers based in China wanted to learn if electroacupuncture would be useful for postoperative ileus after laparoscopic surgery for colorectal cancer. (Postoperative ileus is the failure of the bowel to function properly, a condition that sometimes occurs after surgery for colorectal cancer.) The cohort consisted of 248 patients, with a mean age of 60.2 years, who had laparoscopic surgery for colorectal cancer in one of four tertiary hospitals in China. One hundred and fifty-three of the patients were male. After surgery, the patients were randomly assigned to four sessions of electroacupuncture (n = 125) or four sessions of sham electroacupuncture (n = 123). Both types of acupuncture were administered by licensed acupuncturists. For four consecutive days after surgery, the patients received thirty minutes of electroacupuncture or sham acupuncture. The patients in the electroacupuncture group received treatment at specific acupoints; the patients in the sham acupuncture group received minimally invasive acupuncture at non-acupoints. The researchers learned that, when compared to sham acupuncture, electroacupuncture shortened the duration of postoperative ileus and reduced the incidence of prolonged postoperative ileus following the laparoscopic surgery for colorectal cancer. The researchers commented that electroacupuncture "may provide a reasonable treatment option for patients after colorectal surgery to facilitate GI function recovery."[17]

REFERENCES AND FURTHER READING

Boughanem, H., S. Canudas, P. Hernandez-Alonso et al. "Vitamin D Intake and the Risk of Colorectal Cancer: An Updated Meta-Analysis and Systematic Review of Case-Control and Prospective Cohort Studies." *Cancers* 13 (2021): 2814.

Chan, Doris S., Rosa Lau, Dagfinn Aune et al. "Red and Processed Meat and Colorectal Cancer Incidence: Meta-Analysis of Prospective Studies." *PLoS One* 6, no. 6 (June 2011): e20456.

Chierici, Andrea, Paollo Amoretti, Céline Drai et al. "Does Bariatric Surgery Reduce the Risk of Colorectal Cancer in Individuals with Morbid Obesity? A Systematic Review and Meta-Analysis." *Nutrients* 15 (2023): 467.

Derogar, Maryam, Mark A. Hull, Prashant Kant et al. "Increased Risk of Colorectal Cancer After Obesity Surgery." *Annals of Surgery* 258, no. 6 (December 2013): 983–988.

Gylling, B., R. Myte, J. Schneede et al. "Vitamin B-6 and Colorectal Cancer Risk: A Prospective Population-Based Study Using 3 Distinct Plasma Markers of Vitamin B-6 Status." *American Journal of Clinical Nutrition* 105 (2017): 897–904.

Huang, Chu-Yi, Alinuer Abulimiti, Xin Zhang et al. "Dietary B Vitamins and Methionine Intakes and Risk for Colorectal Cancer: A Case-Control Study in China." *British Journal of Nutrition* 123 (2020): 1277–1289.

Jacobs, Eric J., Cari J. Connell, Alpa V. Patel et al. "Vitamin C and Vitamin E Supplement Use and Colorectal Cancer Mortality in a Large American Cancer Society Cohort." *Cancer Epidemiology, Biomarkers & Prevention* 10 (January 2001): 17–23.

Jafari, F., S. Yarmand, M. Nouri et al. "Ultra-Processed Food Intake and Risk of Colorectal Cancer: A Matched Case-Control Study." *Nutrition and Cancer* 75, no. 2 2023): 532–541.

Jin, D., Y. Lu, W. Wu et al. "Diet-Wide Association, Genetic Susceptibility and Colorectal Cancer Risk: A Prospective Cohort Study." *Nutrients* 15 (2023): 4801.

Leufkens, Anke M., Fränzel J. B. Van Duijnhoven, Peter D. Siersema et al. "Cigarette Smoking and Colorectal Cancer Risk in the European Prospective Investigation into Cancer and Nutrition Study." *Clinical Gastroenterology and Hepatology* 9 (2011): 137–144.

O'Sullivan, Dylan E., R. Liam Sutherland, Susanna Town et al. "Risk Factors for Early-Onset Colorectal Cancer: A Systematic Review and Meta-Analysis." *Clinical Gastroenterology and Hepatology* 20 (2022): 1229–1240.

Papadimitriou, N., E, Bouras, P. A. van den Brandt et al. "A Prospective Diet-Wide Association Study for Risk of Colorectal Cancer in EPIC." *Clinical Gastroenterology and Hepatology* 20, no. 4 (April 2022): 864–873.

Schlussel, Andrew T., Ronald A. Gagliano Jr., Susan Seto-Donlon et al. "The Evolution of Colorectal Cancer Genetics–Part 1: From Discovery to Practice." *Journal of Gastrointestinal Oncology* 5, no. 5 (2014): 326–335.

Shroff, Jennifer, Nirav Thosani, Sachin Batra et al. "Reduced Incidence and Mortality from Colorectal Cancer with Flexible Sigmoidoscopy Screening: A Meta-Analysis." *World Journal of Gastroenterology* 20, no. 48 (December 28, 2014): 18466–18476.

Wang, Yu, Jing-Wen Yang, Shi-Yan Yan et al. "Electroacupuncture vs Sham Electroacupuncture in the Treatment of Postoperative Ileus After Laparoscopic Surgery for Colorectal Cancer: A Multicenter, Randomized Clinical Trial." *JAMA Surgery* 158, no. 1 (2023): 20–27.

Yang, Yunfan, Li Yang, Liping Zhou, and Siyuan Tang. "A Critical Review of the Effect of Dietary Fiber Intake on the Prevention of Colorectal Cancer in Eastern Asian Countries." *Journal of Healthcare Engineering* 2021 (2021): 6680698.

CANCER, ESOPHAGEAL

INTRODUCTION

Esophageal cancer develops in the esophagus, the tube that connects the throat to the stomach and moves food along the first part of the digestive system. Tumors develop in the mucosa, which is the inner lining of the esophagus. A particularly aggressive type of cancer, esophageal cancer occurs when cells in the esophagus mutate and grow much faster than normal cells. The esophagus is very flexible and expands as the tumor grows. Only 25 percent of people with esophageal cancer receive a diagnosis before the cancer has spread.

There are two main types of esophageal cancer. Cancers that begin in the gland cells at the bottom of the esophagus close to the stomach are adenocarcinomas. These are the most common type of esophageal cancer in the United States. Squamous cell carcinoma primarily begins in the upper and middle part of the esophagus. Squamous cells are flat and thin and line the surface of the esophagus. Other types of esophageal cancer tend to be rare. These include small cell carcinoma, sarcoma, lymphoma, melanoma, and choriocarcinoma.

According to an article in *Gastroenterology Clinics of North America*, esophageal cancer was first mentioned in ancient Egypt around 3000 BC. About two thousand years ago, there were reports of this illness in China. Between the sixteenth and nineteenth centuries, there were advances in the visualization and removal of these tumors. And, although there have been many advances since then, because so many cases are diagnosed at an advanced stage, "there have been no substantial overall improvement in outcomes from this insidious disease."[1]

SYMPTOMS, RISKS, AND COMPLICATIONS

Early esophageal cancer tends to have no symptoms. Unfortunately, many of the symptoms associated with esophageal cancer are not evident until the cancer has spread. Still, they are important to note. The most common symptom of esophageal cancer is trouble swallowing (dysphagia). Food may feel as if it is caught in the chest. Some people actually choke on food. Over time, these symptoms tend to worsen, and swallowing may be accompanied with a good deal of discomfort. Another common symptom is pain, pressure, or burning in the middle of the chest. Because eating is so uncomfortable, many people with esophageal cancer lose weight without trying, and they have a persistent cough or hoarseness.

There are different risks associated with each type of esophageal cancer. Chronic acid reflux, gastroesophageal reflux disease (GERD), Barrett's esophagus, and chronic heartburn are risk factors for adenocarcinoma. White people are at increased risk for adenocarcinoma. Heavy alcohol consumption, smoking, and organ transplants increase the risk of squamous cell carcinoma. This type is more often seen in African Americans, American Indians, and Hispanics. Men are more likely than women to develop esophageal cancer, and people with obesity have an increased risk, as do people who have a history of human papillomavirus or prolonged occupational exposure to certain chemicals. Other people at increased risk include those who frequently drink very hot liquids, do not eat adequate amounts of fruits and vegetables, and have a history of radiation treatment to the chest or upper abdomen.

Complications associated with esophageal cancer include obstruction of the esophagus, making it difficult to eat and drink, and bleeding in the esophagus, which may be slow and steady or sudden and intense.

PREVALENCE

Worldwide, esophageal cancer is the seventh most common cancer and the sixth most common cause of cancer deaths. It is highly prevalent in northern China, India, and Southern Africa. In fact, a notable 50 percent of all the worldwide cases occur in China. In the United States, esophageal cancer only makes up about 1 percent of all diagnosed cancers. In 2024, there were about 22,370 cases diagnosed (17,690 men, 4,680 women) in the United States. During the same year, there were about 16,130 deaths from this disease (12,880 men and 3,250 women). In the United States, the lifetime chances of getting esophageal cancer are about one in 127 in men and one in 434 in women. Although recently the rates of esophageal cancer have been slightly lower, the overall prevalence has tended to stay about the same.[2]

DIAGNOSIS AND TREATMENT OPTIONS

The most frequent test used to diagnose esophageal cancer is the esophagogastroduodenoscopy. During this test, a medical provider passes a flexible tube with an attached camera, known as an endoscope, into the esophagus to look for abnormal cells. If the biopsy reveals cancer, then the medical provider may order an ultrasound imaging test known as endoscopic ultrasonography. Other common tests used for people who appear to have esophageal cancer include positron emission tomography (PET) scan, which uses radioactive dye to determine if the cancer has spread to other parts of the body, and CT scan, another type of imaging test that may include a dye. It also helps determine if the cancer has spread.

Most treatment plans for esophageal cancer tend to include a three-pronged approach—radiation, chemotherapy, and surgery. In order to shrink the tumors, treatment tends to begin with radiation and chemotherapy before surgery. But, treatment plans may vary from patient to patient, and they will tend to be associated with the stage of the cancer, the patient's overall health and nutrition status, the location of the tumor, and the patient's personal preferences. An esophagectomy is the most common treatment for early-stage esophageal cancer. It involves removing some or most of the esophagus and the surrounding tissue. Surgeons pull up part of the stomach into the chest and neck to create a new esophagus. This may trigger a problem known as dumping syndrome, in which food passes too quickly through the stomach, causing symptoms, such as nausea, vomiting, diarrhea, stomach cramps, sweating, and/or skin flushing. About half of the people treated for early-stage esophageal cancer are alive five years after diagnosis.

RESEARCH FINDINGS

There Are Some Interesting Differences between Esophageal Cancer in Western and Asian Countries

In an article published in the *Chinese Journal of Cancer*, researchers from China outlined some of the differences between esophageal cancer in Western and Asian countries. According to these researchers, the highest worldwide rates of esophageal cancer are seen in eastern Asia and eastern and Southern Africa. At the same time, the lowest rates are seen in Europe and North America. While the incidence of esophageal squamous cell cancer has been declining, the incidence of esophageal adenocarcinoma has been rising. In some Western countries, such as the United States, approximately half of esophageal cancer cases are adenocarcinoma. In contrast, in Asia, esophageal squamous cell cancer is dominant. The researchers noted that an important explanation for the decline in esophageal squamous cell cancer in the United States is the decrease in tobacco smoking and alcohol consumption. They contend that more than 90 percent of the esophageal squamous cell cancers in the United States and other Western countries are related to tobacco smoking and alcohol consumption. Tobacco smoking and alcohol consumption are also the main risk factors for esophageal squamous cell cancer in Asia, but other important risk factors include drinking hot beverages, family cancer history, poor nutrition, mechanical injuries, and opium use. The researchers contend that the sharp increase in esophageal adenocarcinoma in the United States is related to the increasing number of overweight people and people with obesity. Another important risk factor is the increasing frequency of gastroesophageal reflux disease and Barrett's esophagus. While treatments have improved, the researchers noted that the overall survival rate of people with esophageal cancer remains low, with a range of about 10–15 percent. Women tend to have better outcomes than men. The researchers noted that "ethnic differences should be taken into account in preventive and clinical practices."[3]

Cigarette Smoking Increases the Risk of Esophageal Cancer

In a systematic review and meta-analysis published in the *Japanese Journal of Clinical Oncology*, researchers from Japan examined the association between cigarette smoking and risk of esophageal cancer. The researchers identified four cohort studies and eleven case-control studies that met their criteria. Of the cohort studies, one presented the results by sex and three gave the results only for men. Of the case-control studies, one noted the results by sex, five gave the results for men and women combined, three gave results only for men, and two had the results only for women. All of the cohort studies and eight of the eleven case-control studies showed strong positive associations between cigarette smoking and esophageal cancer. Further, the dose-response relationships between cigarette smoking and risk of esophageal cancer were demonstrated in all of the cohort studies and five case-control studies. Even ever-smokers had a significantly higher risk for esophageal cancer than never smokers. Only one cohort study and one case-control study showed the reversal of risk after smoking cessation. The researchers concluded that "there is convincing evidence that cigarette smoking strongly increases the risk of esophageal cancer in the Japanese population."[4]

But, Smoking Cessation May Only Reduce the Risk of Esophageal Squamous Cell Cancer

In a systematic review and meta-analysis published in the *JNCI Journal of the National Cancer Institute*, researchers from China examined the relationship between smoking cessation and the risk of esophageal cancer. They located fifty-two studies that met their criteria. Forty-one studies addressed smoking data and esophageal squamous cell cancer, and twenty-three studies analyzed smoking data and esophageal adenocarcinoma. Forty-four studies were case-control in design; they had 11,965 esophageal cancer cases and 47,817 controls. The remaining eight studies were cohort in design, with 1,185 new esophageal cancer cases among 1,045,947 cohort members. Twenty-two studies were conducted in Europe, ten in the United States, seven in China or Taiwan, three were in Japan, three in Brazil, three in Uruguay, and one in each of the following—Argentina, Australia, the Czech Republic, and Serbia. Some of the information in a few of the studies overlapped with information from a few of the other studies. The researchers learned that people who stopped smoking greatly reduced their risk of esophageal squamous cell cancer. Compared with current smokers, a strong risk reduction was evident after five or more years and became even stronger after ten or twenty more years. While this association was weak in Asian populations, it was strong in Western populations. At the same time, the risk of esophageal adenocarcinoma did not notably decline after smoking cessation. When compared to current smokers, the risk reduction was only slightly lower among former smokers. And, this risk reduction took twenty years to take effect. The researchers concluded that "the preventive effects of smoking cessation on esophageal cancer shown in this study can help guide future health policy and clinical practice."[5]

Heavy Alcohol Consumption Increases the Risk of Esophageal Cancer in Middle-Aged Men

In a trial published in the journal *Molecular and Clinical Oncology*, researchers from China investigated alcohol consumption among middle-aged men who developed esophageal squamous cell cancer. The cohort consisted of 535 men under the age of sixty years who had esophageal squamous cell cancer; they were all age-matched to a control subject. Almost three-quarters of the subjects were between the ages of fifty and fifty-nine, and slightly more than one-quarter were between the ages of forty and forty-nine. The researchers determined that heavy alcohol consumption, defined as more than 53.3 g ethanol per day, was an important risk factor for esophageal squamous cell cancer in middle-aged Chinese males. Further, heavy alcohol consumption, even for a shorter duration, may lead to the development of esophageal squamous cell cancer at a younger age. In this study, smoking was not identified as a significant risk factor.[6]

Abdominal Obesity Is Associated with an Increased Risk of Esophageal Cancer

In a nationwide population-based cohort study published in the *Journal of Gastroenterology*, researchers from South Korea reviewed the association between abdominal obesity, as measured by waist circumference, and the risk of esophageal cancer. The cohort consisted of 22,809,722 individuals who had regular health check-ups provided by the National Health Insurance Corporation in South Korea, a national insurer managed by the Korean government. Abdominal obesity was defined as a waist circumference greater than 90 cm for men and greater than 85 cm for women. During a median follow-up period of 6.4 years, 12,033 individuals developed esophageal cancer. Compared to the non-abdominal obese people, the researchers learned that the people with abdominal obesity were generally older, more likely to be ex/non-smokers, and less likely to be excessive alcohol consumers. They exercised less frequently, were residents of urban areas, had diabetes and dyslipidemia, higher fasting glucose levels, higher systolic and diastolic pressure, and higher serum total cholesterol. The researchers determined that in the total population studied, abdominal obesity was positively associated with the development of esophageal cancer; it increased the risk by 29 percent. They concluded that "abdominal body fat accumulation might be a risk factor for esophageal cancer."[7]

There Seems to Be an Association between Hot Tea Consumption and Risk of Esophageal Cancer

In a systematic review and meta-analysis published in the journal *Frontiers in Nutrition*, researchers from China evaluated the association between hot tea consumption and risk of esophageal cancer. They identified twenty-three reports on thirty-four individual studies that met their criteria; these included 5,050 cases of esophageal cancer and 10,609 controls. All of the included articles were published in English, and the cases were histologically, pathologically, or cytologically confirmed as esophageal cancer. In the studies, twenty were population-based case-control, eight were hospital-based case-control, and six were prospective cohort in design. Twenty-two studies were conducted in Asia, four were from the Americas, four from Europe, three in Australia, and one in Africa. Twenty-two studies reported results for males and females together, six provided results only for women, and six reported results only for men. The researchers learned that hot tea consumption was associated with a significantly increased risk of esophageal squamous cell cancer; the increased risk for esophageal adenocarcinoma was not significant. The researchers commented that their findings are "consistent with the majority of the literature to date."[8]

There Appears to Be a Relationship between Height, Body Mass Index, and Esophageal Cancer

In a study published in the journal *Cancer Causes and Control*, researchers from Norway examined the association between height, BMI, and esophageal cancer. Over a period of several decades, data were collected on the heights and weights of more than two million Norwegian men and women; during a follow-up of an average of twenty-three years, there were 2,245 histologically verified esophageal cancer cases—1,597 in men and 648 in women. The mean age at diagnosis was sixty-nine and seventy-two in men and women, respectively. In men, 28 percent of cases were adenocarcinomas and 64 percent were squamous cell cancer. In women, the corresponding figures were 20 percent and 73 percent. The mean age at diagnosis for men with adenocarcinoma and squamous cell cancer was seventy and sixty-eight, respectively. The similar figures for women were seventy-six and seventy-one. While 13 percent of the women had obesity, a smaller 6 percent of the men had obesity. The researchers learned that underweight men and women had an increased risk of esophageal cancer. Overweight men and men with obesity had about the same risk of esophageal cancer as normal-weight men, while overweight women had a lower overall risk than normal-weight women. When reviewed more closely, overweight people and people with obesity had a lower risk of esophageal squamous cell cancer than normal-weight individuals, but a higher risk of esophageal adenocarcinoma. Meanwhile, the risk of esophageal cancer decreased with increasing height; the risk in the tallest men was about half the risk in the shortest men. Though the evidence was weaker, similar differences were seen in women. Commenting on their overall results, the researchers noted that low BMI increased the risk of esophageal squamous cell cancer and high BMI increased the risk of esophageal adenocarcinoma. "BMI had opposite relations to the two most common histological groups of esophageal cancer."[9]

Consumption of Red and Processed Meats May Be Related to Risk of Esophageal Squamous Cell Cancer

In a study published in the *Annals of Oncology*, researchers from the Netherlands examined the association between the consumption of red and processed meats and the risk of esophageal cancer. Their cohort consisted of 120,850 people between the ages of fifty-five and sixty-nine years. Their food intake was assessed using a 150-item food frequency questionnaire. After 16.3 years of follow-up, there were 107 cases of esophageal squamous cell cancer and 145 cases of esophageal adenocarcinomas. Compared to the subjects with the lowest intake of red meat, the subjects with the highest intake of red meat were more likely to be smokers, have a slightly higher BMI, a lower education, and be consumers of more energy and alcohol and less fruits and vegetables. Subjects with the highest intake of processed meat were slightly younger, had a higher BMI, were more likely to be smokers, and were less likely to have a family history of esophageal or gastric cancer. Compared to those in the lowest intake, they consumed more energy (calories) and alcohol, and they had less education. The researchers found that among men, processed meat intake was strongly associated with esophageal squamous cell cancer. Their calculations predicted a 2.15 increase in risk per 50 g per day increment in processed meat intake. There did not appear to be an association between intake of red and processed meat and esophageal adenocarcinoma in men. Moreover, the researchers found no association between intake of red and processed meat in women with either type of esophageal cancer. The researchers commented that their findings "underscore the importance of analyzing histological subtypes separately."[10]

Higher Intake of Fruits and Vegetables Is Associated with Lower Rates of Esophageal Squamous Cell Cancer

In a systematic review and meta-analysis published in the *International Journal of Cancer*, researchers from China investigated the association between intake of fruits and vegetables and risk of esophageal cancer. The researchers found thirty-two articles, twenty-seven case-control, and five cohort studies, of 10,037 people with esophageal squamous cell cancer. Seventeen studies were from Asia, four from North America, four from South America, and seven from Europe. Twenty-nine studies reviewed the association between fruit intake and the risk of esophageal squamous cell cancer, and twenty-four studies addressed the relationship between vegetable intake and the risk of esophageal squamous cell cancer. In general, there was an inverse association between intake of these foods and the risk of this type of cancer. The intake of fruits and vegetables was associated with significant reductions in esophageal squamous cell cancer. The researchers noted the need for more research "in well-designed prospective studies with validated questionnaires and good control of confounders."[11]

In a case-control study published in the journal *Diseases of the Esophagus*, researchers from Australia and China also examined the association between the consumption of fruits and vegetables and the risk of esophageal cancer in the north-west region of China, where the population deals with high rates of this disease. The cohort consisted of 359 people with incident esophageal cancer and 380 hospital-based controls. Seventy-two percent of the participants were men, and the cohort had an average age of sixty-one years. About half of the group were smokers who regularly drank alcoholic beverages. Using a validated semi-quantitative food frequency questionnaire, information on fruit and vegetable intake was obtained during face-to-face interviews. The researchers learned that the patients with esophageal cancer consumed significantly less fruits and vegetables than the controls. And, they had a significantly lower intake of vitamin C, vitamin E, niacin, folate, β-cryptoxanthin, potassium, magnesium, and calcium. It is notable that people with the highest intake of fruits and vegetables had more than a 50 percent reduction in risk for esophageal cancer. The researchers concluded that "habitual consumption of fruits and vegetables appeared to be inversely associated with the risk of esophageal cancer for adults in north-west China, together with supportive evidence from the corresponding dietary nutrients."[12]

Post-surgical Vitamin D Supplementation May Help People Dealing with Esophageal Cancer

In a study published in the journal *Scientific Reports*, researchers based in China wanted to determine if postoperative vitamin D supplementation was useful for people with esophageal cancer. The cohort consisted of 303 patients. Of these, forty-nine (16.2 percent) used vitamin D after their surgeries, taking 200 to 400 IU daily. However, 254 (83.8 percent) did not use vitamin D supplementation. After two years, only 181 of these patients were still alive. Thirty-two of these patients were taking vitamin D and 149 were not. Vitamin D users tended to be younger, have attended some college, had a higher income, participated in more physical activity, had a lower fat intake, used less tobacco, and were more likely to suffer from diabetes. They had better social functioning, global health, appetite, and quality of life, as well as less fatigue and appetite loss. The researchers commented that "the association of vitamin D with cancer has been reported by several reviews, which proposed it might have potential role as anticancer drug." Thus, their findings "showed that vitamin D supplement use could serve as a promising intervention to enhance QOL [quality of life] and prolong DFS [disease-free survival] in EC [esophageal cancer]."[13]

Some B Vitamins May Lower the Risk of Esophageal Cancer

In a systematic review and meta-analysis published in the journal *Cancer Management and Research*, researchers from China studied the association between dietary intake of the B vitamins (B1, B2, B3, B5, B6, B9, and B12) and the risk of esophageal cancer. The researchers identified nineteen articles that met their criteria. All of the studies, which were published between 1988 and 2017, were conducted in Asia, Europe, America, and Australia. One study was cohort in design and eighteen were case-control. The researchers determined that dietary intake of vitamins B1, B3, B6, and B9 were associated with a decreased risk of esophageal cancer. In contrast, no such association was seen between dietary vitamins B2 and B5 and esophageal cancer. A statistically significant inverse association was observed for an increase of 100 μg per day in supplemental vitamins B6 and B9 and risk of esophageal cancer. On the other hand, vitamin B12 derived from animal foods may be related to an increased risk of esophageal cancer. The researchers commented that "the reason why vitamin B affects the risk of cancer may be because it is essential for the biosynthesis of nucleotides, replication of DNA, supply of methyl groups, and the growth and repair of cells."[14]

Dietary Vitamin C May Provide Some Protection from Esophageal Cancer

In a systematic review and dose-response meta-analysis published in the *International Journal of Cancer*, researchers from China examined the association between intake of dietary vitamin C and the risk of esophageal cancer. The researchers located fifteen articles reporting on twenty studies that met their criteria; there were 3,955 people with esophageal cancer and 7,063 controls. Nineteen of the studies were case-control in design, and one was a cohort study. Eighteen of the studies came from the United States or Europe. Only two studies were from Asia. The researchers determined that the people with the highest intake of dietary vitamin C had the lowest levels of esophageal cancer. In fact, with the increase in vitamin C intake of 50 mg per day, the risk of esophageal cancer statistically decreased by 13 percent. The researchers concluded that "further well-designed large prospective cohort studies with repeated measurements of dietary vitamin C intake, long follow-up periods, and adjustment for all potential cofounders are needed to verify the association of dietary vitamin C intake with esophageal cancer."[15]

Higher Dietary Vitamin E Intake May Lower the Risk of Esophageal Cancer

In a systematic review and meta-analysis published in the journal *Nutrients*, researchers from China evaluated the association between dietary vitamin E intake and the risk of esophageal cancer. They located twelve articles on fourteen studies that met their criteria, with 3,013 cases of esophageal cancer and 11,384 controls. Among these studies, one was cohort in design and eleven were case-control studies. Most of the studies were conducted in Europe. But, the remainder were from America, Asia, and Oceania. Food frequency questionnaires were used to assess dietary vitamin E intakes. When the researchers compared the highest intake of vitamin E to the lowest intake of vitamin E, they determined that vitamin E appeared to play a role in the prevention of esophageal cancer. People who had the highest intake of dietary vitamin E were the least likely to develop esophageal cancer. This was particularly true for esophageal squamous cell cancer. The researchers concluded that "more large-scale prospective studies and randomized controlled trials are still needed to confirm our results, though our findings could provide certain evidence for esophageal cancer prevention."[16]

Herbal Medicine May or May Not Be Useful for Dumping Syndrome

In a literature review published in the journal *Integrative Cancer Therapies*, researchers from Korea evaluated the usefulness of herbal medicine for the dumping syndrome associated with gastrointestinal surgery. The researchers located three randomized controlled trials with 174 patients with dumping syndrome that met their criteria. The patients were included without any restriction on sex, age, race, country, or onset. All treatments using herbal medicines were included without any limitations on number, administration methods, dosages, and durations of treatment. The control treatments included any type of conventional therapy, placebo therapy, or no treatment. There were no reports of dropouts. The duration of treatments ranged from ten to thirty-five days. All three trials used different herbal medicines that were taken orally. Two of the trials found that the herbal medicine significantly improved the symptoms. But, the researchers concluded that they had too few articles and too small a sample size to draw a definitive conclusion. And, there was concern about the quality of the trials and their potential high risk of bias. Nevertheless, the researchers commented that "using herbal medicine to treat dumping syndrome could be more beneficial than conventional therapy alone."[17]

Traditional Chinese Medicine May Improve Longevity in People with Stage 4 Esophageal Squamous Cell Cancer

In a retrospective study published in the *International Journal of General Medicine*, researchers from China evaluated the use of traditional Chinese medicine (TCM) for people with stage 4 esophageal squamous cell cancer. The cohort consisted of 402 patients with esophageal squamous cell cancer who were treated at one of two hospitals in China from July 2017 to June 2020. Of these, 196 (48.8 percent) were treated with TCM and conventional medicine and 206 were treated only with conventional medicine. During this study period, a fourth of all patients admitted to these hospitals with cancer received a primary diagnosis of esophageal cancer. And, though all of these patients clearly had a poor prognosis, the researchers determined that the patients treated with the combination therapy lived two months longer than those who were only treated with conventional therapy. The researchers concluded, "it is undeniable that in the real world, TCM is useful in the treatment of esophageal cancer, whether in syndrome differentiation or as an adjunct to Western medicine. A comprehensive approach based on TCM may reduce adverse reactions from Western therapies, increase treatment sensitivity, and reduce the change of recurrence."[18]

REFERENCES AND FURTHER READING

Bo, Yacong, Yan Lu, Yan Zhao et al. "Association Between Dietary Vitamin C Intake and Risk of Esophageal Cancer: A Dose-Response Meta-Analysis." *International Journal of Cancer* 138 (2016): 1843–1850.

Cho, Jae Ho, Cheol Min Shin, Kyung-Do Han et al. "Abdominal Obesity Increases Risk for Esophageal Cancer: A Nationwide Population-Based Cohort Study of South Korea." *Journal of Gastroenterology* 55 (2020): 307–316.

Cui, Lingling, Li Li, Yalan Tian et al. "Association Between Dietary Vitamin E Intake and Esophageal Cancer Risk: An Update Meta-Analysis." *Nutrients* 10 (2018): 801.

Engeland, Anders, Steinar Tretli, and Tone Bjørge. "Height and Body Mass Index in Relation to Esophageal Cancer; 23-Year Follow-Up of Two Million Norwegian Men and Women." *Cancer Causes and Control* 15 (2004): 837–843.

Eslick, Guy D. "Esophageal Cancer: A Historical Perspective." *Gastroenterology Clinics of North America* 38, no. 1 (2009): 1–15.

Hong, Seungcheol, Bongki Park, Hyeonseok Noh, and Dong-Jun Choi. "Herbal Medicine for Dumping Syndrome: A Systematic Review and Meta-Analysis." *Integrative Cancer Therapies* 18 (2019): NA.

Keszei, A. P., L. J. Schouten, R. A. Goldbohm, and P. A. van den Brandt. "Red and Processed Meat Consumption and the Risk of Esophageal and Gastric Cancer Subtypes in The Netherlands Cohort Study." *Annals of Oncology* 23 (2012): 2319–2326.

Kumagai, N., T. Wakai, K. Akazawa et al. "Heavy Alcohol Intake Is a Risk Factor for Esophageal Squamous Cell Carcinoma Among Middle-Aged Men: A Case-Control and Simulation Study." *Molecular and Clinical Oncology* 1 (2013): 811–816.

Li, Honglin, Chunzheng Ma, Sisi Chang et al. "Traditional Chinese Medicine Decoctions Improve Longevity Following Diagnosis with Stage IV Esophageal Squamous Cell Carcinoma: A Retrospective Analysis." *International Journal of General Medicine* 15 (2022): 1665–1675.

Liu, Jun, Jian Wang, Ye Leng, and Changxing Lv. "Intake of Fruit and Vegetables and Risk of Esophageal Squamous Cell Carcinoma: A Meta-Analysis of Observational Studies." *International Journal of Cancer* 133 (2013): 473–486.

Luo, Hui and Hong Ge. "Hot Tea Consumption and Esophageal Cancer Risk: A Meta-Analysis of Observational Studies." *Frontiers in Nutrition* 9 (April 2022): 831567.

Ma, Jun-Li, Yan Zhao, Chen-Yang Guo et al. "Dietary Vitamin B Intake and the Risk of Esophageal Cancer: A Meta-Analysis." *Cancer Management and Research* 10 (2018): 5395–5410.

Oze, Isao, Keitaro Matsuo, Hidemi Ito et al. "Cigarette Smoking and Esophageal Cancer Risk: An Evaluation Based on a Systematic Review of Epidemiologic Evidence Among the Japanese Population." *Japanese Journal of Clinical Oncology* 42, no. 1 (2012): 63–73.

Tang, L., A. H. Lee, F. Xu et al. "Fruit and Vegetable Consumption and Risk of Esophageal Cancer: A Case-Control Study in North-West China." *Disease of the Esophagus* 27 (2014): 777–782.

Wang, Lu, Cong Wang, Jiangfeng Wang et al. "Longitudinal, Observational Study on Associations Between Postoperative Nutritional Vitamin D Supplementation and Clinical Outcomes in Esophageal Cancers Patients Undergoing Esophagectomy." *Scientific Reports* 6 (2016): 38962.

Wang, Qiao-Li, Shao-Hua Xie, Wen-Tao Li, and Jesper Lagergren. "Smoking Cessation and Risk of Esophageal Cancer by Histological Type: Systematic Review and Meta-Analysis." *JNCL Journal of the National Cancer Institute* 109, no. 12 (2017): djx115.

Zhang, Han-Ze, Guang-Fu Jin, and Hong-Bing Shen. "Epidemiologic Differences in Esophageal Cancer Between Asian and Western Populations." *Chinese Journal of Cancer* 31, no. 6 (2012): 281–286.

CANCER, LIVER

INTRODUCTION

Liver cancer (hepatocellular carcinoma—HCC) is a primary cancer that forms in the cells of the liver, a large, football-sized organ located in the upper portions of the abdomen. But, a much less common form of liver cancer may occur in the epithelial cells of the bile ducts in the liver. This is termed cholangiocarcinoma. Liver cancer develops when liver cells mutate or have changes in their DNA. These altered cells grow very quickly and eventually form a mass or tumor. HCC is usually seen in individuals with chronic hepatitis B or hepatitis C infections or cirrhosis due to alcohol. Though there are other causes, they are less likely.

Hepatocellular carcinoma is classified into one of four stages. With stage I, there is a single tumor in the liver that measures no more than 2 centimeters, or there is a solitary tumor greater than 2 centimeters without vascular invasion. With stage II HCC, there is a single tumor more than 2 centimeters without vascular invasion or multiple tumors no greater than 5 centimeters. With stage III HCC, there are multiple tumors, at least one of which measures more than 5 centimeters. And, with stage IV HCC, the cancer has spread to adjacent organs or involves the major portal vein or hepatic vein.

However, it is not unusual for cancer cells that form in another part of the body to spread to the liver. This type of cancer is not termed liver cancer. Rather, it is called metastatic cancer.

In the 1960s, while analyzing blood samples from different populations across the world, Baruch Blumberg, MD/PhD, identified the surface antigen of HBV (hepatitis B virus). Blumberg and others found that this antigen was present in those with hepatitis B and that HBV could cause liver cancer. Blumberg received the Nobel Prize in 1976 for his work on HBV.[1]

SYMPTOMS, RISKS, AND COMPLICATIONS

Unfortunately, in the earlier stages, when it is most treatable, HCC tends to have no symptoms. As the cancer progresses, symptoms may include loss of appetite and subsequent weight loss, upper abdominal pain and/or swelling, right-sided abdominal pain, rapid weight gain from the build-up of fluids, a lump below the rib cage, pain near the right shoulder, nausea and vomiting, general weakness and fatigue, dark-colored urine, intense itching, bloating, shortness of breath, yellow discoloration of the skin (jaundice) and the white of the eyes (icterus), fever, a general feeling of being unwell, and chalky, white stools.

Sometimes, HCC secretes hormones. When this occurs, there are additional symptoms. These may include high levels of cholesterol (hypercholesterolemia), low levels of blood sugar (hypoglycemia), diarrhea, male enlarged breasts (gynecomastia), high red blood cell levels (erythrocytosis), and elevated levels of blood calcium (hypercalcemia).

A number of factors increase the risk of HCC. These include chronic infection with the hepatitis B (HBV) or the hepatitis C virus (HCV), cirrhosis or scarring of the liver, certain inherited diseases, diabetes, higher consumption of alcohol, traumatic injury to the liver, exposure to aflatoxins, and nonalcoholic fatty liver disease.

HCC is associated with several complications. These may include bleeding and the subsequent development of anemia, bile duct obstruction, portal hypertension (elevated pressure in the portal vein system) and bleeding into the esophagus, hepatorenal syndrome (kidney failure in advanced liver disease), and hepatic encephalopathy, with symptoms that may initially resemble Alzheimer's disease.

PREVALENCE

In 2024, about 41,630 new cases of liver cancer were diagnosed in the United States; there were 28,000 in men and 13,630 in women. About 29,840 people died from this illness; 19,120 men and 10,720 women. It is most often diagnosed between the ages of fifty-five and sixty-four years. While liver cancer is less common in the United States than in many other countries, the numbers in the United States have been rising. Liver cancer is more often seen in countries in sub-Saharan Africa and Southeast Asia. In these countries, it may be the most frequently seen type of cancer. Each year, throughout the world, more than 800,000 people are diagnosed with liver cancer, and it accounts for more than 700,000 annual deaths.[2] So, it is a type of cancer with a relatively poor prognosis.

DIAGNOSIS AND TREATMENT OPTIONS

Testing for liver cancer begins with blood tests, such as liver function tests, which check liver enzymes, proteins, and other substances. These tests determine whether the liver is healthy and functioning properly or damaged. Blood tests may also look for alpha-fetoprotein (AFP). High levels of AFP may indicate liver cancer. An ultrasound may be used to obtain images of the liver, as may a CT scan. In addition, images may be obtained from a MRI, which uses a large magnet, radio waves, and a computer. An angiogram may be used to examine the blood vessels in the liver. During this test, a dye is injected into an artery. If the healthcare provider suspects cholangiocarcinoma, other tests may be ordered. These include an endoscopic retrograde cholangiopancreatography (ERCP), which uses an endoscope and catheter to examine bile ducts, and a percutaneous transhepatic cholangiography (PTC), which inserts a needle with contrast dye into the bile ducts and liver before X-rays are taken.

Like many other forms of cancer, treatment is most successful during the early stages of the disease. With HCC, this includes focusing on treating hepatitis B and hepatitis C when they are first detected, before they may transform into liver cancer. Once liver cancer is growing, it may be treated with radiation therapy, chemotherapy, immunotherapy, and targeted therapy. There is also surgery to remove part of the liver, and, in some cases, the entire liver may be removed and replaced with a donor liver (liver transplantation). Other treatments include hepatic arterial embolization, which destroys cancer cells by blocking the blood supply; ablation, which kills cancer cells with extreme heat; and cryoablation, which uses extreme cold to destroy cancer cells. Sometimes alcohol or chemotherapy may be injected directly into the liver, or beads filled with radioactive material may be placed in the liver. People with liver cancer often turn to alternative and complementary treatments to ease pain and anxiety and, possibly, improve the prognosis. Though there is little published scientific research on the effectiveness of these treatments for HCC, they may include acupressure, acupuncture, hypnosis, massage therapy, music therapy, and relaxation techniques. With liver cancer, these treatments should never be used as a replacement for conventional medicine.

RESEARCH FINDINGS

Vitamin E Intake May Lower the Risk of Liver Cancer

In a study published in the *Journal of the National Cancer Institute*, researchers from Nashville, Tennessee, and China evaluated the association between vitamin E intake from diet and supplements and the risk of liver cancer. The cohort consisted of 132,837 men and women from the Shanghai Men's Health Study and the Shanghai Women's Health Study. Interviews were conducted using a validated food frequency questionnaire, and data were collected. Follow-ups included in-person interviews. After the first two years of follow-up were excluded, there were 5.5 years of follow-up in the men's study and 10.9 years of follow-up in the women's study. During that time, 149 men and 118 women developed liver cancer. The participants who developed liver cancer were older and more likely to have a lower education level. They were more likely to have a history of viral hepatitis, chronic liver disease and cirrhosis, cholelithiasis or cholecystectomy, and a family history of liver cancer in first-degree relatives. In the men's survey, the men who developed liver cancer were more likely to have a lower family income, a history of diabetes, and higher fat intake. In the women's survey, the women who developed liver cancer were more likely to have a higher body mass index. The researchers determined that vitamin E intake, including supplement use, was inversely associated with liver cancer risk. This association was consistent among participants with or without self-reported liver disease or a family history of liver cancer. (It should be noted that when the study only included data from the men, the association was not significant.) Nevertheless, the findings are still notable. The "high intake of vitamin E either from diet or supplements was related to lower risk of liver cancer in middle-aged or older people from China."[3]

Physical Activity Seems to Offer Some Protection from Liver Cancer

In a systematic review and meta-analysis published in the *International Journal of Environmental Research and Public Health*, a researcher from South Korea examined the ability of physical activity to reduce the risk of liver cancer and liver cancer mortality. The researcher identified ten prospective cohort studies that met the established criteria. Four of the studies were conducted in the United States, three were from Japan, one from Taiwan, one from South Korea, and one was a multinational study that had subjects from several countries. In total, there were 8,283,426 subjects, and the average follow-up was 11.35 years. The levels of physical activity were divided into three groups—high (three or more hours per week), moderate (two to three hours per week), and low (less than two hours per week). The researcher determined that high and moderate amounts of physical activity were associated with a 75 percent decreased risk of liver cancer. And, those who participated in high amounts of physical activity had a 25 percent lower risk of liver cancer mortality; moderate participation was associated with a 19 percent reduction in liver cancer mortality. According to the researcher, "risks and mortality of liver cancer were associated with the amount and intensity of physical activity." The researcher concluded that there is a need for more studies to confirm these results.[4]

And, Although Exercise Appears to Be Useful for Those Who Already Have Liver Cancer, Very Few People with Liver Cancer Actually Exercise

In a trial published in the journal *Scientific Reports*, researchers from China wanted to learn if participating in exercise would benefit those already diagnosed with liver cancer. The cohort consisted of 207 subjects with an average age of 55.4 years. Recruited from a tertiary cancer hospital, the subjects completed nurse-administered questionnaires that assessed their medical and demographic variables, exercise habits, and cancer-related fatigue. The patients were classified as active or insufficiently active. The researchers determined that only 6.8 percent of the subjects met the requirements for exercise, and 30.4 percent exercised one or two times per week; 26.6 percent exercised for less than thirty minutes, and 77.8 percent conducted light exercise. About 45 percent maintained or increased their exercise after diagnosis, while 35.3 percent stopped exercising and 19.3 percent reduced the amount of exercise. While the subjects were aware of the benefits of exercise, they tended to encounter different obstacles after receiving treatment. And, according to the researchers, this was a widespread problem. As a result, the researchers advised that "more measures, including clinical education and research, should be taken to improve the knowledge and management of exercise in patients. Hospitals and communities should properly conduct supervised sports interventions, strengthen the establishment of rehabilitation sites for patients with cancer, and provide suitable sports sites for discharged patients."[5]

Vitamin D Deficiency Is Associated with an Increased Risk of Liver Cancer

In a systematic review and meta-analysis published in the *Asian Pacific Journal of Cancer Prevention*, researchers from China assessed the association between levels of vitamin D in the blood and the risk of liver cancer. The researchers identified eleven studies that met their criteria. There were six case-control studies and five cohort studies with a total of 12,895 incident cases. Four studies were conducted in Europe, five in Asia, and two in Egypt. The researchers determined that people with a vitamin D deficiency had a significantly higher risk of liver cancer. In fact, the overall pooled relative risk increased by 2.16 percent. The researchers concluded that their findings "support the hypothesis that vitamin D deficiency status is related to a higher risk of liver cancer, and thus maintenance of sufficient serum vitamin D levels could be beneficial for prevention of liver cancer."[6]

Smoking Is an Independent Risk Factor for Hepatocellular Cancer

In a study published in the *British Journal of Cancer*, researchers from Singapore, Minneapolis, Minnesota, and Los Angeles, California, evaluated the association between smoking and the risk of HCC in the Singapore Chinese Health Study, a prospective cohort with a low intake of alcohol. In this study, which included 63,257 men and women between the ages of forty-five and seventy-four years, information on cigarette smoking and alcohol intake was obtained through structured in-person enrollment interviews. From this cohort, the researchers evaluated 61,321 subjects who had no history of invasive cancer at enrollment. During a mean follow-up of 11.5 years, there were 394 incident cases of HCC. Almost all of the cases were diagnosed histologically. After they adjusted for alcohol consumption and other potential confounders, the researchers determined that current smokers had a statistically significant higher risk of HCC that was dose- and duration-dependent. So, those who smoked more and those who smoked for longer periods of time had an increased risk. The researchers concluded that their findings "provided the strongest epidemiologic evidence to date that tobacco smoking is a causal factor for HCC development in humans."[7]

Another Study Found an Association between Tobacco Smoking and the Use of Solid Fuels for Cooking and the Risk of Liver Cancer

In a prospective cohort study of half a million Chinese adults published in the *International Journal of Cancer*, researchers from China examined the association between tobacco smoking, cooking with solid fuels, and the risk of liver cancer. Data were obtained from the China Kadoorie Biobank (CKB) study, which recruited slightly more than half a million people between the ages of thirty and seventy-nine years from ten areas across China during a four-year period of time. They had a mean age of 51.5 years, and 59 percent were female. At baseline, the subjects reported on their smoking and fuel use. During an 11.1-year median follow-up period, there were 2,997 recorded cases of liver cancer. Overall, 29.4 percent were current smokers. Among those who cooked at least once per month, 48.8 percent always used solid fuels, such as coal or wood, for cooking. Current smokers and solid fuel users had less education and lower income, were less likely to be nonmanual workers, and more likely to drink alcohol, to use solid fuels for heating, and to have poorer kitchen ventilation. Compared to those who always used clean fuels for cooking, solid fuel users were more likely to be rural residents, current smokers, and to have exposure to environmental tobacco smoke. The researchers learned that tobacco smoking and solid fuel use were each associated with an increased risk of liver cancer. Compared with never smokers, current smokers had a 28 percent higher risk of developing liver cancer. The researchers concluded that "tobacco smoking and solid food use for cooking were each independently associated with higher risk of liver cancer incidence." And, they added that their findings "reinforce the importance of smoking cessation and promotion of access to clean energy, especially in less-developed areas."[8]

Hepatitis B and Hepatitis C Are Major Worldwide Causes of Liver Cancer

In a systematic review published in the journal *Hepatology*, researchers from France evaluated the worldwide association between hepatitis B, hepatitis C, and liver cancer. The researchers located 260 studies with a total of 119,006 HCC cases from fifty countries. Study sizes varied substantially and so did the contributions from each country. The majority of cases were from eastern Asia (39.2 percent), followed by North America (27.8 percent) and Europe (6.5 percent). Most European and American countries showed a preponderance of HCV over HBV, and Asian and African countries generally showed mostly HBV. The number of HCV-positive HCC cases was "substantial" in Taiwan, Mongolia, Japan, and Pakistan, as well as in Western-Central Asia and Northern Africa. Since the year 2000, the United States, Brazil, and Germany showed evidence of a high prevalence of HCV in HCC. At the same time, Japan and Italy had a decline in the proportion of HCV-positive HCC. No eligible studies were available for large parts of Africa, Eastern Europe, Central Asia, and Oceania. The researchers concluded that HBV and HCV are major causes of HCC "in virtually all world areas, with a growing fraction of HCC cases in several countries attributable to HCV." Improvements in the treatment of HBV and HCV may help stem this tide, "but limited access and high cost of mass viral screening and new drugs are major challenges for secondary prevention." That is why the focus must be on preventing these infections, emphasizing "universal vaccination against HBV, safe injections and blood transfusion practices, and avoidance of parenteral treatment when oral alternatives are available."[9]

Moderate to Heavy Alcohol Consumption Increases the Risk of Liver Cancer

In a systematic review and meta-analysis published in the journal *Gut and Liver*, researchers from South Korea reviewed the association between varying levels of alcohol consumption and the risk of liver cancer. The researchers identified six nested case-control studies and twenty-two cohort studies that met their criteria. These included 4,899 incident cases and 10,859 liver cancer-related deaths. Eighteen studies were from Asia, five were from the United States, and five were from Europe. The researchers determined that moderate and heavy drinkers—women who drank one or more drinks per day and men who drank two or more drinks per day—had pooled odds ratios of 1.418 for liver cancer and 1.167 for liver cancer mortality. So, people who drank more than light drinkers had a 42 percent increased risk of liver cancer and a 17 percent increase in liver cancer death. Compared to those who drank less alcohol, the liver-related mortality rate was 3.2 fold higher in moderate drinkers. The researchers noted that most previous studies had been conducted on people who drank more than 40 to 60 g per day of alcohol. Thus, according to these researchers, even smaller amounts of alcohol, such as one or two drinks per day, may have an adverse effect on health. The researchers concluded that "more than light alcohol consumption should be considered harmful as it not only increases the incidence of liver cancer but also increases liver disease and overall mortality."[10]

Following a Hepatectomy, the Outcomes of Younger Patients Are Better than Older Patients

In a study published in the journal *Liver Cancer*, researchers from Japan examined the safety of a hepatectomy (the removal of all or part of the liver) for people in their seventies and eighties. The researchers identified 27,094 patients who had a hepatectomy for liver cancer over a five-year period of time. The patients were divided into the following five categories: fifty-nine years and under, sixty to sixty-nine years, seventy to seventy-nine years, eighty to eighty-four years, and eighty-five years and older. The groups had, respectively, the following number of patients—5,099, 8,809, 10,805, 2,011, and 370. Patients between the ages of seventy and seventy-nine were most likely to have two or more comorbidities, but, interestingly, the proportion of patients without comorbidity was lowest among those between the ages of eighty and eighty-four. The researchers learned that compared to patients in their seventies, the patients who were fifty-nine years or younger had significantly lower mortality rates. However, there were no significant differences observed in those aged eighty to eighty-four and those over the age of eighty-five. The researchers noted that the operative risks for a hepatectomy gradually increased with age until seventy years. Morbidity and mortality tended to reach a plateau among those in their 70s, and there was no difference in the short-term outcomes after the surgery between those in their 70s and those in their 80s. It was evident that the selection was "unconsciously self-regulated in patients aged over 80 years by selecting a more favorable case and implementing a less invasive procedure, such as limited resection or laparoscopic hepatectomy." As a result, surgeons were able to obtain good results even in patients in their seventies, eighties, and nineties.[11]

Statin Use May Lower the Risk of Hepatocellular Cancer in People at Increased Risk

In a longitudinal nationwide nested case-control study published in the *Journal of Hepatology*, researchers from South Korea assessed the association between the use of statin medications and the risk of HCC. Data were obtained from the National Health Insurance Service Physical Health Examination Cohort. Based on the time of the follow-up, sex, and age, individuals diagnosed with HCC were matched to controls. In total, 1,642 cases of HCC were matched to 8,210 controls from 514,866 participants. The mean follow-up time was 7.5 years. The subjects were predominantly male (83.6 percent), and 69.4 percent were between the ages of fifty and sixty-nine years. The researchers determined that compared to the controls, the people with HCC had more elevated liver enzymes, liver cirrhosis, chronic viral hepatitis, alcohol-related disorders, less frequent aspirin use, and less frequent use of a statin, such as atorvastatin, lovastatin, pitavastatin, and rosuvastatin. When compared to non-users, the subjects who used statins had a significantly lower rate of HCC. And, with the cumulative increases in statin doses, there was a trend toward greater risk reduction. And, this benefit may be even stronger in those with diabetes mellitus and liver cirrhosis: people who have an even higher risk of HCC.[12]

And, Statin Use after Diagnosis of Hepatocellular Cancer Is Associated with a Decreased Mortality from This Disease

In a retrospective study published in the journal *Clinical Gastroenterology and Hepatology*, researchers from Houston, Texas wanted to learn if the use of statins after a diagnosis of HCC would reduce the mortality from the disease. The researchers analyzed data from 15,422 patients with HCC in the Veterans Administration Central Cancer Registry; they were diagnosed from 2002 to 2016. Among all of these patients, the median survival time following diagnosis was only 17.24 months. Yet, some patients tended to live longer than others, and one of the reasons appeared to be statins. After identifying statin prescriptions that were filled before and after the cancer diagnosis, they determined that statin use after diagnosis was recorded for 14.9 percent of the patients with HCC. Moreover, post-diagnosis statin use was associated with a decreased risk of cancer-specific death and all-cause mortality. The patients who used statins after their HCC diagnosis had a 15 percent lower risk of cancer-specific diagnosis mortality and an 11 percent lower risk of all-cause mortality. So, it appears that a large number of patients with HCC would benefit from beginning a statin medication after their diagnosis. This benefit seemed evident for those on higher and lower statin doses and continued across a range of "lag periods." At the same time, in this particular cohort, there did not appear to be a notable association between the use of statins before diagnosis and mortality. The researchers concluded that they found "a strong and statistically significant inverse association between postdiagnosis use [of statins] and risk of mortality."[13]

Intense Nursing Care May Improve the Anxiety, Depression, and Quality of Life of People Undergoing a Liver Resection because of a Diagnosis of Liver Cancer

In a systematic review and meta-analysis published in the journal *Medicine*, researchers from China reviewed the role that nursing may play in the recovery from liver resection surgery for liver cancer. The researchers located five studies that met their criteria. Four were observational studies, and one was a randomized trial. The studies included 1,205 patients with liver cancer who were enrolled between 2010 and 2018. Of these, 667 patients were assigned to receive intensive care nursing, and 538 received conventional nursing care. The mean age of the patients ranged from 50.1 to 58.8 years; males were the majority in all of the studies, ranging from 54.76 percent to 87.13 percent. The percentage of patients who were smokers ranged from 47.62 percent to 70 percent. The researchers learned that most of the patients who were assigned to an intense nursing intervention were significantly very satisfied with their quality of life. A minority of patients who were not assigned to intensive nursing care were still satisfied. However, patients who were not assigned to intense nursing care were significantly dissatisfied with their quality of life. Moreover, the patients who did not receive intense nursing care had significantly higher rates of anxiety and depression. And, physical function and total activity score were also significantly better in those patients who received intense nursing care. The researchers emphasized the need for more studies, noting that their findings "should further be confirmed in larger nursing related studies based on patients with liver cancers."[14]

There Seems to Be an Association between Adherence to a Low-Fat Diet and a Reduced Risk of Liver Cancer

In a prospective study published in the journal *Frontiers in Nutrition*, researchers from China analyzed the association between a low-fat diet and the risk of liver cancer. Data were obtained from the Prostate, Lung, Colorectal, and Ovarian Screening Trial, which was administered by the National Cancer Institute; the cohort that the researchers used included 98,455 subjects. Among the data collected was information on dietary history from a 137-item food frequency questionnaire. The higher the score, the more closely a subject followed a low-fat diet; people in the highest quartile were those who most closely adhered to a low-fat diet. Other information on demographics, lifestyle factors, and medical history was also collected, and data were obtained on individuals diagnosed with liver cancer from self-reports, family reports, death certificates, and other methods. During 872,639.5 person-years of follow-up, there were ninety-one documented cases of liver cancer, with an overall incidence rate of 0.01 cases per one hundred person-years. So, the rate was incredibly low. Still, the researchers found that subjects in the highest quartile had a significantly lower rate of liver cancer than those in the lowest. There was a clear association between the consumption of a diet low in fat and the risk of liver cancer. People who ate the least amount of dietary fat had the lowest risk of liver cancer. The researchers concluded that a "low-fat diet is associated with a reduced risk of liver cancer in the US population." That is why, "adherence to a low-fat diet is helpful for the prevention of liver cancer."[15]

Acupuncture May Be Useful for the Anxiety, Depression, and Insomnia Associated with Liver Cancer

In a pilot study published in the *Journal of Korean Oriental Medicine*, researchers based in South Korea evaluated the use of acupuncture to relieve the symptoms of anxiety, depression, and insomnia that are often associated with liver cancer. The cohort only consisted of eight patients with liver cancer who were dealing with anxiety and depression; there were four men and four women. They ranged in age from forty-seven to seventy-six years, with a mean age of 59.75 years. The patients were treated three times a week for eight weeks, thus receiving a total of twelve treatments. The treatments were directed to nine acupuncture points, and the needles were inserted for a total of twenty-five minutes. The patients' anxiety, depression, and insomnia were measured by the National Cancer Center score on visits one, four, seven, ten, and thirteen. This scoring system consisted of two questions for each of the three symptoms. To evaluate the safety of the acupuncture treatments, the researchers measured body temperature, blood pressure, pulse, and body weight at each visit. During the study, other tests, such as biochemical tests and abdominal CTs, were periodically conducted. And, the researchers carefully monitored the patients to ensure that the treatments were not further impairing their health. The researchers learned that the subjects experienced "remarkable" improvements in their symptoms, without causing any side effects or negatively impacting their liver cancer. The researchers concluded that their findings suggest that acupuncture treatments are "beneficial for liver cancer patients to reduce anxiety, depression and insomnia."[16]

REFERENCES AND FURTHER READING

de Martel, C., D. Maucort-Boulch, M. Plummer, and S. Franceshi. "World-Wide Relative Contribution of Hepatitis B and C Viruses in Hepatocellular Carcinoma." *Hepatology* 62 (2015): 1190–1200.

Kim, Gyuri, Suk-Yong Jang, Chung Mo Nam, and Eun Seok Kang. "Statin Use and the Risk of Hepatocellular Carcinoma in Patients at High Risk: A Nationwide Nested Case-Control Study." *Journal of Hepatology* 68 (2018): 476–484.

Koh, W.-P., K. Robien, R. Wang et al. "Smoking as an Independent Risk Factor for Hepatocellular Carcinoma: The Singapore Chinese Health Study." *British Journal of Cancer* 105 (2011): 1430–1435.

Lee, Chang-Hyeong, Byung-Seok Kim, Ji-Suk Kim et al. "The Effects of Acupuncture on the Insomnia, Anxiety and Depression of Liver Cancer Patients: Pilot Study." *Journal of Korean Oriental Medicine* 33, no. 2 (2012): 34–46.

Lee, Junga. "Associations Between Physical Activity and Liver Cancer Risks and Mortality: A Systematic Review and Meta-Analysis." *International Journal of Environmental Research and Public Health* 17 (2020): 8943.

Li, Juan, Qinqin Cheng, Xiangqian Zhu et al. "The Relationship of Exercise and Cancer-Related Fatigue in Patients with Advanced Liver Cancer: A Cross-Sectional Study." *Scientific Reports* 13 (2023): 17341.

Okinaga, Hiroko, Hideo Yasunaga, Kiyoshi Hasegawa et al. "Short-Term Outcomes Following Hepatectomy in Elderly Patients with Hepatocellular Carcinoma: An Analysis of 10,805 Septuagenarians and 2,381 Octo- and Nonagenarians in Japan." *Liver Cancer* 7 (2018): 55–64.

Park, Hana, Seung Kak Shin, Ijin Joo et al. "Systematic Review and Meta-Analysis: Low-Level Alcohol Consumption and the Risk of Liver Cancer." *Gut and Liver* 14, no. 6 (2020): 792–807.

Peng, L., L. Xiang, Z. Xu et al. "Association Between Low-Fat Diet and Liver Cancer Risk in 98,455 Participants: Results from a Prospective Study." *Frontiers in Nutrition* 9 (2022): 1013643.

Thrift, A.P., Y. Natarajan, Y. Liu, and H. B. El-Serag. "Statin Use After Diagnosis of Hepatocellular Carcinoma is Associated with Decreased Mortality." *Clinical Gastroenterology and Hepatology* 17 (2019): 2117–2125.

Wen, Q., K. H. Chan, K. Shi et al. "Tobacco Smoking and Solid Fuels for Cooking and Risk of Liver Cancer: A Prospective Cohort Study of 0.5 Million Chinese Adults." *International Journal of Cancer* 151 (2022): 181–190.

Yi, Zhenghui, Linjie Wang, and Xiangqun Tu. "Effect of Vitamin D Deficiency on Liver Cancer Risk: A Systematic Review and Meta-Analysis." *Asian Pacific Journal of Cancer Prevention* 22, no. 4 (April 2021): 991–997.

Zhang, Qiao, Rong Wan, and Changdan Liu. "The Impact of Intense Nursing Care in Improving Anxiety, Depression, and Quality of Life in Patients with Liver Cancer." *Medicine* 99 (2020): 34.

Zhang, Wei, Xiao-Ou Shu, Honglan Li et al. "Vitamin Intake and Liver Cancer Risk: A Report from Two Cohort Studies in China." *Journal of the National Cancer Institute* 104 (2012): 1173–1181.

CANCER, ORAL

INTRODUCTION

Also known as mouth cancer, oral cancer affects the inner lips and the first part of the tongue, the roof and floor of the mouth, as well as the oropharynx or the last part of the tongue, the tonsils, and the sides and back of the throat. It includes the gums, the lining inside the cheeks, and the area immediately behind the wisdom teeth. The vast majority of oral cancers begin in the squamous cells in the oral cavity; these cells are flat, and when their DNA changes, the cells begin growing and multiplying much faster than normal.

People who are diagnosed with early oral cancer have an excellent prognosis. Their overall five-year survival rate is 84 percent. If the cancer has spread to nearby tissues, organs, or lymph nodes, the five-year survival rate drops to 65 percent. Most cancers of the mouth are related to tobacco use, alcohol consumption, or both; most throat cancers are caused by the human papilloma virus (HPV). In recent years, the incidence of HPV-positive oral cancer has been rising.

Oral cancer may be traced to ancient civilizations, including ancient Egypt and ancient Greece. For example, references to the Egyptian medical and surgical practices from 3000 to 2500 BC have been found in papyri and hieroglyphics located in ancient ruins. At that time, treatment focused on the surgical removal of the abnormal masses and trying to reduce bleeding with cauterization.[1]

SYMPTOMS, RISKS, AND COMPLICATIONS

Unlike most problems of the mouth that may surface for a few days or weeks before they resolve, oral cancer tends to appear as white, gray, or red patches or sores, or patches of white and red, that bleed and do not disappear. Oral cancer may also be found in rough spots or crusty areas on the inner lips, gums, or inside the mouth. People with oral cancer may have bleeding inside the mouth for no obvious reason; they may have numbness, pain, or tenderness on the face or neck. They may have a persistent sore throat. Chewing and/or swallowing may be difficult, and people may have problems with moving their jaw or tongue. Dentures that previously fit well may no longer be comfortable. Sometimes, there is unintentional weight loss, persistent ear pain, and/or unexplained bad breath.

The vast majority of people who develop oral cancer have at least one of the following factors. They smoke cigarettes, cigars, and/or pipes; use smokeless tobacco products, such as chewing tobacco; drink excessive amounts of alcohol; have human papillomavirus (HPV); and/or have a family history of oral cancer. It is believed that there is an association between poor diet and oral cancer. Still, some people without any obvious risk factors develop this disease. Left untreated, oral cancer tends to spread throughout the mouth and throat and then to other areas of the head and neck.

PREVALENCE

Oral cancer is the most common form of head and neck cancer; it typically affects people who are fifty years or older. In the United States, oral cancer accounts for about 3 percent of all cancers diagnosed annually; in 2022, there were about 54,000 new cases.[2] Worldwide, it is the sixteenth most common malignancy and the fifteenth leading cause of death.[3] Men have a higher risk than women, as do Caucasians. Overall, about eleven people out of every one hundred thousand will develop oral cancer. And, about one-third of the people who have oral cancer develop a new cancer. So, periodic follow-ups are highly recommended.

DIAGNOSIS AND TREATMENT OPTIONS

Oral cancers are frequently first observed by dentists and/or dental hygienists during a regular check-up and/or cleaning. Dentists and dental hygienists are trained to know the appearance of a healthy mouth, and they check for abnormalities. (But, it is important to know that people may also use a bright light and a mirror to conduct their own periodic self-exams at home. Take a few extra minutes to look closely at the entire oral cavity and to feel for any lumps or bumps in the neck and under the lower jaw.) If oral cancer is suspected, the dentist will suggest a consultation with a specialist, such as a head and neck surgeon, also known as a maxillofacial surgeon. The surgeon, in turn, may want to biopsy the area in question. If the area is fairly small, the surgeon will remove tissue with an excisional biopsy. If the area is larger, the surgeon may want to use an endoscope to examine more of the throat and mouth. (An endoscope is a thin, flexible tube with an attached light and viewing lens.) To detect cancer that may have spread, the surgeon may order other tests including a CT scan, a MRI test, an ultrasonography, or a PET scan.

The surgeon will then stage the cancer. Oral cancers are staged using the TNM system. T stands for the size and location of the tumor; N indicates whether the cancer has spread to the lymph nodes; and M denotes whether the cancer has spread to other parts of the body (metastasized). A T1 oral cancer measures 2 centimeters or less, a T2 oral cancer measures 2–4 centimeters, and a T3 oral cancer is larger than 4 centimeters.

Several factors play a role in the therapy or therapies that are recommended. These include the type of cancer and if it has spread, as well as the patient's age and general health.

The three main treatments for oral cancer are surgery, radiation, and chemotherapy. On occasion, immunotherapy (biological therapy) may be recommended. It improves the immune function of the body, enabling the body to better fight the cancer cells. Another type of treatment is called targeted therapy. It uses drugs to precisely attack cancer cells.

RESEARCH FINDINGS

People with Oral Cancer May Have a Host of Different Symptoms before and after Surgery

In a longitudinal study published in the *Asia-Pacific Journal of Oncology Nursing*, researchers from China wanted to identify the symptoms experienced by people with oral cancer, both before and after their surgery. The cohort consisted of 197 patients with oral cancer. They had a mean age of 52.6 years, and 86.8 percent were male; at diagnosis, 47.7 percent had an advanced stage of oral cancer. Of the patients, 27.4 percent had comorbidities, including hypertension and diabetes, and 23.4 percent had a post-surgical tracheotomy. The researchers learned that the most common pre-surgery symptom was pain. That was followed by difficulty swallowing/chewing and mouth/throat sores. One week after surgery, the most common problem was difficulty swallowing/chewing, followed by problems with voice/speech and problems with mucus. One month after surgery, the patients experienced several equally difficult symptoms, including numbness or tingling, difficulty swallowing/chewing, and impaired voice/speech. The researchers learned that the symptoms changed over time "with the symptom burden being heaviest about seven days after surgery." Further, the researchers noted that certain patients tended to have more symptoms. These included patients who were self-employed, had additional medical problems, later stage cancer, adjuvant therapy, and greater nutritional problems. On the positive side, pain was greatly reduced one month after surgery. The researchers concluded that their findings "demonstrated the importance and urgency of symptom management in patients undergoing oral cancer surgery."[4]

Some Dental Students and Dental Residents Appear to Need More Training on How to Recognize Oral Cancer

In a cross-sectional trial published in the journal *Medicina*, researchers from Romania assessed the level of oral cancer awareness among dental students and dental residents. The cohort consisted of 197 fourth- and fifth-year dental students as well as first-year residents in general dentistry. There were seventy-seven fourth-year students, sixty-three fifth-year students, and fifty-seven first-year residents. They ranged in age from twenty-one to forty-three years, with a mean age of twenty-five years, and there were seventy-one males and 126 females. To determine their level of knowledge, the researchers created a twenty-two-question questionnaire about the risk factors for oral cancer, with a focus on HPV infection. Most of the students and residents correctly identified smoking, alcohol, and HPV as risk factors, as well as white and red patches/lesions. Chronic mucosal irritation was identified by most of the fifth-year students, dietary factors were noted by 23.5 percent of the residents, and older age was only mentioned by 9.5 percent of the fifth-year students. The highest number of correct answers concerning potentially malignant lesions was noted by the fifth-year students. They also knew the most about the potential locations of oral cancers, such as the tongue, the floor of the mouth, the lips, and the buccal mucosa (inner lining of the cheeks). And, most of the students and residents did not conduct a complete clinical examination. For example, though more than 85.7 percent examined the oral mucosa, far fewer palpated the lymphatic nodules, with the highest number, 41.6 percent, among the fourth-year students. The researchers concluded that their findings "highlighted the need for adaptation of the academic curriculum and continuous post-academic medical training, mainly practical, with a focus on building the necessary skills for the correct screening of oral cancer."[5]

Exposure to Secondhand Smoke Increases the Risk of Oral Cancer

In a systematic review and meta-analysis published in the BMJ journal *Tobacco Control*, researchers from Portugal, the UK, Spain, and Chestnut Hill, Massachusetts investigated the association between secondhand smoke and oral cancer. They located five case-control studies that met their criteria; three were conducted in Asia, one in Europe, and one was a multicenter study from North America, Latin America, and Europe. The eligible studies included 1,179 cases and 5,798 controls, with exposure to secondhand smoke in 3,452 individuals; 3,525 individuals had not been exposed to secondhand smoke. Four studies included men and women; one study was only with women. The researchers found a statistically significant association between exposure to secondhand smoke and an increased risk of oral cancer. Moreover, there was a direct association between duration of exposure and increased risk; people who were exposed for longer periods of time—more than ten or fifteen years—have an even higher risk for oral cancer. The researchers concluded that their findings "could provide guidance to public health professionals, researchers, and policymakers to further support effect SHS [secondhand smoke] exposure prevention programs worldwide."[6]

There Is an Association between Alcohol Consumption and Risk of Oral Cancer

In a population-based cohort study published in *JAMA Network Open*, researchers from Korea evaluated the association between the reduction, cessation, or increase of alcohol consumption and the development of alcohol-related cancers and all cancers. According to the researchers, several types of cancers have a direct association with alcohol consumption. These include cancers of the mouth, pharynx, and larynx. The cohort consisted of more than 4,513,746 Koreans, with a mean age of 53.6 years; 51.5 percent were men and 48.5 percent were women. They were studied for two years and the follow-up averaged 6.45 years. During that time, the incident rate of cancer was 7.7 per one thousand person-years. The participants were categorized based on their alcohol consumption. One beer or one glass of wine was categorized as having 14 g of alcohol; a shot had 1.5 ounces. Alcohol consumption was then defined as none (0 g per day), mild (less than 15 g per day), moderate (fifteen to 29.9 g per day), and heavy (30 or more g per day). That means that moderate drinking was one to two drinks per day, and heavy drinking was more than two drinks per day. A little more than one-quarter of the cohort were mild drinkers, 9.6 percent were moderate drinkers, and 8.6 percent were heavy drinkers. The researchers determined that compared to individuals who do not drink, those who drink moderately had a 10 percent higher chance of developing cancer, and those who drink heavily had a 34 percent higher risk. Interestingly, "quitting was not associated with a lower incidence of alcohol-related cancer, but if abstinence was maintained over time, the incidence of alcohol-related and all cancers tended to decrease." Still, "reducing drinking from heavy to moderate or mild levels was associated with a decreased risk of alcohol-related and all cancers."[7]

People Who Smoke More and Drink Higher Amounts of Alcohol Know More about Oral Cancer

In a cross-sectional study published in the journal *BMC Oral Health*, researchers from Wisconsin wanted to assess the current knowledge, awareness, and behaviors of patients concerning oral cancer. So, they distributed a twenty-one-question survey to patients in the waiting rooms of a large integrated medical-dental health system serving north-central Wisconsin. Five hundred and four dental patients and 306 medical patients completed the survey; of these, 62.2 percent were female and 92 percent were Caucasian. Study participation was voluntary and anonymous. Thirty-four percent of the participants reported current use of both smoking and smokeless tobacco, and another 39 percent reported use of these products in the past. Twenty-two percent of the participants had been exposed to passive smoke. Sixty-three percent of the participants said they used alcohol. Slightly more than a third said that they drank alcohol less than once per week; 16.3 percent drank alcohol one to two times a week; 6.1 percent drank three or four times per week; 2 percent drank five to six times per week, and 2.9 percent drank alcohol every day. At the same time, 37.3 percent never drank alcohol. About 40 percent of the participants noted that their healthcare providers educated them about oral cancer, and about 22 percent noted that their healthcare providers educated them about the association between HPV and oral cancer. Ninety-four percent of the participants correctly identified that smoking was a risk factor for oral cancer, and 82 percent also knew that secondhand smoke was a risk factor. Seventy-nine percent were aware that alcohol increased the risk, and 50 percent indicated that ill-fitting dentures were risky. In descending order, the participants said that the following could be symptoms of oral cancer—abnormal mass/lump in the mouth, a mouth sore that does not heal, white/red patches in the mouth, difficulty chewing or swallowing, and a change in voice quality. About 23 percent reported smoking and drinking alcohol. Of these, 39 percent were aware that alcohol contributed to oral cancer risk, and almost all knew that tobacco increased the risk. Interestingly, the participants who smoked twenty or more cigarettes per day knew more about the oral cancer risk than those who smoked nineteen or fewer cigarettes per day. And, participants who drank alcohol knew more about the oral cancer risk from alcohol and tobacco than those who did not drink alcohol. The researchers commented that the participants who knew less about the risk factors of oral cancer had a "greater risk for first presenting with disease at an advanced stage."[8]

YouTube Videos on Oral Self-Examination to Detect Oral Cancer May Be Well Done but Much of the Information May Be Incorrect

In a study published in the *Journal of International Society of Preventive and Community Dentistry*, researchers from India investigated the quality, reliability, and comprehensiveness of YouTube videos on oral self-examination to detect oral cancer and precancerous lesions. After analyzing 800 videos, the researchers found twenty-four that met their inclusion criteria; these videos were all in English. Eighty-seven percent of the videos were uploaded by a healthcare group, and the remainder were uploaded by a non-healthcare group. The researchers classified the videos from one to five, with one being very poor quality and five being excellent quality. The videos ranged in duration from one minute one second to twelve minutes one second, with an average duration of 3.89 minutes. In the visibility assessment, the most seen video had 237,056 views and the least seen had forty views. The most popular video received 1,453 likes and the most unpopular one had 127 dislikes. In general, the videos uploaded by the healthcare groups had better visibility, quality, reliability, and comprehensiveness than those uploaded by the non-healthcare groups. But, the difference in these characteristics between those uploaded by healthcare and non-healthcare groups are not statistically significant. Yet, the accuracy of the information may be problematic. In fact, the researchers found only one video that "provided viewers with correct information about oral self-examination." All the other videos "either did not use a proper technique or they showed only a few steps of the oral self-examination." The most common mistake the videos made was failing to mention the need to remove dentures before beginning a self-examination. The researchers concluded that it is the responsibility of "healthcare professionals, academic institutions, and professional organizations to improve YouTube content and refer patients to scientifically reliable content sources."[9]

Certain Factors Are Associated with Poorer Oral Cancer Outcomes

In a retrospective, cross-sectional study published in the journal *Frontiers in Oral Health*, researchers from Rwanda wanted to determine what factors increase the risk of an adverse outcome from oral cancer treatment. The cohort consisted of 311 patients who were cared for at the Oral and Maxilla Facial Surgery department of a large military hospital in Rwanda between January 1, 2007, and December 31, 2019. The hospital was the only one in the city providing this type of care, and people come from the entire country to be treated. Almost three-quarters of the patients were from rural areas, and almost four out of every five patients drank alcohol. The researchers learned that most of the patients were between the ages of forty-one and sixty years, with an average age of 50.6 years. Fifty-six percent were male; more than 80 percent were married, and about two-thirds were Catholic. Almost 60 percent never smoked tobacco. The researchers found that certain factors appeared to play a role in the outcome. Among these are educational background and religion. For example, compared to a person with a higher education, a patient with no formal education had almost three times the risk of having an oral cancer adverse outcome and death. And, compared to Catholics, Muslims had almost seven times the risk of a bad outcome. Factors such as age, gender, marital status, residence, primary site of infection, and wealth index were found not to significantly impact the outcome. The researchers concluded that "these parameters need to be taken into account for the individualized therapy management of patients with OC [oral cancer]."[10]

Smokeless Tobacco Use Is Associated with a Higher Risk of Oral Cancer in Women than in Men

In a systematic review and meta-analysis published in the journal *BMC Cancer*, researchers from China estimated the risk associated with the use of smokeless tobacco and oral cancer in women and compared it to the risk in men. They located nineteen studies with 6,593 cases of oral cancer that met their criteria. Fifteen studies were case-control or case-conference studies, and the remaining four were cohort studies. Thirteen studies were conducted in India, two in Pakistan, two in Sweden, one in the United States, and one in Central and Southeast Asia. Sample sizes for the individual studies ranged from 258 to 279,897; cases of oral cancer ranged from eighty-four to 1,401. The researchers found that the use of smokeless tobacco was associated with an increased risk of oral cancer in both men and women, but women had a "much higher risk" than men. The researchers underscored the need for more research on this association. "Further, large-scale prospective cohort studies should be conducted to verify sex-based difference in specific smokeless products."[11]

There Is an Association between Naswar, a Smokeless Tobacco, and the Incidence of Oral Cancer

In a case-control study published in the online journal *PLoS ONE*, researchers from Germany and Pakistan assessed the risk associated with chewing Naswar, a brand of smokeless tobacco, and the incidence of oral cancer in Khyber Pakhtunkhwa, Pakistan, which has a population of 17.5 million. The majority of the population lives in rural areas, and agriculture and trade are the primary earning resources. According to the researchers, Pakistan has an extraordinarily high prevalence of oral cancer. It is the most frequent cancer among males and the second most common cancer among both sexes. For the study, people with oral cancer were recruited at three tertiary care centers. There were eighty-four people with oral cancer, 62 percent of whom were male; there were 174 age- and sex-matched controls. The most common primary sites of oral cancer were the gums and the buccal mucosa. Ninety-five percent of the patients and 92 percent of the controls were in a low or middle economic strata. The researchers learned that when compared to people who had never used Naswar, people who had "ever" used Naswar had more than a twenty-fold higher risk of oral cancer. Even though more males developed oral cancer than females, females who use Naswar have a higher risk of oral cancer than males. From their calculations, the researchers noted that in Pakistan, Naswar is associated with 68 percent of the cases of oral cancer in men and 38 percent of the cases in women. The researchers commented that their findings "are highly relevant for South and Central Asia, where Naswar use is common." Unfortunately, because Naswar is much cheaper than smoking cigarettes, more people may use this smokeless alternative. "Although still requiring further validation through independent studies, these findings may be used for smokeless tobacco control in countries where Naswar use is common."[12]

Electronic Cigarettes May Be Associated with Increased Risk of Oral Cancer

In an article published in the *British Journal of Oral and Maxillofacial Surgery*, researchers from the UK examined the association between e-cigarettes and oral cancer. They noted that there has been an "exponential" rise in their use in the UK since they became available in 2005. Yet, there is little evidence about their safety. The electronic nicotine delivery systems or ENDS includes e-cigarettes, electronic vaporizers, and vape pens. They all have a battery-powered heating element that is used to aerosolize a liquid, which is then inhaled. Their contents include nicotine, flavoring chemicals, tobacco alkaloids, formaldehyde, glycerol, and heavy metals. Apparently, the amount of nicotine and toxins varies from brand to brand. Though e-cigarettes have fewer carcinogens than regular cigarettes, they may still damage DNA, cause oral inflammation, periodontal disease, deterioration of dental and gingival health, and changes to the oral microbiome. And, there are case reports of heavy users of e-cigarettes developing oral cancers. The researchers commented that e-cigarettes should not be considered safe.[13]

Two such case reports were included in an article in the journal *Otolaryngology*. According to the authors of the article, who were researchers from Ohio and Vietnam, the first case report described a sixty-six-year-old male who had unintended weight loss, difficulty swallowing, and a dry mouth. His immunization records were up-to-date for HPV, varicella zoster virus, and hepatitis B virus. His medical history was unremarkable except for the use of e-cigarettes about twenty times per day for the past thirteen years. After viewing his oral cavity, the otolaryngologist suspected either an infection or oral cancer. Following a biopsy, a diagnosis of basaloid squamous cell carcinoma was made. In a second case, a fifty-nine-year-old man came to the otolaryngologist's office with an ulceration of the lower lip that had failed to heal for nine months. While the man did not have pain or discomfort, he did have some difficulty swallowing and a dry mouth. The man said that he had no history of trauma to the oral area, and he denied a history of alcohol use. However, the man did report using thirty e-cigarettes per day for the past thirteen years. No other abnormal oral cavity findings were observed. A biopsy was conducted, and the patient was informed that he had the same diagnosis as the previous man, basaloid squamous cell carcinoma. The authors of the case studies noted that "tobacco cigarette smoking is a known risk for cancers, including oral cancers. Patients and clinicians (physicians, dentists, and nurses) need to be aware that the use of electronic cigarettes (E-cigarettes) or other electronic nicotine delivery systems (ENDS) may also be associated with an increased risk of oral cancer."[14]

There Appears to Be an Association between Low Levels of Vitamin D and Oral Cancer

In a trial published in the journal *Clinical and Experimental Dental Research*, researchers from Saudi Arabia evaluated the serum vitamin D levels of patients with oral squamous cell carcinoma (oral cancer) and compared them to controls who did not have cancer. The cohort consisted of fifty-one patients with oral cancer (twenty-two males and twenty-nine females) and 113 cancer-free controls (thirty-six males and seventy-seven females). The mean age of the cancer patients was 59.33 years, and the mean age of the controls was 49.24 years. Forty-five percent of the oral cancers were located on the tongue. Only five patients with cancer were below the age of forty years. Among the cancer patients, 74.51 percent had moderate to severe vitamin D deficiencies; a much smaller 20.35 percent of the control group had moderate vitamin D deficiency. No one in the control group had severe vitamin D deficiency. As a result, the researchers concluded that it may be necessary for them to assess the vitamin D status of "patients attending our medical and dental outpatient clinics and to prescribe vitamin D supplements to subjects with moderate to severe deficiencies."[15]

People with Oral Cancer May Also Have Lower Intakes of Dietary Fiber and Vitamin C

In a trial published in the journal *Frontiers in Public Health*, researchers from China reviewed the relationship between intake of dietary fiber and vitamin C and the incidence of oral cancer. The cohort consisted of 382 patients who were newly diagnosed with oral cancer; they were matched in age and sex to 382 controls. The median ages of the cancer and control groups were 49 and 56 years, respectively. A food frequency questionnaire assessed pre-diagnostic consumption of dietary fiber and vitamin C. The researchers determined that the cancer group had a higher proportion of participants with alcohol consumption and a family history of cancer. Compared with the controls, the intake of dietary fiber and vitamin C was significantly lower among those with oral cancer. The researchers concluded that there is a link between the incidence of oral cancer and low intake of dietary fiber and vitamin C. "Further well-designed particularly large-scale cohort studies are need to corroborate our findings."[16]

REFERENCES AND FURTHER READING

Cameron, Alice, Hao Meng Yip, and Montey Garg. "E-Cigarettes and Oral Cancer: What Do We Know So Far?" *British Journal of Oral and Maxillofacial Surgery* 61 (2023): 380–382.

Gulve, N. D., P. R. Tripathi, S. D. Dahivelkar et al. "Evaluation of YouTube Videos as a Source of Information About Oral Self-Examination to Detect Oral Cancer and Precancerous Lesions." *Journal of International Society of Preventive and Community Dentistry* 12 (2022): 226–234.

Inchingolo, F., L. Santacroce, A. Ballini et al. "Oral Cancer: A Historical Review." *International Journal of Environmental Research and Public Health* 17 (2020): 3168.

Khan, Z., S. Dreger, S. M. H. Shah et al. "Oral Cancer via the Bargain Bin: The Risk of Oral Cancer Associated with a Smokeless Tobacco Product (Naswar)." *PLoS One* 12, no. 7 (2017): e0180445.

Mariano, Lorena C., Saman Warnakulasuriya, Kurt Straif, and Luis Monteiro. "Secondhand Smoke Exposure and Oral Cancer Risk: A Systematic Review and Meta-Analysis." *Tobacco Control* 31, no. 5 (2022): 597–607.

Mu, G., J. Wang, Z. Liu et al. "Association Between Smokeless Tobacco Use and Oral Cavity Cancer Risk in Women Compared with Men: A Systematic Review and Meta-Analysis." *BMC Cancer* 21 (2021): 960.

Murariu, Alice, Elena-Raluca Baciu, Livia Bobu et al. "Knowledge, Practice, and Awareness of Oral Cancer and HPV Infection Among Dental Students and Residents: A Cross-Sectional Study." *Medicina* 58 (2022): 806.

Ndayisabye, H., A. Ndagijimana, E. Biracyaza, and A. Umubyeyi. "Factors Associated with Ora; Cancer Adverse Outcome at the Rwanda Military Hospital, a Retrospective Cross-Sectional Study." *Frontiers in Oral Health* 3 (March 2022): 844254.

Nguyen, Hoang, Joseph P. Kitzmiller, Kieu Tho Nguyen et al. "Oral Carcinoma Associated with Chronic Use of Electronic Cigarettes." *Otolaryngology* 7, no. 2 (2017): 304.

Ou, Meijun, Guifen Wang, Yixia Yan et al. "Perioperative Symptoms Burden and Its Influencing Factors in Patients with Oral Cancer: A Longitudinal Study." *Asia-Pacific Journal of Oncology Nursing* 9 (2022): 100073

Shimpi, Neel, Monica Jethwani, Aditi Bharatkumar et al. "Patient Awareness/Knowledge Towards Oral Cancer: A Cross-Sectional Survey." *BMC Oral Health* 18 (2018): 86.

Udeabor, Samuel E., Abdullah M. Albejadi, Waleed A. K. Al-Shehri et al. "Serum Levels of 25-Hydroxy-Vitamin D in Patients with Oral Squamous Cell Carcinoma: Making the Case for Chemoprevention." *Clinical and Experimental Dental Research* 6 (2020): 428–432.

Wang, Jing, Yi Fan, Jiawen Qian et al. "Relationship Between Dietary Fiber and Vitamin C Intake and Oral Cancer." *Frontiers in Public Health* 10 (2022): 880506.

Yoo, J. E., K. Han, D. W. Shin et al. "Association Between Changes in Alcohol Consumption and Cancer Risk." *JAMA Network Open* 5, no. 8 (2022): e2228544.

CANCER, PANCREATIC

INTRODUCTION

Pancreatic cancer is a type of cancer that begins as a growth of cells in the pancreas, an organ in the abdomen, between the spine and the stomach, that makes enzymes and hormones. The enzymes, such as lipase, protease, and amylase, help digest food, and the hormones, such as insulin, are needed to manage blood sugar. Pancreatic cancer occurs when cells in the pancreas change their DNA and begin to multiply very quickly, eventually forming a mass. The tumor invades and destroys healthy cells and may spread to other organs.

More than 95 percent of pancreatic cancers are pancreatic ductal adenocarcinomas, which begin in the cells that line the ducts that carry digestive enzymes out of the pancreas. The main pancreatic duct, the duct of Wirsung, connects the pancreas to the common bile duct. Much less often, cancer forms in the hormone-producing cells of the neuroendocrine cells of the pancreas. These types of cancer are called pancreatic endocrine cancer or pancreatic neuroendocrine tumors.

Unfortunately, pancreatic cancer is rarely diagnosed in its earlier stages, when treatment may be more effective. Early pancreatic cancer does not appear on imaging tests. It often does not cause symptoms until it has spread to other organs, when it is much harder to treat. In the United States, the five-year survival rate is 11 percent. That means that five years after diagnosis, only eleven of every one hundred pancreatic cancer patients are still alive.[1]

According to an article in the *Chinese Journal of Cancer Research*, in his 1761 publication "The Seats and Causes of Disease," Italian anatomist Giovanni Battista Morgagni reported several cases of pancreatic "scirrhus," which appears to be the first account of pancreatic ductal adenocarcinoma.[2]

SYMPTOMS, RISKS, AND COMPLICATIONS

While they may not appear until the disease is more advanced, there are a number of symptoms associated with pancreatic cancer. These include fatigue, weakness, loss of energy, loss of appetite and weight, abdominal pain that spreads to the sides or back, diarrhea, nausea, bloating, gas, yellowing of the skin and whites of the eyes (jaundice), light-colored or floating stools, dark-colored urine, pain in the middle of the back, itchy skin, a new diagnosis of diabetes or diabetes that is becoming harder to control, recent onset of pancreatitis (inflammation of the pancreas), and pain or swelling in an arm or leg which may be caused by a clot.

A number of factors increase the risk of pancreatic cancer. These include a family history of pancreatic cancer, smoking cigarettes, type 2 diabetes, cirrhosis of the liver, cystic fibrosis, pancreatitis, pancreatic cysts, obesity, older age, exposure to certain chemicals such as pesticides and petrochemicals, hereditary syndromes, and drinking excessive amounts of alcohol.

There are a few complications that may appear with pancreatic cancer. People with pancreatic cancer tend to lose weight from the nausea or vomiting associated with the pancreas pressing against the stomach or the cancer treatments. Also, since the pancreas may not be producing enough enzymes, the body may have trouble obtaining nutrients from foods. Pancreatic cancer that blocks the bile ducts may cause jaundice. When this occurs, a medical provider may do a procedure known as an endoscopic retrograde cholangiopancreatography to examine the bile and pancreatic ducts and possibly insert a stent to hold the bile duct open. During this procedure, a long tube with a tiny camera is inserted into the mouth, down the esophagus, into the stomach, and the upper part of the intestines. A dye is placed into the pancreatic and bile ducts. After imaging tests are taken, the stent is positioned in the correct spot. Pancreatic cancer tends to spread to nearby blood vessels, lymph nodes, the liver, peritoneum (the lining of the abdominal cavity), and the lungs. By the time these are diagnosed, most pancreatic cancers are hard to effectively treat.

Still another potential complication is pain, which may be caused by a growing tumor pressing against nerves. Treatments that shrink the tumor and pain medications may be useful. If these are not effective, a medical provider may suggest a celiac plexus block, which uses a needle to put alcohol into the nerves that control pain in the abdomen. This stops the nerves from sending pain signals to the brain. If pancreatic cancer grows into or presses on the first part of the small intestine, a blockage may occur. Since this prevents the flow of food into the small intestine, it may require placing of a stent to hold the small intestine open or surgery to insert a feeding tube or attach the stomach to the lower part of the intestines where the cancer is not causing a blockage.

PREVALENCE

Fortunately, in the United States, pancreatic cancer is not a common form of cancer. It accounts for about 3 percent of all cancers and about 7 percent of all cancer deaths. It is the tenth most common cancer in men and people assigned male at birth, and the eighth most common cancer in women and people assigned female at birth.[3] In the United States, the average lifetime risk of pancreatic cancer is about one in fifty-six for men and one in sixty for women. In 2024, about 66,440 (34,530 men and 31,910 women) were diagnosed with pancreatic cancer. About 51,750 (27,270 men and 24,480 women) died of this disease.[4]

DIAGNOSIS AND TREATMENT OPTIONS

A number of different tests may be used to detect pancreatic cancer. Initial blood work may be ordered for liver and pancreatic function. Also, blood tests detect tumor markers. For pancreatic cancer, high levels of carbohydrate antigen (CA 19-9), a type of protein released by pancreatic cancer cells, might indicate a tumor. Imaging tests may begin with a transabdominal ultrasound or a CT scan. Subsequent testing may include an MRI and a PET. These enable your medical provider to obtain images of the pancreas and other nearby organs. An endoscopic ultrasound (EUS) may be ordered to obtain another view. During this procedure, a thin tube known as an endoscope is inserted into the mouth, down the esophagus, into the stomach, and pancreas and high-frequency sound waves produce detailed images of the digestive tract and surrounding organs. Tissue samples are normally taken. A staging laparoscopy may be used to determine the extent of the pancreatic cancer. During this procedure, a surgeon makes a few small incisions into the abdomen and inserts a long tube with a camera at the end to look for abnormalities.

Surgical resection offers the only chance of a cure for pancreatic cancer. Treatment options may also include chemotherapy, radiation, other types of surgery, or a combination of these and other therapies. Healthcare providers rank pancreatic tumors into four different categories. A resectable tumor is a tumor that is confined to the pancreas and does not involve any nearby vessels or organs. A surgeon will remove this entire tumor. A borderline resectable tumor is a tumor that is in the pancreas and some nearby blood vessels. A surgeon will also remove this type of tumor. A locally advanced pancreatic tumor has significant involvement in the nearby blood vessels and is probably unsafe to remove. And, metastatic pancreatic tumor has spread to other parts of the body and will not be removed.

There are a few different types of pancreatic cancer surgery. If the tumor is in the widest part of the pancreas, near the small intestine, a surgeon may recommend a pancreaticoduodenectomy or a Whipple procedure. During this surgery, the surgeon removes the widest part of the pancreas, the duodenum, the gallbladder, a portion of the bile duct, and nearby lymph nodes. The remaining bile duct and pancreas are attached to the small intestine. If the tumor is at the end of the pancreas, a surgeon may perform a distal pancreatectomy. In this surgery, the end of the pancreas and the spleen are removed. If the cancer is located in several parts of the pancreas, a total pancreatectomy may be performed. In this surgery, the pancreas, gallbladder, spleen, and part of the stomach and small intestine are removed. After the pancreas is removed, people need to take insulin shots and digestive enzymes.

Chemotherapy, which kills cancer cells, may be delivered in a pill form or as an intravenous solution. In people with advanced pancreatic cancer, it may be the only treatment offered. Radiation therapy uses high-energy X-rays to kill cancer cells and relieve some of the symptoms of pancreatic cancer. Targeted treatments use drugs that target certain proteins that control how cancer cells grow and spread. These are normally combined with other treatments. Frequently used targeted therapies for pancreatic cancer include erlotinib, olaparib, larotrectinib, and entrectinib. People with pancreatic cancer often have a good deal of pain. So, these treatments may be combined with medications or treatments for pain.

RESEARCH FINDINGS

Higher Consumption of Fruits and Vegetables May or May Not Be Associated with a Lower Risk of Pancreatic Cancer

In a clinic-based case-control study published in the *Journal of Gastrointestinal Cancer*, researchers from Rochester, Minnesota, Bethesda, Maryland, and Minneapolis, Minnesota reviewed the association between consumption of fruits and vegetables and the risk of pancreatic cancer. The cohort consisted of 384 people with pancreatic cancer and 983 controls, who were matched by age, sex, and region of residence. All of the subjects provided demographic information and completed a 144-item food frequency questionnaire. The researchers learned that the patients with pancreatic cancer were more likely to be male, older, and ever-smokers. They were more likely to have a history of pancreatitis and diabetes, especially the recent onset of diabetes. When male and female cases were compared, males were slightly younger, had a higher than usual BMI, and were more likely to have ever smoked and to have a personal history of pancreatitis or diabetes. The researchers found a significant inverse association between pancreatic cancer and nutrient supplement groupings in a dose-dependent manner, including magnesium, potassium, selenium, alpha-carotene, beta-carotene, beta-cryptoxanthin, lutein and zeaxanthin, niacin, total alpha-tocopherol, total vitamin A activity, vitamin B6, and vitamin C. And, they concluded that the "nutrients obtained from eating a diet high in fruits and vegetables (and to a lesser degree nutrient supplements) are associated with decreased risk of developing pancreatic cancer, and that this reduction occurs in a dose dependent manner." That is why, "it is essential from a prevention standpoint to promote a diet rich in fruits and vegetables which contain numerous potentially beneficial nutrients."[5]

In a prospective study published in the journal *Cancer Epidemiology Biomarkers & Prevention*, researchers from Sweden examined the association between consumption of fruits and vegetables and the risk of pancreatic cancer. The cohort consisted of 81,922 men and women in the Swedish Mammography Cohort and the Cohort of Swedish Men. The median consumption of total fruits and vegetables was 4.7 servings per day for women and 3.6 servings per day for men. Men and women with high fruit and vegetable consumption were younger, smoked less, exercised more, consumed more alcohol, and were more likely to have a post-secondary education and to use multivitamin supplements. During an average follow-up of 6.8 years, there were 135 incident cases of pancreatic cancer—seventy-four in men and sixty-one in women. The researchers found no significant association between the consumption of total fruits and vegetables, total fruits, or total vegetables and the risk of pancreatic cancer. However, they observed a non-significant inverse association between the consumption of cruciferous vegetables and the risk of pancreatic cancer. When the various cruciferous vegetables were studied separately, only cabbage consumption had a statistically significant inverse association with pancreatic cancer. While there was no association between citrus fruit or green leafy vegetable consumption and pancreatic cancer, the subjects who consumed one or more servings per week of spinach had a statistically non-significant lower risk of pancreatic cancer. The researchers concluded that their findings "do not support a strong role for fruit and vegetable consumption in the prevention of pancreatic cancer." Still, they added that their findings "do not rule out the possibility of a protective role for specific fruit or vegetable subgroups, such as cruciferous vegetables, or for specific nutrients or phytochemicals."[6]

Adherence to the Mediterranean Diet Appears to Reduce the Risk of Pancreatic Cancer

In a study published in the *British Journal of Cancer*, researchers from Italy and the Netherlands analyzed data from two case-control studies on the association between adherence to the Mediterranean diet and the risk of pancreatic cancer. The cohort from the two studies included 688 people with pancreatic cancer and 2,204 hospital controls. When compared to the controls, the researchers learned that the patients with pancreatic cancer were more likely to be female and somewhat older. They had a lower BMI, were more often a heavy smoker, and tended to have a history of diabetes. No difference was observed in alcohol consumption and education. The researchers determined that there was a significant inverse association between the Mediterranean diet and the risk of pancreatic cancer. The more people adhered to a Mediterranean diet, the more their risk of pancreatic cancer decreased. So, those who closely followed the tenets of the Mediterranean diet had the lowest rates of pancreatic cancer. The researchers commented that "the combination of the favourable fatty acid profile, high fibre content, antioxidants, and phytochemicals typical of the Mediterranean diet, and their synergistic effect, appear to have a beneficial role on pancreatic, as on other cancers." And, they concluded that "the consistency of the results of the two studies, conducted in different calendar periods and using different dietary questionnaires gives further support to the finding of a beneficial role of the Mediterranean diet on pancreatic cancer."[7]

Consumption of Meat and Fat Seems to Increase the Risk of Pancreatic Cancer

In a multiethnic cohort study published in the *Journal of the National Cancer Institute*, researchers from Los Angeles, California, and Honolulu, Hawaii, analyzed data from the prospective multiethnic cohort study in Hawaii and Los Angeles to learn more about the association between the intake of meat, other animal products, fat, and cholesterol and the risk of pancreatic cancer. The cohort consisted of 190,545 subjects who were African American, Latino, Japanese-American, Native Hawaiian, or Caucasian. About 45 percent were male. During the seven years of follow-up, there were 482 incident cases of pancreatic cancer. Pancreatic cancer patients were, on average, five years older than the nonpatients and included a higher percentage of men. There was a statistically significant association between current smoking, a prior diagnosis of diabetes mellitus, a family history of pancreatic cancer, and a diagnosis of pancreatic cancer. There were also statistically significant differences in the ethnic distributions. Higher percentages of people with pancreatic cancer were seen among African Americans, Japanese Americans, and Native Hawaiians. Dietary intake was assessed with a quantitative food frequency questionnaire. The researchers determined that the strongest association was seen between processed meat and pancreatic cancer; when compared to those in the lowest quartile, those in the fifth quartile of daily intake had a 68 percent increased risk of pancreatic cancer. Comparing the highest with the lowest quartile, intakes of pork and of total red meat were both associated with a 50 percent increase in risk. There were no associations of pancreatic cancer risk with the intake of poultry, fish, dairy products, eggs, total fat, or cholesterol. Interestingly, intake of total and saturated fat from meat was associated with statistically significant increases in pancreatic cancer risk but intake of saturated fat from dairy products was not. The researchers concluded that people may be able to reduce their risk of pancreatic cancer "by reducing consumption of red and processed meat." Still, "because the fat components of the meats did not seem to account for these findings, other compounds in these foods that are responsible for the association need to be identified."[8]

Low Levels of Vitamin D May Increase the Risk of Pancreatic Cancer

In a study published in *Cancer Epidemiology, Biomarkers & Prevention*, researchers from several locations, but based in Boston, wanted to determine if pre-diagnostic levels of serum vitamin D were associated with the risk of pancreatic cancer. That is why they conducted a pooled analysis of nested case-control studies with 451 cases of pancreatic cancer and 1,167 controls from five cohorts—Health Professionals Follow-Up Study, Nurses' Health Study, Physicians' Health Study, Women's Health Initiative-Observational Study, and the Women's Health Study. Incident cases of pancreatic cancer were identified by self-report or during follow-up of a participant's death. Deaths were ascertained from next-of-kin or the postal service and by searching the National Death Index. The researchers determined that the patients with pancreatic cancer had lower levels of serum vitamin D than the controls. In fact, plasma levels of vitamin D were inversely associated with the risk of pancreatic cancer, and this association was statistically significant. A similar inverse association was seen across a wide variety of subgroups including whites, women, and men. Further, the inverse association was similar regardless of whether the blood was drawn in months with low or high ultraviolet light exposure. Those subjects with "sufficient" levels of vitamin D had about a 30 percent lower risk for pancreatic cancer than those with "insufficient" levels. The researchers commented that "in light of the high prevalence of vitamin D insufficiency in the population, further studies should examine whether increasing vitamin D levels impacts the incidence of this highly lethal malignancy."[9]

In a retrospective review published in the *Journal of Translational Medicine*, researchers from St. Louis, Missouri, examined the vitamin D status of patients with pancreatic adenocarcinoma who were treated at the Siteman Cancer Center. The researchers collected data on demographic information, clinical staging at the time of the vitamin D assessment, vitamin D levels, and survival status of 178 patients with pancreatic adenocarcinoma. Ninety percent were fifty years or older, and 87 percent were Caucasian. Forty-six percent were female, and 54 percent were male. Sixty-four percent had stage 3 or 4 pancreatic cancer. Of the 178 patients, eighty-seven (49 percent) had vitamin D deficiency and forty-four (25 percent) had vitamin D insufficiency. Only forty-seven (26 percent) had sufficient levels of vitamin D. The researchers learned that the median vitamin D levels were significantly lower among nonwhite patients and among patients with stage 1 and stage 2 disease. Only thirteen patients (20 percent) with stage 1 and 2 pancreatic adenocarcinoma had sufficient vitamin D levels, while thirty-four patients (30 percent) of stage 3 or 4 pancreatic adenocarcinoma had sufficient levels of vitamin D. Low levels of vitamin D were found to be associated with a poor prognosis in patients with stage 3 and stage 4 disease. The researchers recommended "the systematic screening of patients with pancreatic cancer for vitamin D deficiency and the rigorous monitoring of these patients while they are receiving oral supplementation."[10]

Vitamin C Intake May Be Associated with the Risk of Pancreatic Cancer

In a systematic review and meta-analysis published in the journal *Scientific Reports*, researchers from China evaluated the association between vitamin C intake and the risk of pancreatic cancer. They identified seventeen observational studies with 4,827 cases of pancreatic cancer that met their criteria. There were four cohort studies and thirteen case-control studies. Four studies were conducted in the United States, two in Canada, nine in Europe, one in Japan, and one in Australia. The quality of the studies was generally good. While no significant association was reported in nine studies, eight of the studies found an inverse association between vitamin C intake and the risk of pancreatic cancer. Still, when they pooled the results, the researchers observed that compared to the lowest intake of vitamin C, the highest intake of vitamin C seemed to be associated with a significantly lowered risk of pancreatic cancer. And, these associations were evident in Caucasians, Asians, and mixed populations. No publication bias was noted. The researchers commented that "the higher intake of vitamin C could reduce the risk of pancreatic cancer."[11]

Vitamin B6 May Lower the Risk of Pancreatic Cancer

In a systematic review and meta-analysis published in *Nutrition Journal*, researchers from China evaluated the use of vitamin B6, vitamin B12, and methionine, an amino acid, to risk the risk of pancreatic cancer. The researchers identified eighteen studies that met their criteria. These studies were published between 1991 and 2020; there were eleven prospective studies and seven case-control studies. Six studies were performed in the United States, six in Europe, five in Asia, and one in Australia. Ten studies examined the association between pancreatic cancer risk and the dietary intake of vitamins B6 and B12 and methionine, and eight studies assessed blood levels of the vitamins and methionine. Though the results from the studies on vitamin B6 intake and pancreatic cancer were inconsistent, all of the studies on the association between blood levels of vitamin B6 and pancreatic cancer risk showed a statistically significant inverse association. Higher rates of vitamin B6 in the blood were directly associated with lower rates of pancreatic cancer. There did not appear to be an association between the intake of vitamin B12 or methionine and pancreatic cancer. "Considering that vitamin B6 is present in a wide variety of foods such as beef, liver, tuna, and bananas, this research is expected to offer novel avenues for the primary prevention and control of pancreatic cancer." Nevertheless, the researchers cautioned that their findings were obtained primarily from case-control studies, "and the data for the high level of dietary vitamin B6 intake were sparse."[12]

Exercise May Be Useful for People with Pancreatic Cancer

In a literature review published in the journal *Cancers*, researchers from Germany investigated the use of exercise as a supportive therapy for people dealing with pancreatic cancer. The researchers located seven randomized controlled trials with 396 patients that prescribed home-based or supervised exercise programs with aerobics or resistance training. There were 207 patients in the intervention groups and the remaining patients in the control groups. The studies were published between 2012 and 2023. The number of subjects in each of the studies ranged from twenty-eight to 151, and they had a mean age of 51.9 years and 66.5 years, respectively. The duration of the interventions ranged from twelve weeks to twelve months. The majority of the patients were diagnosed with pancreatic ductal adenocarcinoma. Nearly, all of the patients had surgery. The researchers learned that exercise was feasible and safe for people dealing with pancreatic cancer. In addition, exercise was associated with improved quality of life. For example, the subjects who exercised had better cognitive functioning, role functioning, sleep, social functioning, and mental health. They had less cancer-related fatigue and better muscle strength. Still, the researchers cautioned that there are only a limited number of studies on this topic, and there is very little research on the use of exercise for people with more advanced pancreatic cancer. That is why they emphasized the need for more randomized controlled trials "with larger sample sizes."[13]

Chinese Herbal Medicine May Be Useful for Some People with Pancreatic Cancer

In a trial published in the journal *Integrative Cancer Therapies*, researchers from Hong Kong wanted to learn if Chinese herbal medicine could prolong the lives of people diagnosed with pancreatic cancer. The cohort consisted of 182 patients who were diagnosed with pancreatic cancer. At recruitment, the patients were thirty to eighty-seven years old, with a mean age of fifty-six years. All of them were treated with Chinese herbal medicine with or without conventional treatments, such as surgery, chemotherapy, or radiation. Overall survival rates ranged from four months to 9.6 years, with a mean survival of 29.6 months and a median survival of 15.2 months. Seventy-six percent of the patients were alive one year after diagnosis. The researchers commented that the Chinese herbal medicine treatments appeared to prolong life and improve the quality of life. And, they concluded that their findings "support a better prognosis for pancreatic cancer patients who receive CHM [Chinese herbal medicine] treatment compared with conventional treatment alone."[14]

In a systematic review and meta-analysis published in the journal *Evidence-Based Complementary and Alternative Medicine*, researchers from China examined the beneficial and adverse effects of the combination of conventional and Chinese herbal medicine to treat inoperable pancreatic cancer. The researchers located twenty-nine studies with 1808 patients that met their criteria for inclusion. Twenty-seven studies were published in Chinese and two in English. All but one of the studies was conducted in China; the remaining study was conducted in Japan. All of the studies exhibited comparable baseline patient characteristics, including age, gender, and stage of pancreatic cancer. The researchers determined that compared to the non-Chinese herbal medicine regimens, the treatments with Chinese herbal medicine significantly improved the one-year survival rates. In addition, the Chinese herbal medicine increased the role of antitumor therapies and improved the quality of life of the patients. The researchers concluded that Chinese herbal medicine "is a promising strategy as an adjunctive therapy in treating unresectable and advanced pancreatic cancer and that TCH [traditional Chinese medicine] in combination with conventional therapy is useful for overcoming this stubborn disease."[15]

Spiritual Meditation May Be Useful for People with Pancreatic Cancer

In a pilot trial published in the journal *Complementary Medicine Research*, researchers from Germany evaluated the usefulness of spiritual meditation for people with advanced pancreatic cancer. They focused on using spiritual meditation to decrease pain, improve quality of life, reduce stress, and alleviate negative emotions. The initial cohort consisted of twenty patients, eleven women and nine men, with a mean age of sixty-two years. Eighteen patients were referred by their physicians and two by their meditation practitioner. All of the patients had either advanced or metastatic pancreatic cancer. They were instructed to practice daily meditation at home either with the help of an audio recording or with the guidance of a friend or family member using a written script. Nine patients survived the study year. Still, at the final one-year visit, data were only available for seven patients. The researchers determined that the patients who regularly practiced meditation had improvements in their pain, quality of life, stress, and negative emotions/anxiety, while depression scores remained stable. Because spiritual meditation appeared to help these patients, the researchers proposed that such support should be provided to patients with advanced pancreatic cancer as part "of a comprehensive patient care from the time of diagnosis." And, they concluded that their findings "demonstrated the acceptability and feasibility of spiritual meditation in patients with PDAC [advanced pancreatic ductal adenocarcinoma]."[16]

REFERENCES AND FURTHER READING

Bosetti, C., F. Turati, A. Dal Pont et al. "The Role of Mediterranean Diet on the Risk of Pancreatic Cancer." *British Journal of Cancer* 109 (2013): 1360–1366.

Cho, May, Parvin F. Peddi, Kevin Ding et al. "Vitamin D Deficiency and Prognostics Among Patients with Pancreatic Adenocarcinoma." *Journal of Translational Medicine* 11 (2013): 206.

Eggers, Christine, Elisabeth Olliges, Stefan Boeck et al. "Exploring Pain, Quality of Life, and Emotional Well-Being in Patients with Advanced Pancreatic Cancer Practicing Spiritual Mediation: A Pilot Study." *Complementary Medicine Research* 30 (2023): 289–298.

Fan, Hua, Jiantao Kou, Dongdong Han et al. "Association Between Vitamin C Intake and the Risk of Pancreatic Cancer: A Meta-Analysis of Observational Studies." *Scientific Reports* 5 (2015): 13973.

Griffin, James F., Katherine E. Poruk, and Christopher L. Wolfgang. "Pancreatic Cancer Surgery: Past, Present, and Future." *Chinese Journal of Cancer Research* 27, no. 4 (August 2015): 332–348.

Jansen, Rick J., Dennis P. Robinson, Rachael Z. Stolzenberg-Solomon et al. "Nutrients from Fruits and Vegetable Consumption Reduce the Risk of Pancreatic Cancer." *Journal of Gastrointestinal Cancer* 44, no. 2 (June 2013): 152–161.

Larsson, Susanna C., Niclas Håkansson, Ingmar Näslund et al. "Fruit and Vegetable Consumption in Relation to Pancreatic Cancer Risk: A Prospective Study." *Cancer Epidemiology Biomarkers & Prevention* 15, no. 2 (February 2006): 301–305.

Li, Bin, Run Gan, Quanjun Yang et al. "Chinese Herbal Medicines as a Adjunctive Therapy for Unresectable Pancreatic Cancer: A Systematic Review and Meta-Analysis." *Evidence-Based Complementary and Alternative Medicine* 2015 (2015): 350730.

Nöthlings, Ute, Lynne R. Wilkens, Suzanne P. Murphy et al. "Meat and Fat Intake as Risk Factors for Pancreatic Cancer: The Multiethnic Cohort Study." *Journal of the National Cancer Institute* 97, no. 19 (October 5, 2005): 1458–1465.

Rosebrock, Kim, Marianne Sinn, Faik G. Uzunoglu et al. "Effects of Exercise Training on Patient-Specific Outcomes in Pancreatic Cancer Patients: A Scoping Review." *Cancers* 15 (2023): 5899.

Wei, Dan-Hong and Qi-Qi Mao. "Vitamin B6, Vitamin B12 and Methionine and Risk of Pancreatic Cancer: A Meta-Analysis." *Nutrition Journal* 19 (2020): 111.

Wolpin, Brian M., Kimmie Ng, Ying Bao et al. "Plasma 25-Hydroxyvitamin D and Risk of Pancreatic Cancer." *Cancer Epidemiology, Biomarkers & Prevention* 21, no. 1 (January 2012): 82–91.

Wong, Wendy, Bing Zhong Chen, Allyson Kin Yan Lee et al. "Chinese Herbal Medicine Effectively Prolongs the Overall Survival of Pancreatic Cancer Patients: A Case Series." *Integrative Cancer Therapies* 18 (2019): NA.

CANCER, STOMACH

INTRODUCTION

Also known as gastric cancer, stomach cancer is cancer that begins in the cells that line the stomach, which is in the upper middle part of the abdomen, just below the ribs. While stomach cancer may originate in any part of the stomach, in most parts of the world, it occurs in the stomach body or the main part of the stomach. In the United States, stomach cancer is most likely to begin at the gastroesophageal junction or the area where the esophagus meets the stomach.

Stomach cancer starts to form when a trigger, such as an infection, years of acid reflux, or diets that contain too many salty foods, damages the cells in the inner lining of the stomach. This causes changes in the cells' DNA, and the newly developing cancer cells grow much faster than the normal cells. In time, the cells form a mass.

There are a few different types of stomach cancer. Adenocarcinoma forms in the cells that produce mucus in the innermost lining of the stomach; this is the most common type of stomach cancer. Gastrointestinal stromal tumors (GIST) form in nerve cells found in the walls of the stomach and other digestive organs; it is a type of soft-tissue sarcoma. Carcinoid tumors begin in the neuroendocrine cells, and lymphoma begins in the cells of the immune system. Most lymphomas that start in the stomach are a type of non-Hodgkin's lymphoma.

Stomach cancer was described as early as 3000 BC in hieroglyphic inscriptions and papyri manuscripts from ancient Egypt. Using data collected in Verona, Italy from 1760 to 1839, the first major statistical analysis of cancer incidence and mortality was compiled. It showed that during that time period stomach cancer was the most common and lethal type of cancer.[1]

SYMPTOMS, RISKS, AND COMPLICATIONS

In the earliest stages, stomach cancer does not always cause symptoms. Still, there are a host of different symptoms associated with stomach cancer. These include abdominal pain, difficulty swallowing, a bloated feeling after eating, feeling full after eating small amounts of food, lack of hunger even at normal meal times, heartburn, indigestion, nausea and vomiting, weight loss, fatigue, and stools that look black.

There are several factors that increase the risk of stomach cancer. These include gastroesophageal reflux disease (GERD), a diet high in salt, salt-preserved foods, and cured meats, a diet low in fruits and vegetables, Helicobacter pylori infection, gastritis, smoking, stomach polyps, family history of stomach cancer, and a family history of genetic syndromes that increase the risk of stomach cancer. Obesity, smoking, and a history of gastric surgery are also associated with an increased risk for gastric cancer.

Stomach cancer may easily cause a loss of appetite and weight. It is not uncommon for people dealing with stomach cancer to become thin. Stomach cancer has been associated with ascites, a condition in which fluid builds up in the abdomen, leading to feelings of pressure and shortness of breath. Unless it is diagnosed in the earlier stages, stomach cancer may easily spread to the lungs, liver, and bones.

PREVALENCE

In the United States, stomach cancer is not a common cancer. It accounts for only 1.5 percent of all new cancers diagnosed in the United States each year. It has been estimated that in 2024 there will be about 16,160 new cases in men and 10,730 new cases in women. During the same year, there were about 6,490 deaths in men and 4,390 deaths in women. Stomach cancer mostly affects older people. About half of the people diagnosed every year are 65 years or older.[2] While it is very uncommon in the United States, primarily because of reductions in rates of Helicobacter pylori bacteria and improved refrigeration, stomach cancer is common in other parts of the world, such as East Asia. There, it is a frequent cause of cancer-related death. Worldwide, stomach cancer is the fifth most common type of cancer.[3]

DIAGNOSIS AND TREATMENT OPTIONS

There are several tests that may be used to diagnose stomach cancer. The most frequently used test is the upper gastrointestinal endoscopy with a biopsy. During that test, a medical provider inserts an endoscope—thin, lighted tube—into the mouth, down the esophagus, and into the stomach. Tissue samples are taken for biopsy. Another frequently used test is the barium swallow. During this test, the patient drinks a liquid that contains a silver-white metallic compound known as barium, and X-rays are taken. A computerized tomography or CT scan may be used with or without dye to take images of areas inside the body. If stomach cancer is diagnosed, a few other tests may be used to stage the cancer or to determine how far the cancer may have spread. These include an endoscopic ultrasound, a procedure in which an endoscope is inserted into the mouth, esophagus, and stomach. A probe at the end of the tube bounces high-energy sound waves off internal organs and makes echoes. Another test, the PET-CT scan, combines images from a PET scan and a CT scan. They are done at the same time on the same machine. For the PET scan, a small amount of radioactive glucose may be injected into a vein; for the CT scan, a small amount of dye may be injected into a vein or swallowed.

These tests will enable the medical provider to stage the cancer. Stage 0 cancer is very small and only on the inside surface of the stomach. In this stage, there is no evidence of a primary tumor. A stage 1 cancer has grown into the inner layers of the stomach. In stage 2 and stage 3, the cancer has grown deeper into the walls of the stomach, and it may well have spread to the nearby lymph nodes. Stage 4 cancer has spread beyond the stomach to nearby organs. People with stage 0 and stage 1 have an overall better prognosis than those with stages 2, 3, and 4.

Normally, treatment for stomach cancer begins with surgery. Small cancers may be surgically removed during a procedure known as an endoscopic mucosal resection. A tube is passed from the mouth, through the esophagus, and into the stomach. Then, special cutting tools are used to remove the cancer. If the tumor is larger, part of the stomach may be removed; this is known as a subtotal gastrectomy. Larger tumors require the removal of the entire stomach—a total gastrectomy. With stage 4 stomach cancer, the stomach and other nearby organs may be removed. If there are distant metastases or the invasion of major blood vessels or some other structures by the tumor, then surgery may not be advised. While chemotherapy may not be necessary for early, localized stomach cancer, it may well be advised for the more advanced stages. In some cases, chemotherapy is used before surgery. The most common type of chemotherapy travels throughout the entire body; this is known as systemic chemotherapy. In some cases, however, chemotherapy is directed only to the stomach area. Given immediately after surgery, this type of treatment is known as hyperthermic intraperitoneal chemotherapy (HIPEC). To make this form of chemotherapy more effective, it will be heated. Though radiation therapy may not be advised for the lowest stages of stomach cancer, it may well be combined with chemotherapy. When radiation is used before surgery, it is called neoadjuvant radiation; when it is used after surgery, it is called adjuvant radiation. Other therapies tend to be used for more advanced stomach cancer. These include targeted therapy, immunotherapy, and palliative care. Targeted treatments use medications to attack specific chemicals within cancer cells; immunotherapy boosts the immune system, enabling it to better fight the cancer cells, and palliative care provides treatments that keep patients as comfortable as possible.

As has been noted, treatment for stomach cancer is more likely to be successful if the cancer is confined to the stomach. The prognosis for people with small stomach cancers is quite good. Unfortunately, many stomach cancers are not found until the cancer is more advanced. Stomach cancer that has grown through the stomach wall or has spread to other parts of the body is more difficult to treat. When cancer has spread to another part of the body, it may cause symptoms specific to where it has spread.

RESEARCH FINDINGS

People Who Eat More Vegetables Lower Their Risk of Gastric Cancer

In a pooled analysis of four cohort studies published in the journal *Annals of Oncology*, researchers from Japan assessed the association between the intake of fruits and vegetables and the risk of gastric cancer among the Japanese population. The studies had a total of 191,232 subjects; there were 87,771 men and 103,461 women. During 2,094,428 person-years of follow-up, 2,995 cases of gastric cancer were identified. The researchers found a "marginally significant" reduction in the risk of gastric cancer that was associated with the consumption of vegetables and green-yellow vegetables but not fruit among men and women. This was especially true for the risk of distal gastric cancer among men. In a more specific analysis, the researchers determined that this risk reduction could be around 20 percent.[4]

But, Different Results Were Obtained from Another Study

In a systematic review and meta-analysis published in the *European Journal of Cancer*, researchers from China also investigated the association between fruits and vegetables and the risk of stomach cancer. They identified seventeen articles on twenty-four studies that met their criteria. In total, there were more than 2.4 million subjects, and during a median follow-up of ten years, there were 6,632 cases of gastric cancer. Of the seventeen articles, eight were from Asia, five from America, and four from Europe. The majority of the studies were of high quality, and there was no indication of publication bias. Thirteen articles with nineteen studies examined the association between vegetable intake and gastric cancer risk, and sixteen articles with twenty-two studies reviewed the association between total fruit intake and gastric cancer risk. The researchers determined that the consumption of fruit, but not vegetables, was inversely associated with the risk of gastric cancer. The greatest reduction in risk was seen at the lower range of fruit intake—about 100 g per day. "Thus, from a public health perspective, targeting individuals and populations with a low intake of fruit might be most effective for GC [gastric cancer] prevention."[5]

But, Another Study Found Both Fruits and Vegetables Useful against Gastric Cancer

In a systematic review and dose-response meta-analysis published in the journal *Frontiers in Nutrition*, researchers from Iran analyzed the association between fruit and vegetable consumption and the risk of gastric cancer. They identified seventeen articles containing eighteen prospective studies that met their criteria; there were 1,527,911 participants between the ages of eighteen and ninety years. Sample sizes ranged from 742 to 490,802. During the follow-up periods that ranged from 4.5 to twenty-one years, there were 8,477 cases of gastric cancer. Of the seventeen articles, ten described studies in Western countries, including the United States and Europe, and the remaining seven were conducted in Asian countries. Except for three articles, the studies used food frequency questionnaires. In all of the studies, gastric cancer was diagnosed using data obtained from medical records and cancer registries. Ten articles containing fifteen studies with 1,445,175 participants and 7,075 cases of gastric cancer assessed the link between vegetable intake and gastric cancer. Twelve articles and sixteen studies with a total sample size of 1,465,515 participants and 7,330 cases of gastric cancer examined fruit intake and gastric cancer. Six publications (nine studies) entered the total intake of fruits and vegetables in their analyses. These studies had 1,256,299 participants and 4,591 cases of gastric cancer. The researchers determined that a higher intake of total fruit and total fruit and vegetables was associated with a 13 and 25 percent lower risk of gastric cancer, respectively. Further, in the linear dose-response analysis, each 100 g per day increase in total fruit intake and a 200 g per day increase in total fruit and vegetable intake were associated with a 5 and 6 percent lower risk of gastric cancer, respectively. The researchers concluded that "further studies should examine the associations of individual fruits and vegetables with gastric cancer risk."[6]

High Adherence to the Mediterranean Diet Is Associated with a Reduced Risk of Gastric Cancer

In a systematic review and dose-response meta-analysis published in the journal *Frontiers in Nutrition*, researchers from China evaluated the association between high adherence to the Mediterranean diet and the risk for gastric cancer. The researchers identified five prospective cohort studies and six case-control studies with a total of 1,366,318 participants and 5,708 cases of gastric cancer that met their criteria. The included studies were published between 2010 and 2023; all of the participants were at least eighteen years old. The studies were conducted in the United States, Spain, Italy, Afghanistan, Sweden, the Netherlands, Jordan, and other European countries. In all of the studies, dietary intake was measured with food frequency questionnaires. The number of study participants ranged between 270 and 494,968. When compared to those with the lowest adherence to the Mediterranean diet, the researchers learned that those with the highest adherence had a 29 percent reduction in the risk for gastric cancer. In addition, in the ten studies that were included in the dose-response analysis, a linear dose-response analysis found that each one-score increment in the Mediterranean diet was associated with a 5 percent lower risk of gastric cancer. The researchers commented that their findings "provide further scientific evidence supporting the adoption of adherence to the Mediterranean diet for the primary prevention of gastric cancer."[7]

People Who Smoke Increase Their Risk for Gastric Cancer

In a systematic review and meta-analysis published in the journal *Cancer Causes & Control*, researchers from Portugal assessed the association between cigarette smoking and gastric cancer. They located forty-two articles that met their criteria for the systematic review, and thirty-two studies (twenty-seven cohort and five nested case-control) met their criteria for at least one of the meta-analyses. Of the initial forty-two studies, twenty were from Asia, twelve were from Europe, and ten were from the United States. The mean follow-up time was 8.5 years, with the actual times ranging from 1.5 to twenty-five years. The researchers learned that males who smoke have a 60 percent higher risk for gastric cancer than males who never smoked; in females, the risk is increased by 20 percent. While there was a good deal of heterogeneity between the studies, the researchers commented that "the large majority of the studies found a positive association between smoking and gastric cancer." And, they made a truly notable conclusion. They said that their findings "provide solid evidence to classify smoking as the most important behavioral risk factor for gastric cancer."[8]

Higher Levels of Serum Vitamin D Are Associated with Reduced Risk for Stomach Cancer

In a retrospective, single-center, case-control study published in the *World Journal of Gastroenterology*, researchers from Elmhurst, New York examined the association between stomach cancer and levels of serum vitamin D. The cohort consisted of forty-nine patients who were diagnosed with gastric adenocarcinoma at Elmhurst Hospital Center; all of these patients had documented levels of vitamin D. The cohort was matched to a control group of subjects who had no known history of cancer but also had documented levels of vitamin D. The researchers found that the average age of patients with gastric adenocarcinoma and documented vitamin D levels was sixty-four years. When compared to the controls, the prevalence of vitamin D insufficiency in patients with gastric adenocarcinoma was significantly higher than in patients with normal vitamin D levels. There were forty-one gastric adenocarcinoma patients with vitamin D insufficiency compared to eighteen patients with normal vitamin D levels without gastric adenocarcinoma. The researchers determined that patients with lower levels of vitamin D had an increased risk for gastric adenocarcinoma. There was, however, no correlation between the severity of vitamin D deficiency and the stage of gastric adenocarcinoma.[9]

Vitamin C Also Reduces the Risk of Stomach Cancer

In a study published in the *World Journal of Gastroenterology*, researchers from Korea examined the effects of dietary vitamin C on the risk for stomach cancer. The cohort consisted of 415 patients with stomach cancer and 830 controls; there were 810 men and 435 women. Using self-administered questionnaires, data were collected on demographics, medical history, and dietary and nutrient intake. Compared to the control group, the men and women in the stomach cancer group had less education, a lower-level job, less household income, and more tobacco use. They performed less regular exercise and had a higher rate of H. pylori infection. The men in the case group had a higher family history of gastric cancer. The researchers learned that the subjects with stomach cancer had a lower intake of vitamin C. They consumed less foods such as cabbage, lettuce, strawberries, orange juice, watermelon, apples, and bananas. At the same time, vitamin C intake did not offer any stomach cancer protection for those infected with H. pylori. According to the researchers, this finding is supported by many other studies. "The total fruit consumption and some vitamin C contributing foods showed a negative association with gastric cancer."[10]

Intake of Vitamin B12 Does Not Appear to Increase the Risk of Stomach Cancer

In a systematic review and meta-analysis published in the journal *Nutrition and Cancer*, researchers from China reviewed the relationship between vitamin B12 consumption and the risk of stomach cancer. They located nine studies with 3,494 cases of gastric cancer and 611,638 participants that met their criteria. There were three prospective cohort studies, two nested case-control studies, and four retrospective case-control studies. All of the studies were published in English. Three were conducted in the United States, three in China, and one each in Australia, Finland, and Denmark. The researchers determined that the intake of vitamin B12 did not increase the risk of gastric cancer. In a related analysis, the researchers found that a high intake of vitamin B12 may increase the risk of gastric cancer in people who are positive for H. pylori and decrease the risk in people who are H. pylori negative. Further, a high intake of vitamin B12 is associated with a decreased risk of gastric cancer in non-smokers but an increased risk in smokers. The researchers concluded that there is "no significant association between vitamin B12 intake and the risk of gastric cancer."[11]

Folate and Vitamin B6, as well As Methionine, Do Not Increase the Risk of Gastric Cancer

In a study published in the journal *Cancer Prevention Research*, researchers from Japan evaluated the association between folate, vitamins B6 and B12, and methionine, an essential amino acid, and the risk for stomach cancer. They included data from 86,820 Japanese individuals (40,563 men and 46,257 women) who completed a validated food frequency questionnaire with 138 food items in the Japan Public Health Center-Based Prospective Study. During a median of 15.4 years of follow-up, there were 2,269 cases of stomach cancer. The researchers found no association between the intake of the vitamins and methionine and the risk of stomach cancer. However, there was an increased risk of gastric cancer for the highest dietary intake of folate among participants with high sodium intake. The researchers commented that their findings were consistent with several studies conducted in the United States, Australia, and China. The researchers concluded that "future studies should investigate the effect of folate supplementation on the risk of gastric cancers in patients with precancerous lesions such as atrophic gastritis or gastric dysplasia."[12]

Garlic Intake May or May Not Lower the Risk of Gastric Cancer

In a systematic review and meta-analysis published in the journal *Gastroenterology*, researchers from China reviewed the association between the consumption of allium vegetables, such as garlic, onions, shallots, leeks, and chives, and the risk of gastric cancer. They located nineteen case-control studies and two cohort studies, with 543,220 subjects, that met their criteria. Of the case-control studies, eleven were population-based and eight were hospital-based. Of the twenty-one studies, ten were conducted in Europe, six in China, and one each in Japan, Korea, Iran, Venezuela, and Uruguay. Sample sizes ranged from 210 to 521,787. And the number of gastric cancer cases varied from ninety-eight to 1,124. The researchers learned that high allium consumption was associated with a reduced risk of gastric cancer. According to the case-control studies, an increase in allium vegetable consumption of 20 g per day, about the weight of one garlic bulb, was associated with a statistically significant 9 percent decrease in the risk of gastric cancer. The researchers concluded that there is now strong evidence that increased consumption of allium vegetables is associated with reductions in the risk of gastric cancer. "Further study is needed to confirm this finding and to explore which constituents in allium vegetables play a significant role in gastric cancer prevention."[13]

In a study published in the *International Journal of Cancer*, researchers from Boston, Massachusetts, New Haven, Connecticut, and Korea evaluated the relationship between the consumption of garlic and the risk of stomach cancer. They used data obtained from 77,086 women in the Nurses' Health Study and 46,398 men in the Health Professionals Follow-Up Study. Garlic intake was assessed with a validated semi-quantitative food frequency questionnaire that was periodically administered. Gastric cancer cases were identified by self-report or the national death index. In the Nurses' Health Study, there were 138 cases of gastric cancer during thirty years of follow-up, and in the Health Professionals Follow-Up Study, there were 154 cases during twenty-eight years of follow-up. Participants with higher garlic intake tended to be nonwhite, physically active, ever-smokers, drinkers of more alcohol, and consumers of more fruits, vegetables, and coffee. They were also more likely to be diabetic. But, there did not appear to be an association between the use of garlic and the risk of stomach cancer. The researchers concluded that they found "no evidence that high intake of garlic reduces gastric cancer risk."[14]

There May or May Not Be an Association between Red and Processed Meat Consumption and Gastric Cancer

In a systematic review and meta-analysis published in the journal *Oncotarget*, researchers from China studied the relationship between the consumption of red and processed meat and risk of gastric cancer. They identified forty-two studies that met their criteria. Twenty-four studies addressed red meat (twenty case-control and four cohort) and thirty-three dealt with processed meat (twenty-five case-control and eight cohort). The red meat included beef, pork, lamb, mutton, beef burgers, veal, horse, liver, and others. The processed meat included bacon, lunch meat, ham, sausage, salami, hot dogs, smoked meat, salted meat, and others. The case-control studies found that the consumption of red and processed meat increased the risk of gastric cancer, but this association was not evident in the cohort studies. When dose-response analyses were conducted, the researchers noted a negative association for red meat and a positive association for processed meat. The researchers concluded that there is a need for "further well-designed prospective studies."[15]

In a systematic review and meta-analysis of epidemiological observational studies published in the online journal *PLoS One*, researchers from China also evaluated the association between red and processed meat and gastric cancer. The researchers located twelve cohort and thirty case-control studies that met their criteria. There were twelve cohort studies for processed meat, five for red meat, and five for red and processed meat. Additionally, there were seven case-control studies for red meat, twelve case-control studies for processed meat, and eleven for red and processed meat. The twelve cohort studies consisted of a total of 2,343,450 participants and 5,118 cases of gastric cancer. The thirty case-control studies involved 11,680 cases and 67,544 controls. Eleven studies were conducted in Asia, sixteen in Europe, eleven in North America, and four in Latin America. Two of the studies included only men, and two had only women. The researchers found significant associations between the consumption of both red and processed meat and risk of gastric cancer. Positive findings were also observed for beef, bacon, and ham, but not pork. However, when the studies were analyzed by design, the association was significant in the case-control studies but not in the cohort studies for red meat. At the same time, most subgroup analyses confirmed a significant association between processed meat intake and risk for gastric cancer. So, while the results may differ, they tend to point to the fact that the consumption of red and processed meat "contributes to increased gastric cancer risk." Still, the researchers underscored the need for more research on this association. "These findings from our study need to be confirmed in future research in well-designed cohort or interventional studies."[16]

Higher Salt Intake Increases the Risk of Gastric Cancer

In a systematic review and meta-analysis published in the journal *Nutrients*, researchers from China evaluated the association between salt intake and the risk of gastric cancer. They identified thirty-eight case-control studies with 37,225 subjects that met their criteria. There was significant heterogeneity between the studies, and publication bias was detected. Eleven studies were from China, four were from Korea, four from Italy, two from Iran, two from Turkey, and one each from France, England, Spain, Japan, Puerto Rico, Sweden, Mexico, Thailand, Uruguay, Colombia, Portugal, Serbia, Canada, Ecuador, and Poland. In all of the studies, the dietary salt intake was estimated by a frequent food questionnaire or relevant tests. The researchers found a significant positive association between high salt intake and gastric cancer, and this association was not significantly different between geographic regions, estimation methods of dietary salt intake, and the source of controls. The researchers concluded that people who prefer salty foods "need to receive dietary education and diet management for the prevention of gastric cancer."[17]

Obesity during Adolescence Increases the Risk of Gastric Cancer

In a multicenter case-control study published in *Cancer Causes & Control*, researchers from Korea evaluated the association between obesity during adolescence and the risk of gastric cancer. The cohort consisted of 1,492 incident cases of gastric cancer and 1,492 age- and sex-matched controls. The mean age of the cases was 58.6 years in men and 56.3 years in women. There were more ever-smokers among men with gastric cancer, which was not observed in women. Men with gastric cancer were more likely to be drinkers; again, this was not observed in women. Both men and women with gastric cancer were less likely to be regular exercisers. The BMI at age eighteen was calculated using weights and heights from a questionnaire. The researchers determined that the BMI at adolescence was a strong risk factor for gastric cancer. A high BMI was significantly associated with the risk of gastric cancer; in both men and women, there was a nonlinear threshold effect beginning at 25.3 kg/m^2. The researchers concluded that there appears to be an association between overweight status and obesity in adolescence and several types of cancer. They noted that their findings "may shed light to the public health, stressing the importance of weight control in childhood in the development of gastric cancer."[18]

REFERENCES AND FURTHER READING

He, J., H. Fu, C. Li et al. "Association Between Vitamin B12 and Risk of Gastric Cancer: A Systematic Review and Meta-Analysis of Epidemiological Studies." *Nutrition and Cancer* 74, no. 9 (2022): 3263–3273.

Hoang, B. V., J. Lee, I. J. Choi et al. "Effect of Dietary Vitamin C on Gastric Cancer Risk in the Korean Population." *World Journal of Gastroenterology* 22, no. 27 (July 21, 2016): 6257–6267.

Khairan, Paramita, Tomotaka Sobue, Ehab Salah Eshak et al. "Association of B Vitamins and Methionine Intake with the Risk of Gastric Cancer: The Japan Public Health Center-Based Prospective Study." *Cancer Prevention Research* 15 (2022): 101–110.

Kim, Hanseul, NaNa Keum, Edward L. Giovannucci. Et al. "Garlic Intake and Gastric Cancer Risk: Results from Two Large Prospective US Cohort Studies." *International Journal of Cancer* 143, no. 5 (September 1, 2018): 1047–1053.

Ladeiras-Lopes, Ricardo, Alexandra Kirchhofer Pereira, Amanda Nogueira et al. "Smoking and Gastric Cancer: Systematic Review and Meta-Analysis of Cohort Studies." *Cancer Causes & Control* 19 (2008): 689–701.

Naemi Kermanshahi, M., E. Safaei, H. Tutunchi et al. "Fruit and Vegetable Intake in Relation to Gastric Cancer Risk: A Comprehensive and Updated Systematic Review and Dose-Response Meta-Analysis of Cohort Studies." *Frontiers in Nutrition* 10 (2023): 973171.

Shimazu, T., K. Wakai, A. Tamakoshi et al. "Association of Vegetable and Fruit Intake with Gastric Cancer Risk Among Japanese: A Pooled Analysis of Four Cohort Studies." *Annals of Oncology* 25 (2014): 1228–1233.

Song, Minkyo, Ji-Yeob Chai, Jae Jeong Yang et al. "Obesity at Adolescence and Gastric Cancer Risk." *Cancer Causes & Control* 26 (2015): 247–256.

Vyas, Neil, Rafael Ching Companioni, Melik TIba et al. "Association Between Serum Vitamin D Levels and Gastric Cancer: A Retrospective Chart Analysis." *World Journal of Gastrointestinal Oncology* 8, no. 9 (September 15, 2016): 688–694.

Wang, Q., Y. Chen, X. Wang et al. "Consumption of Fruit, But Not Vegetables, May Reduce Risk of Gastric Cancer: Results from a Meta-Analysis of Cohort Studies." *European Journal of Cancer* 50 (2014): 1498–1509.

Wu, X., L. Chen, J. Cheng et al. "Effects of Dietary Salt Intake on Risk of Gastric Cancer: A Systematic Review and Meta-Analysis of Case-Control Studies." *Nutrients* 14 (202): 4260.

Zhao, Z., Z. Yin, and Q. Zhao. "Red and Processed Meat Consumption and Gastric Cancer Risk: A Systematic Review and Meta-Analysis." *Oncotarget* 8, no. 18 (017): 30563–30575.

Zhou, Y., W. Zhuang, W. Hu et al. "Consumption of Large Amounts of *Allium* Vegetables Reduces Risk for Gastric Cancer in a Meta-Analysis." Gastroenterology 141 (2011): 80–89.

Zhu, H., X.. Yang, C. Zhang et al. "Red and Processed Meat Intake Is Associated with Higher Gastric Cancer Risk: A Meta-Analysis of Epidemiological Observational Studies." *PLoS One* 8, no. 8 (2013): e70955.

Zhu, Qin, Long Shu, Feng Zhou et al. "Adherence to the Mediterranean Diet and Risk of Gastric Cancer: A Systematic Review and Dose-Response Meta-Analysis." *Frontiers in Nutrition* 10 (September 8, 2023): 1259453.

CELIAC DISEASE

INTRODUCTION

Also known as gluten-sensitive enteropathy, celiac disease is a disorder in which the consumption of gluten, a protein found in wheat, barley, rye, and sometimes oats, triggers an immune response in the small intestine. Over time, this reaction damages the villi in the small intestine and prevents these tiny hairlike projections from properly absorbing nutrients, a condition called malabsorption.

Unfortunately for those with celiac disease, gluten is found in many of the foods in the standard Western diet, from cereals to breads to pasta and baked goods. In addition, gluten may be an additive in food products and supplements. Although there are a few types of gluten-free beer, the vast majority of beer products contain some form of gluten from barley or rye.

For decades before there were adequate labeling laws, finding the actual ingredients in processed foods could be challenging. Fortunately, in the United States, there are now labeling laws that require the listing of common allergens on the labels of processed foods. People with celiac disease must become comfortable reading labels. When the information on a label is insufficient, they need to learn to telephone, email, and text companies to ask about the content of their products. The safest processed foods tend to be those that are listed "certified gluten-free."

Though often misdiagnosed, people have probably suffered from celiac disease for thousands of years. It is known that the Greek physician and medical writer Aretaeus of Cappadocia wrote the first description of the disease. In the 1800s, Matthew Baillie, a British physician and pathologist, described a diarrheal disorder that improved with a rice-based diet. In 1887, Samuel Gee, an English physician, detailed the parameters of celiac disease and suggested that it might be treated with diet. Decades later, in 1924, American pediatrician Sidney Haas treated children with celiac disease with his banana diet. But, it was the Dutch physician, Willem Dicke, who realized that when bread became unavailable during the Second World War, the mortality rate for celiac disease dropped to zero. It was Dicke who hypothesized that wheat protein may be a key cause of celiac disease.[1]

SYMPTOMS, RISKS, AND COMPLICATIONS

The intestinal damage caused by the consumption of gluten results in a wide range of symptoms, including diarrhea, fatigue, unintended weight loss, bloating, flatulence, abdominal pain, constipation, and foul-smelling stools. However, more than half of those with celiac disease have non-digestive related symptoms. These include iron deficiency anemia, reduced bone density, dermatitis herpetiformis (an itchy, blistery skin rash), mouth ulcers such as cankers, headaches and fatigue, nervous system problems, brain fog, bone or joint pain, irritability (children), depression, reduced functioning of the spleen (hyposplenism), and elevated liver enzymes. Children with celiac disease may have nausea and vomiting, chronic diarrhea, a swollen belly, constipation, gas, and pale, foul-smelling stools. Malabsorption problems in children may lead to failure to thrive, damage to tooth enamel, weight loss, anemia, irritability, short stature, delayed puberty, and neurological problems such as attention-deficit/hyperactivity disorder (ADHD).

While it is known that celiac disease tends to run in families and has some form of genetic basis, the exact cause is unknown. Some contend that celiac disease is related to infant feeding practices, gastrointestinal infections, or gut bacteria, but none of these causes has been proven. Celiac disease tends to occur more often in people who have type 1 diabetes, Down syndrome, William syndrome, Turner syndrome, autoimmune thyroid disease, and Addison's disease. It may also be seen in individuals with gastroesophageal reflux disease, inflammatory bowel disease, and eosinophilic esophagitis. Celiac disease is most often seen in people assigned female at birth (AFAB). Over the years, there have been anecdotal reports from healthcare providers that celiac disease frequently occurs when there is some type of physical and/or emotional stress, such as surgery, sickness, or death in the family. While celiac disease most often appears during two times in the life cycle—early childhood and mid-life, it may occur at any time after gluten is introduced into an infant's diet. People with celiac disease had an increased risk of developing another autoimmune disorder, and this risk increases the longer celiac disease is untreated.

When not managed or treated, celiac disease may lead to serious complications, such as serious malnutrition, bone weakening, infertility and miscarriage, lactose intolerance, intestinal lymphoma, small bowel cancer, seizures, osteomalacia, osteopenia and osteoporosis, permanent dental enamel defects, and peripheral neuropathy. Children may fail to grow and develop normally.

PREVALENCE

While celiac disease is most often seen in people who are of Northern European descent, it may also be seen in individuals from North Africa, the Middle East, India, and northern China. Celiac disease affects about 1 percent of the population in Europe and North America. The incidence is much higher for those who have a first-degree relative with celiac; their risk increases to 10 percent. Almost everyone who is diagnosed with celiac disease is white and has a gene mutation known as HLA-DQ2 or HLA-DQ8. But, not everyone who has this gene mutation develops celiac disease.

DIAGNOSIS AND TREATMENT OPTIONS

People with gastrointestinal problems, especially those with family members who had been diagnosed with celiac disease, often correctly suspect they may have the disorder. And, they may want to try a gluten-free diet. Still, before eliminating gluten from the diet, be sure to consult a medical provider. In order to obtain accurate testing results, gluten must still be consumed. People who stop or even reduce their intake of gluten may alter their test results.

There are two main ways to test for celiac disease. The first and easiest is a simple blood test that looks for gluten antibodies; people with celiac disease produce these antibodies when gluten is consumed. The second is an upper endoscopy. A gastroenterologist passes a long, thin tube through the mouth, down the esophagus, into the stomach, and then into the small intestine to take biopsies of tissue. Once both tests are completed and celiac disease is confirmed, more blood tests will be ordered to test for specific vitamin and mineral deficiencies.

At present, there is only one treatment for celiac disease—adhering to a completely gluten-free diet. Anything that is consumed by mouth—whether it is food, drink, supplements, or medication—must be completely gluten-free. Even products that are not consumed but are used in the mouth, such as toothpaste, must be gluten-free. And, when gluten-free food is prepared next to gluten-containing food, there is always the risk of cross-contamination. However, not everyone responds to a gluten-free diet. Some people have celiac symptoms even many months after going gluten-free; this is called refractory celiac disease. This condition may be caused by other factors, including bacterial overgrowth in the intestine, microscopic colitis, pancreatic insufficiency or the poor functioning of the pancreas, irritable bowel syndrome, or difficulty digesting the sugar in dairy products (lactose), table sugar (sucrose), or the type of sugar found in honey and fruits (fructose).

RESEARCH FINDINGS

Adhering to a Gluten-Free Diet Tends to Improve the Gastrointestinal Symptoms of People with Celiac Disease

In a study published in the *American Journal of Clinical Nutrition*, researchers from Iowa City, Iowa, and Rochester, Minnesota, examined the effect of a gluten-free diet on the gastrointestinal symptoms of a cohort of US patients with celiac disease. The cohort consisted of 160 females and 55 males with celiac disease. The ages at diagnosis ranged from one year to ninety years. At diagnosis, many of the subjects had the common gastrointestinal symptoms of diarrhea, steatorrhea (excessive fat in the stools), and weight loss. All of the subjects received similar dietary instructions on how to follow a gluten-free diet, and they were encouraged to join local and national celiac support groups. A scripted follow-up survey was conducted by nurses not involved in the care of these patients. The researchers determined that after the subjects began a gluten-free diet, they tended to experience notable improvement in their gastrointestinal symptoms. For example, within days or weeks, chronic diarrhea, the most common complaint, stopped. The researchers concluded that "with a gluten-free diet, patients have substantial and rapid improvement in symptoms."[2]

Vitamin and Mineral Deficiencies Are Very Common in People with Celiac Disease

In a trial published in the journal *Nutrients*, researchers from the Netherlands assessed the vitamin and mineral status of adults with newly diagnosed celiac disease. The cohort consisted of eighty adults (fifty-two females and twenty-eight males) with a mean age of 42.8 years, who, until the trial began, consumed a gluten-containing Dutch-Western diet. They were compared to twenty-four healthy adults (comparable for sex, age, and BMI). The researchers noted that the mean daily gluten intake in the Netherlands is around 13 g. Analyses were made of several vitamins and nutrients. As a result, the researchers learned that 87 percent of the subjects with celiac disease were deficient in at least one nutrient. Ten of the subjects with celiac disease (12.5 percent) were not deficient in any of the tested vitamins and minerals. Specifically, 7.5 percent of the subjects were deficient in vitamin A; 14.5 percent were deficient in vitamin B6; 20 percent were deficient in folic acid; 19 percent were deficient in vitamin B12; 7.5 percent were deficient in vitamin A; 4.5 percent were deficient in vitamin (25-hydroxy) D; a notable 67 percent were deficient in zinc; 46.2 percent were deficient in iron stores and 32 percent had anemia. Seventeen percent were malnourished, and 22 percent of the women were underweight—they had lost more than 10 percent of their bodyweight during the previous six months or more than 5 percent in the previous month, prior to diagnosis. At the same time, 29 percent were overweight; 26 percent of the overweight subjects had obesity. With the exception of vitamin B12, there were very few vitamin and mineral deficiencies in the healthy controls. The researchers noted that these vitamin and mineral deficiencies appeared to be "unrelated to severity of clinical presentation, nutritional status or (semi-qualified) histopathological damage (score)." That is why, "nutritional parameters should be an integral part of celiac disease treatment."[3]

In a prospective observational study published in the journal *JGH Open*, researchers based in India examined the prevalence and etiology of iron deficiency anemia in people with celiac disease. The cohort consisted of 103 patients with celiac disease; forty-eight were male and fifty-five were female. All of them had detailed clinical assessments that included examinations and tests and a complete anemia work-up. Anemia was detected in ninety-six patients, and the degree of anemia increased with the severity of the villous atrophy. Iron deficiency was seen in eighty-four patients; vitamin B12 deficiency was seen in fourteen patients, and folate deficiency was seen in eleven patients. Seventeen patients had anemia caused by mixed nutritional deficiencies, and four had anemia of chronic disease. The researchers concluded that "anemia in patients with CD is multifactorial. Even though iron deficiency is the most common cause, other nutrient deficiencies should always be explored."[4]

Young Female Adults with Newly Diagnosed Celiac Disease Appear to Be at Increased Risk for Bone Mineral Density Problems

In a systematic literature review published in the journal *Calcified Tissue International*, researchers from Denmark wanted to learn more about the bone mineral density status of young adults with newly diagnosed celiac disease. They located one cross-sectional study and two longitudinal studies that met their criteria; in total, there were 188 female subjects between the ages of 29 and 37 years old. Samples ranged in size from ten to 110. The researchers found that the women tended to have low levels of bone mineral density and higher rates of osteoporosis. Since the researchers were unable to locate similar studies on men, they could not determine if newly diagnosed young adult men would also have these problems. The researchers concluded that "it may be crucial to assess BMD [bone mineral density] at time of diagnosis in young women." Furthermore, "there is a lack of robust evidence to demonstrate that nutritional supplements or antiresorptive agents are beneficial in the prevention of fragile bones in this age group."[5]

Children and Adolescents with Celiac Disease May Also Have Suboptimal Bone Health

In a systematic review and meta-analysis published in the *Journal of Clinical Densitometry*, researchers from Tuscaloosa, Alabama, Elon, North Carolina, and Philadelphia, Pennsylvania, compared the differences in bone health and stature among children and adolescents with celiac disease to healthy controls. The researchers located twelve studies published between 1996 and 2017 that met their criteria; in all of the studies, the diagnosis was based on biopsy or serological analysis. The researchers determined that the children and adolescents with celiac disease had lower bone mineral content and density than the healthy controls. Thus, they had "poorer bone health" than their healthy peers. Likewise, they tended to have a shorter stature and lower body weight. The researchers commented that "further work is needed regarding the etiology and long-term ramifications of the skeletal deficits in childhood celiac disease given that bone mass acquisition during the growing years is a major determinant of osteoporosis and fracture in childhood."[6]

Men and Premenopausal Women with Celiac Disease May Be More Likely to Have Osteopenia and Osteoporosis, but There Needs to Be More Research on the Topic

In a systematic review published in the *Nutrition Journal*, researchers based in Iran examined the incidence of osteopenia and osteoporosis in men and premenopausal women with celiac disease. The researchers located eight cross-sectional studies with 563 subjects from the UK, Brazil, India, Hungary, and Poland that met their criteria. All of the studies were in English, but only one had a control group. The study with the largest sample size had twenty-three males and 105 females; the smallest sample size was twenty-four. Although the studies varied markedly, a few found a significant difference between people with celiac disease and the general population or control group. But, in other studies, there was no discernable difference between the groups. The researchers concluded that there is insufficient data on the association between men and premenopausal women with celiac disease and osteopenia and osteoporosis. Still, it was generally evident that these groups probably have a higher risk for these medical problems. According to these researchers, their findings "suggest that bone loss is more prevalent in celiac disease and can be associated with increased risk of fracture." There is a need for "more case-control studies with more sample size and consideration of cofounding factors."[7]

For Women with Celiac Disease, Adhering to a Gluten-Free Diet May or May Not Improve Bone Mineral Density

In a retrospective study published in the journal *Revista Espanõla de Enfermedades Digestivas*, researchers from Brazil examined the value of a gluten-free diet in a group of Brazilian women with celiac disease. The cohort consisted of forty-one patients with celiac disease; they ranged in age from thirteen to seventy-six years, with a mean age of 46.1 years. At their first densitometry, 14.6 percent had normal bone mass, 56.1 percent had osteopenia, and 29.2 percent had osteoporosis. The women were followed for one to thirteen years, with a median time of five years. During the time they were followed, 12.1 percent began menopause, and four of the twelve osteoporotic patients developed a low-impact fracture. The verified fractures were of the hip, rib, wrist, and ankle. At the second densitometry, 12.8 percent of the women had normal bone mass, 58.9 percent had osteopenia, and 28.2 percent had osteoporosis. The researchers concluded that their cohort of women had "notably impaired" bone health at baseline, "especially in those with a diagnostic delay." Adhering to a gluten-free diet, "modestly improved BMD [bone mineral density] with low impact fractures occurring in one third of the patients during the follow-up period."[8]

People with Idiopathic Osteoporosis May or May Not Need to Be Screened for Celiac Disease

In a case-control trial published in the journal *Gastroenterology and Hepatology from Bed to Bench*, researchers from Iran wanted to determine if it is necessary for people with idiopathic (unknown cause) osteoporosis to be screened for celiac disease. The cohort consisted of 560 subjects, 460 with osteoporosis and one hundred healthy subjects. Among the osteoporotic subjects, 250 were female and 140 were postmenopausal. Sixty-four of the healthy subjects were female. The subjects with positive serologic tests had upper endoscopy testing and duodenum biopsies. The clinical findings were evaluated in both groups and compared with each other. The researchers determined that five (1.08 percent) of the subjects (three females and two males) with osteoporosis and one (1 percent) of the subjects (female) without osteoporosis had celiac disease. The researchers concluded that the prevalence of celiac disease in their cohort was too low to justify screening everyone with osteoporosis for celiac disease. However, people with osteoporosis who have symptoms associated with celiac disease, such as iron deficiency anemia, chronic dyspepsia and bloating, constipation or diarrhea, and recurrent aphthous lesions (canker sores), should be tested for celiac disease.[9]

Fish Oil Supplementation and Aerobic Exercise Appear to Reduce Inflammation in People with Celiac Disease

In a trial published in the *Journal of Nutrition and Metabolism*, researchers from Brazil wanted to learn if twelve weeks of daily fish oil supplementation or daily fish oil supplementation and exercise would reduce levels of inflammation in people with celiac disease. The cohort consisted of nineteen adults with celiac disease and eleven healthy adults without celiac disease. All of the subjects with celiac disease had a good adherence to a gluten-free diet. The subjects with celiac disease were divided into two groups: eleven subjects took fish oil supplementation alone and eight subjects took fish oil supplementation and participated in three sessions per week of sixty minutes of mostly aerobic exercise. Testing for levels of C-reactive protein and interleukin-6 was used to detect levels of inflammation. The researchers learned that the combination of fish oil supplementation and exercise resulted in a significant reduction in inflammation. And, they concluded that "the associated interventions showed a corrective and preventive potential in relation to disorders associated with chronic inflammation."[10]

Undiagnosed and Untreated Celiac Disease May Alter a Women's Reproductive Health

In a nationwide matched cohort study published in the journal *Human Reproduction*, researchers from Denmark wanted to learn how celiac disease influences women's reproductive health both before and after the diagnosis. Through linkage to several national health registries, the researchers identified all of the women diagnosed with celiac disease between 1997 and 2016. They then identified an age and sex-matched comparison cohort and obtained data on reproductive outcomes for both cohorts. The celiac disease cohort contained 6,319 women and the matched cohort had 63,166 women. Slightly more than 60 percent of the women were diagnosed during reproductive age and 15 percent under age fifteen. At the index date, the average number of pregnancies in the two cohorts was similar (1.1 per woman), and the mean age at first pregnancy was also approximately the same. The researchers learned that the women diagnosed with celiac disease were similar to women who did not have celiac disease in a number of important ways. They had a similar chance of pregnancy, a similar live birth rate and risk of stillbirth, a similar chance of molar and ectopic pregnancy, and a similar risk for spontaneous abortion (miscarriage). However, women with undiagnosed celiac disease had higher rates of spontaneous abortion and stillbirths, and they had fewer pregnancies during the two years before diagnosis. Apparently, after women with undiagnosed celiac disease are diagnosed and begin a gluten-free diet, their reproductive problems seem to resolve. The researchers concluded that their findings underscored the need for an "early diagnosis" of this medical problem.[11]

An Interesting Case Report from Iran Appears to Support These Findings

In a case report published in the *Iranian Journal of Reproductive Medicine*, researchers from Iran presented the case of a twenty-six-year-old married woman who had been trying to become pregnant for two years. The initial evaluation of her and her husband found no reason for this problem. However, for twelve months, she had been dealing with "intermittent, non-bloody and osmotic diarrhea" and a three kg (6.61 pound) weight loss. She also had iron deficiency anemia. After undergoing an upper endoscopy, the woman was diagnosed with celiac disease. Three months after beginning a gluten-free diet, her celiac-related symptoms were gone, and she was pregnant. The researchers concluded that "screening for silent or subtle CD especially among suspicious cases such as unexplained infertility seems to be a cost-effective action and in time administration of a gluten-free diet can lead to an almost complete cure."[12]

People with Celiac Disease Appear to Have an Increased Risk for Blood Clots Developing in the Veins

In a systematic review and meta-analysis published in the *Journal of Gastroenterology and Hepatology*, researchers from Thailand and several locations in the United States, but based in Rochester, Minnesota, wanted to learn if people with celiac disease have an increased risk of blood clots developing in the veins, a condition known as venous thromboembolism. A literature search yielded two retrospective cohort studies, one case-control study, and one cross-sectional study that met their criteria. The researchers found a statistically significant increased risk of venous thromboembolism among people with celiac disease "with 25 percent excess risk compared with those without celiac disease." Only one of the four studies investigated the risk over a ten-year period, and this study determined that the risk was highest during the first year after diagnosis. While there is no clear explanation of why this association exists, the researchers suggested that there are a few possible reasons, such as the fact that people with celiac disease tend to have chronic inflammation and vitamin deficiencies. The researchers concluded that since celiac disease is a common disorder in Western populations, "this finding could have a significant impact on public health."[13]

Many Healthcare Providers in Central Europe Need to Learn More about Celiac Disease

In a study published in the *Journal of Pediatric Gastroenterology and Nutrition*, researchers from central European countries but based in Slovenia wanted to determine if healthcare providers in central Europe knew a sufficient amount about celiac disease. Healthcare questionnaires on celiac disease were completed by 1,381 healthcare professionals and 2,262 celiac disease patients or their caregivers from Slovenia, Croatia, Hungary, Germany, and Italy. The questionnaire for healthcare providers had twenty-two questions and was divided into three subsections—epidemiology and clinical presentation, diagnostic procedure, and treatment with follow-up. The questionnaire for celiac patients had fourteen questions and was divided into two subsections—epidemiology, clinical presentation, and diagnostic, and treatment with follow-up. Most of the healthcare professionals were pediatricians, followed by general practitioners, internal medicine specialists, and others. Forty-three percent of the healthcare professionals had a friend or distant relative with celiac disease and 10 percent had a close relative with celiac disease. As might be expected, gastroenterologists knew more about celiac disease than other medical providers. But, healthcare providers were generally not well-versed on the topic. The mean score achieved by all the healthcare professionals was only 50.9 percent. Only 14 percent of all healthcare professionals and 18 percent of pediatricians achieved more than 70 percent of the maximal score. Even the patients or caregivers did not do well on their questionnaire. Their mean score was 56.4 percent. A total score higher than 50 percent was achieved by 58 percent of celiac patients or caregivers and 18 percent achieved more than 70 percent of the maximal score. The researchers noted that both healthcare professionals and patients and caregivers do not have a "satisfactory" level of knowledge about celiac disease. The researchers were particularly dismayed by the relatively low scores of pediatricians and general practitioners in the epidemiology and clinical presentation subsection, "as they represent the first contact point for potential CD patients." Such inadequate knowledge "lead to the disease being underdiagnosed and add to the long diagnostic delays that . . . [have been] observed in many studies."[14]

Celiac Disease May or May Not Increase the Risk of Cancer

In a national cohort study published in the journal *Clinical Gastroenterology and Hepatology*, researchers from New York City, Sweden, and Norway wanted to determine the association between celiac disease and the risk of cancer. From 2015 to 2017, the researchers obtained gastrointestinal histologic report data on 2.1 million Swedish individuals who were biopsied between 1965 and 2016. Data were retrieved from Sweden's twenty-eight pathology departments and were part of the Epidemiology Strengthened by Histopathology Reports in Sweden cohort. It was determined that there were 47,241 people with celiac disease; they were each matched with up to five Swedish controls who did not have celiac disease. Matching factors were based on age, sex, calendar years, and country. The researchers determined that after a median follow-up of 11.5 years, the cancer incidence in people with celiac disease versus people from the general population was 6.5 and 5.7 per one thousand person-years, respectively. While the risk for cancer overall was only significantly increased during the first year after celiac diagnosis, the risk for hematologic, hepatobiliary, and pancreatic cancers continued beyond that one-year timeline. The risk was highest in those who were diagnosed with celiac disease after the age of sixty years and was not increased in those diagnosed before the age of forty. The cancer risk was similar in those diagnosed before and after the year 2000.[15]

In a study published in the *American Journal of Medicine*, researchers from New York City, Chicago, Illinois, and Atlanta, Georgia examined the incidence of cancer among patients seen at a celiac referral center in New York City. The cohort consisted of 381 individuals over the age of eighteen; they had all been diagnosed with celiac disease. About two-thirds of the cohort were female. Forty-three individuals were diagnosed with cancer—nine after a diagnosis of celiac disease, seven within one month of the diagnosis, and twenty-seven before the diagnosis. The mean age at diagnosis was fifty-eight years. The most common type of cancer was non-Hodgkin's lymphoma, followed by melanoma, breast cancer, small bowel cancer, colon cancer, esophageal cancer, lung cancer, chronic lymphocytic leukemia, ovarian cancer, and cervical cancer. There were single cases of liver cancer, prostate cancer, bladder cancer, thyroid cancer, endometrial cancer, and Hodgkin's disease. The researchers noted that when compared with expected rates of cancer, the risks of small bowel adenocarcinoma, esophageal cancer, non-Hodgkin's lymphoma, and melanoma were significantly higher in those with celiac disease. The majority of these cancers occurred before the celiac disease diagnosis. In fact, the incidence of non-Hodgkin's lymphoma was rather dramatic. Patients had a ninefold increased risk of that illness, and this risk "persists beyond the first few years after the diagnosis of celiac disease, despite a gluten free diet."[16]

REFERENCES AND FURTHER READING

Berry, Neha, Jahangeer Basha, Neelam Varma et al. "Anemia in Celiac Disease is Multifactorial in Etiology: A Prospective Study from India." *JGH Open* 2 (2018): 196–200.

Costa, Allysson and Gleisson A. P. de Brito. "Aerobic Exercise Associated with Fish Oil Supplementation Decreases C-Reactive Protein and Interleukin-6 in Celiac Disease Patients. *Journal of Nutrition and Metabolism* 2022 (2022): 3908675.

Fedewa, Michael V., JessicaL. Bentley, Simon Higgins et al. "Celiac Disease and Bone Health in Children and Adolescents: A Systematic Review and Meta-Analysis." *Journal of Clinical Densitometry* 23, no. 2 (2020): 200–211.

Ganji, Reza, Meysam Moghbeli, Ramin Sadeghi et al. "Prevalence of Osteoporosis and Osteopenia in Men and Premenopausal Women with Celiac Disease: A Systematic Review." *Nutrition Journal* 18 (2019): 9.

Ghadir, M., A. Iranikhah, M. Jandaghi et al. "Unexplained Infertility as Primary Presentation of Celiac Disease, a Case Report and Literature Review." *Iranian Journal of Reproductive Medicine* 9, no. 2 (Spring 2011): 135–140.

Green, Peter H. R., Aaron T. Fleischauer, Govind Bhagat et al. "Risk of Malignancy in Patients with Celiac Disease." *American Journal of Medicine* 115, no. 3 (August 15, 2003): 191–195.

Grode, L., B. H. Bech, O. Plana-Rippoll et al. "Reproductive Life in Women with Celiac Disease: A Nationwide, Population-Based Matched Cohort Study." *Human Reproduction* 33, no. 8 (2018): 1538–1547.

Kotze, Lorete M. S., Thelma Skare, Antonella Vinholi et al. "Impact of a Gluten-Free Diet on Bone Mineral Density in Celiac Patients." *Revista Espanõla de Enfermedades Digestivas* 108, no. 2 (2016): 84–88.

Lebwohl, Benjamin, Peter H. R. Green, Louise Emilsson et al. "Cancer Risk in 47,241 Individuals with Celiac Disease: A Nationwide Cohort Study." *Clinical Gastroenterology and Hepatology* 20 (2022): e111–e131.

Mosca, Caterina, Fanney Thorsteinsdottir, Bo Abrahamsen et al. "Newly Diagnosed Celiac Disease and Bone Health in Young Adults: A Systematic Literature Review." *Calcified Tissue International* 110 (2022): 641–648.

Murray, J. A., T. Watson, B. Clearman, and F. Mitros. "Effect of a Gluten-Free Diet on Gastrointestinal Symptoms in Celiac Disease." *American Journal of Clinical Nutrition* 79 (2004): 669–673.

Riznik, Petra, Luigina De Leo, Jasmina Dolinsek et al. "The Knowledge About Celiac Disease Among Healthcare Professionals and Patients in Central Europe." *Journal of Pediatric Gastroenterology and Nutrition* 72, no. 4 (April 1, 2021): 552–557.

Shahbazkhani, B., N. Aletaha, A. Khonche et al. "Is It Necessary to Screen for Celiac Disease in Adult Idiopathic Osteoporosis?" *Gastroenterology and Hepatology from Bed to Bench* 8, no. 2 (2015): 140–145.

Ungprasert, Patompong, Karn Wijarnpreecha, and Pansakorn Tanratana. "Risk of Venous Thromboembolism in Patients with Celiac Disease: A Systematic Review and Meta-Analysis." *Journal of Gastroenterology and Hepatology* 31, no. 7 (July 2016): 1240–1245.

Wierdsma, Nicolette, Marian A. E. van Bokhorst-de van der Schueren, Marijke Beerkenpas et al. "Vitamin and Mineral Deficiencies Are Highly Prevalent in Newly Diagnosed Celiac Disease Patients." *Nutrients* 5 (2013): 3975–3992.

COLON POLYPS

INTRODUCTION

Colon polyps are growths or small benign clumps of cells that form in the mucous lining of the colon (large intestine) or rectum and project into the colon. They vary in shape and size, ranging from less than a quarter-inch in diameter to several inches. They are caused by genetic mutations in the DNA that spontaneously occur when the cells in the colon lining replace themselves. Since they have no positive function, they are routinely removed during a colonoscopy. While usually harmless, over time, colon polyps have the potential to grow cancer cells.

There are a few different classifications of colon polyps. If a polyps looks like a mushroom with a head and a stalk, it is termed "pedunculated." If it does not have a stalk and appears more like a raised lump with a broad base, it is termed a "sessile." There are also different types of polyps. These include adenomatous polyps, serrated polyps, and hamartomatous polyps. Healthcare providers further classify colon polyps into neoplastic or non-neoplastic polyps. Neoplastic polyps, which include all adenomatous polyps (adenomas), sessile serrated lesions, and traditional serrated adenomas, may all grow into cancer. Non-neoplastic polyps, such as hyperplastic polyps and inflammatory pseudopolyps, do not grow into cancer.

While the medical literature does not mention when colon polyps were first observed, it was probably thousands of years ago. It is known that by the 1800s, several syndromes were identified that predisposed people to higher risks of colon polyps. Of course, today medical professionals are well aware of the association between colon polyps and colorectal cancer.

SYMPTOMS, RISKS, AND COMPLICATIONS

Most colon polyps do not cause any symptoms. By the time some may cause symptoms, they may have developed into cancer that may even have spread. Though uncommon, especially in the earlier stages, symptoms include rectal bleeding or bleeding in bowel movements. Because of the bleeding, people may develop iron deficiency anemia and feel weak or tired. People may also experience changes in their bowel habits, suddenly developing chronic diarrhea or chronic constipation, or changes in the color of the stool. They may also begin having excess mucus in their bowel movements, and if the colon polyp is large, it may cause crampy abdominal pain.

Most colon polyps appear to occur randomly. But some people have hereditary syndromes that cause large numbers of certain types of colon polyps, and they may well have a higher risk of cancerous polyps. Examples of these syndromes are familial adenomatous polyposis, serrated polyposis syndrome, and juvenile polyposis syndrome. And it is known that people who have a close relative, such as a sibling or parent, with colon polyps have an increased risk. Other factors that appear to foster the growth of colon polyps include aging, smoking, heavy alcohol use, high-fat or low-fiber diets, a lack of exercise, obesity, diabetes, and inflammatory bowel disease, such as Crohn's disease and ulcerative colitis.

The vast majority of colon polyps never cause any problems or create any complications. However, since some may become cancerous and develop into colorectal cancer, they have the potential to cause a whole range of problems that are outlined in the entry on colorectal cancer. These include abdominal pain, blood in the stool, and a change in bowel habits. As it was explained in the colorectal cancer entry, early colorectal cancer may be treated with surgery, radiation, chemotherapy, or other medical interventions. Once the cancer has spread, it becomes far more aggressive and the various treatments are less effective.

PREVALENCE

Colon polyps are incredibly common, especially as people age. They affect about 20 percent of adults and about 40 percent of those over the age of fifty, as well as 6 percent of children. Though people of all ethnicities may develop colon polyps, they are slightly more common in Western countries. Most colon polyps have the potential to become cancer, but when they are removed in a timely fashion during a colonoscopy, they rarely do. Around 75 percent of colorectal cancers start from adenomatous polyps, and about 80 percent of all colon polyps are adenomas. But only about 5 percent of adenomas are actually malignant. The risk of a random, average-sized colon polyps becoming cancerous is estimated to be 8 percent over ten years and 24 percent over twenty years.

DIAGNOSIS AND TREATMENT OPTIONS

The best way to diagnose colon polyps is with a colonoscopy. During this procedure, your healthcare provider (usually a gastroenterologist) passes a thin tube through the anus into the rectum and then into the entire colon. Your healthcare provider removes any suspicious-looking tissue for further study. Since a colonoscopy involves a preparation that cleanses the colon and the use of anesthesia, some healthcare providers may begin with easier-to-administer screening tools, such as blood and stool tests. Imaging procedures, such as a virtual colonoscopy (a type of CT scan) or a capsule endoscopy (a pill-size video camera that is swallowed), may be ordered. Colon polyps may also be seen in a lower GI X-ray exam, also known as a barium enema.

Normally, unless there are only non-neoplastic polyps, which may be left intact, colon polyps are removed during a colonoscopy. This is a procedure known as polypectomy.

Removing neoplastic polyps reduces the risk of developing colorectal cancer by 80 percent. Still, once people have had colon polyps, they are likely to have more.

RESEARCH FINDINGS

Adherence to the Foods in a Mediterranean Diet Is Inversely Associated with Advanced Colorectal Polyps

In a case-control study published in the *World Journal of Gastroenterology*, researchers from Israel examined the association between the patterns and components of the Mediterranean diet and advanced colorectal polyps. The cohort consisted of 206 subjects with advanced polyps, 192 subjects with non-advanced adenomas, and 385 control subjects. The subjects were between the ages of forty and seventy years; they completed food frequency questionnaires. Compared to the controls, the cases were older, and they had higher BMI and a higher percentage of men, smokers, and users of some medications. The Mediterranean diet scores were calculated by reviewing the intake of ten components—vegetables and legumes, fruit, nuts and seeds, whole grains, fish, ratio of monounsaturated fatty acids to saturated fatty acids, poultry, red meat, alcohol, and sugar-sweetened beverages. The researchers learned that greater adherence to the components of the Mediterranean diet was inversely associated with a diagnosis of advanced polyps in a dose-response manner. So, those who ate the most components of a Mediterranean diet were the least likely to have advanced colorectal polyps. Specifically, the researchers determined that a low intake of sugar-sweetened beverages and red meat and a high intake of fish were inversely associated with advanced polyps. The researchers concluded that "better adherence to the MD [Mediterranean diet], specifically low intake of sugar-sweetened beverages and red meat as well as high intake of fish, is related to lower odds of advanced polyps."[1]

The Intake of Higher Fiber Foods Appears to Be Associated with a Lower Risk of Colorectal Polyps

In a study published in the journal *Gastrointestinal Cancer Research*, researchers from Loma Linda, California, examined the association between higher fiber intake and the risk of colorectal polyps. The cohort, which was obtained from two studies, consisted of 2,818 men and women who had undergone a colonoscopy. Dietary and lifestyle information was obtained from each of the patients. During an approximate twenty-six-year follow-up, a total of 441 incident cases of colon polyps were identified. In general, those who developed colon polyps were older and had a higher BMI, and more men had colon polyps than women. Those who developed colon polyps tended to be less physically active, use more alcohol, and consume more meat. After adjusting for age, sex, body mass index, physical activity, education, and alcohol and meat consumption, the researchers learned that total fiber intake from vegetables was inversely associated with the risk of colon polyps. This association had a dose-response effect. Fiber intake from fruits and grains did not show a statistically significant effect on colon polyps, though they had some protective qualities.

The researchers stressed that "more complete dietary information throughout the follow-up is needed."[2]

People with Gastroesophageal Reflux Disease (GERD) Appear to Have an Increased Risk for Colon Polyps

In a study published in the journal *Digestive Disease and Sciences*, researchers from Oregon and Texas wanted to learn if there was an association between colon polyps and GERD. (See chapter on GERD.) They used data obtained from the Miraca Life Sciences Database, a large national electronic repository of histopathologic records of patients throughout the United States. Approximately, 1,500 individual gastroenterologists contributed to the database. The study included 228,506 subjects who had bidirectional endoscopy, which represented 14.4 percent of the entire Miraca database. The control group consisted of 92,947 patients without any type of colorectal neoplasm. The endoscopies were performed at private, community-based endoscopy centers or multispecialty surgery centers. Twenty-eight percent of the patients were covered by Medicare, 3 percent were covered by Medicaid, 69 percent by private insurance, and less than 1 percent were self-payers. The researchers determined that the patients with polyps were significantly older than the control subjects, and the patients with polyps were significantly more likely to have GERD. So, in this large sample, there was a significant positive association between the presence of colon polyps and GERD. This relationship applied to different forms of colon polyps and different forms of GERD and remained significant after adjusting for the confounding influences of other factors, such as age, sex, and H. pylori infection. The researchers commented that patients with colon polyps and GERD shared a similar set of environmental factors such as obesity, alcohol consumption, and smoking. The researchers concluded that this "positive association merits further investigation in other data sets. If confirmed, it may provide important clues about the pathophysiology of colorectal neoplasms."[3]

People with Obesity Seem to Have a Higher Risk for Colon Polyps

In a case-controlled study published in the journal *Annals of Medicine & Surgery*, researchers from Iran reviewed the association between higher BMIs and the risk of colon polyps. The cohort consisted of 266 subjects. During the colonoscopies that were administered to all the subjects, it was determined that 141 of the subjects had colon polyps and 125 had none. Demographic data were registered. Measurements of the patients' height and weight were performed the morning of the colonoscopy, and those figures were used to calculate the patients' BMIs. The researchers learned that people with higher BMIs had an increased risk for higher grade, neoplastic, tubular, and high-grade dysplasia of colorectal polyps. In fact, their data demonstrated that overweight patients with higher BMIs increased their risk of colon polyps even if they did not have obesity. And they concluded that "elevated BMI from its normal range, whether defined as overweight or obese, is associated with a higher incidence rate of development of colorectal polyps." Further, the most commonly seen colorectal polyps in overweight people and people with obesity were the adenomatous type with high-grade dysplasia. "Even little changes in BMI further than the normal values can independently increase the risk of developing dysplastic adenomatous colorectal polyp(s) significantly."[4]

There Seems to Be an Association between Adenomatous Colon Polyps and Coronary Calcifications

In a population-based, cross-sectional retrospective study published in the journal *Clinics and Research in Hepatology and Gastroenterology*, researchers from Korea examined the association between adenomatous colon polyps and coronary calcifications. The cohort consisted of 1,637 Korean adults; there were 981 men and 656 women, between the ages of eighteen and eighty-two years. The average age was 51.7 years. The mean BMI was 23.5, and 32.6 percent of patients were current smokers. Computed tomography coronary angiography was used to determine degrees of coronary calcification and colonoscopies detected colon polyps. The researchers found that adenomatous colon polyps appeared to be associated with a high risk of coronary artery atherosclerosis in Korean adults. And this association remained significant even after adjusting for potential confounding factors, such as age, sex, smoking status, BMI, blood pressure, fasting glucose level, and total cholesterol. The researchers determined that people with higher levels of coronary calcification had a higher risk of developing adenomatous polyps of the colon. As a result, these people may have an increased risk for colorectal cancer. The researchers concluded that their "findings suggest that people at high risk for coronary atherosclerosis through MDCT [multi-detected row computed tomography] should be considered for further evaluation of adenomatous polyps." And, they underscored the need for more research to understand the association between coronary atherosclerosis and colon polyps.[5]

There May Be an Association between Colon Polyps and Glycemic Status

In a cross-sectional study published in the *Journal of Gastroenterology*, researchers from Taiwan assessed the association between colon polyps and glycemic status. The cohort consisted of 6,348 participants, with 3,777 men and 2,571 women, with a mean age of 50.5 years. They all had health check-ups and colonoscopies. The subjects were then classified into four groups—polyp-free (n = 5,074), non-neoplastic polyps (n = 590), non-advanced polyps (n = 529), and advanced adenomatous polyps (n = 155). The researchers found that there were significant differences in the prevalence of diabetes and pre-diabetes among the groups with different kinds of colon polyps. In addition, there were significant differences in age, gender, total cholesterol, BMI, triglycerides, HDL-C, fasting plasma glucose, and the prevalence of hypertension, obesity, current smoking, and alcohol drinking. The researchers learned that diabetes mellitus was independently related to both non-advanced adenomatous polyps and advanced adenomatous polyps, while pre-diabetes was only related to non-advanced adenomatous polyps. Further, advanced adenomatous polyps were related to age, male gender, and hypertension, while non-advanced adenomatous polyps were related to age, male gender, and current smoking. Meanwhile, obesity, current smoking, and hypertension were the independently associated factors of non-neoplastic polyps. The researchers concluded that "diabetes, but not pre-diabetes, was associated with a higher risk of advanced adenomatous polyps." And, "both diabetes and pre-diabetes were important associated factors of no-advanced adenomatous polyps."[6]

Vitamin D Supplementation Does Not Appear to Increase the Risk of Colorectal Adenomas or Serrated Polyps

In a trial published in the journal *Clinical Gastroenterology and Hepatology*, researchers from Boston, Massachusetts evaluated the relationship between vitamin D supplementation and the risk of colorectal adenomas or serrated polyps. The cohort consisted of 25,871 adults who had no history of cancer or cardiovascular disease; there were 12,786 men who were fifty years or older and 13,085 women who were fifty-five years or older. (This was known as the VITAL trial.) The mean age of the subjects was sixty-seven years; 51 percent were female, and 20 percent were African American. The subjects were randomly placed on 2,000 IU vitamin D3 and 1 g marine n-3 fatty acid per day or a placebo. During a median follow-up period of 5.3 years, there were 308 cases of conventional adenomas in 12,927 subjects in the vitamin D group and 287 cases in 12,944 subjects in the placebo group. There were 172 cases of serrated polyps in the vitamin D group and 169 cases in the placebo group. The researchers found that vitamin D supplementation was not associated with an increased risk of either conventional adenomas or serrated polyps. The researchers concluded that this was "a potential benefit for individuals with low baseline level of vitamin D."[7]

There Seems to Be a Link between Elevated Levels of Homocysteine and the Risk of Colon Polyps

In a systematic review and meta-analysis published in the journal *Bioscience Reports*, researchers from China analyzed the relationship between folate, vitamin B12, and homocysteine, a type of amino acid that the body makes, and colon polyps. (At higher levels, homocysteine may increase the risk of coronary artery disease, blood clots, and strokes.) The researchers identified thirteen case-control studies that met their criteria. Six case-control studies with 241 cases and 623 controls examined serum folate and colon polyps and 790 cases and 1268 controls reviewed red blood cell folate and colon polyps. The researchers noted that they also studied the very limited data on the effect of vitamin B12 on colon polyps and could find no significant difference between the cases and controls. Thirteen case-control studies involving 879 cases and 1818 controls evaluated the association between levels of homocysteine and colon polyps. A pooled analysis of the data in these studies showed a negative correlation between the risk of colorectal polyps and the levels of serum folate, red blood cell folate, and vitamin B12. On the other hand, elevated levels of homocysteine may increase the risk of colon polyps. "Quantitative synthesis data provide evidence regarding the role of an elevated homocysteine level in the developing colorectal polyp risk." Larger sample sizes of folate and vitamin B12 are needed to confirm the exact role that they may play.[8] (It should be parenthetically noted that vitamins B6, B12, and folic acid naturally lower levels of homocysteine in the body. It should also be added that folate is a naturally occurring substance, and folic acid is manmade and often used in supplements and fortified foods.)

Smoking Increases the Risk of Colon Polyps

In a case-control study published in the *Journal of Clinical Gastroenterology*, researchers from Israel assessed the association between lifetime smoking habits and colorectal polyps. The cohort consisted of 828 consecutive subjects between the ages of forty and seventy years who were having a screening or diagnostic colonoscopy at the Department of Gastroenterology and Hepatology at the Tel Aviv Medical Center. Polyps were stratified according to histological factors (serrated or adenomatous) and location. Smoking status was defined as never smokers, ever-smokers, current smokers, and past smokers. Smoking intensity was defined as the number of daily cigarettes. The researchers learned that all levels of smoking intensity were associated with colorectal polyps; all of the groups of smoking intensity, including the minimal category of one to five daily cigarettes, were positively associated with all of the polyp groups. In an analysis of polyp types, smoking intensity categories were associated with higher odds of both adenomas and serrated polyps, but the association was stronger for serrated polyps. Smoking for twenty years or longer was strongly associated with distal polyps or polyps that were located in the descending colon, the sigmoid colon, or the rectum. All associations were stronger for distal serrated polyps. In their discussion of their findings, the researchers noted that "current smoking, past smoking, and smoking intensity were positively associated with colorectal polyps, after adjustment for a wide range of potential confounding variables, including other lifestyle parameters and BMI." And they concluded that there may be a "need to incorporate smoking history and details of smoking habits into screening guidelines."[9]

In a trial published in the journal *Cancer Causes & Control*, researchers from Los Angeles, California, Chapel Hill, North Carolina, Minneapolis, Minnesota, and Toronto, Canada evaluated the association between cigarette smoking and the risk of colon polyps. They used individual-level data from 2,915 patients participating in three colonoscopy-based clinical trials. All three trials were randomized, double-blind, and placebo-controlled. A little more than 70 percent of the subjects were male, and the overall mean age of the subjects was 59.7 years. All of the patients had one or more adenomas removed at baseline and were followed for up to four years. Using questionnaires, information on personal characteristics, medical history, smoking habits, and other lifestyle factors were collected at baseline. In all three studies, polyp occurrence was determined during a colonoscopy. Compared to non-smokers, the researchers determined that the smokers had a slightly higher risk for adenomas and a greater risk for serrated polyps. For both adenomas and serrated polyps, the risks associated with smoking were stronger in the left colorectum. The researchers commented that they found strong evidence that cigarette smoking is associated with the development of serrated polyps but only weak evidence between cigarette smoking and conventional adenomas.[10]

Red and Processed Meat Intake May or May Not Raise the Risk of Colon Polyps

In a cross-sectional study published in the *American Journal of Clinical Nutrition*, researchers from Germany evaluated the association between the consumption of meat and the risk of colon polyps. The cohort consisted of 15,950 participants aged fifty-five years or older who had a screening colonoscopy. The researchers determined that 3,340 participants

(20.4 percent) had non-advanced adenomas, 1,643 (10 percent) had advanced adenomas, and 189 (1.2 percent) had colorectal cancer. Participants with neoplasms were more likely to be older men and current smokers who drank more alcohol. They had higher intakes of red and processed meat, higher BMIs, and a family history of colorectal cancer. Participants without neoplasms had significantly higher intakes of poultry, fruit, and vegetables, and they were more likely to have had a previous colonoscopy and a higher level of physical activity. There was no difference between the two groups with respect to the current use of nonsteroidal anti-inflammatory drugs and years of education. Interestingly, the researchers were unable to observe any overall statistically significant association between red or processed meat consumption and the prevalence of any adenomas or advanced adenomas. However, in a subgroup analysis, red meat was positively associated with the prevalence of advanced adenomas in participants aged sixty-five years and older. In addition, when the researchers conducted a site-specific analysis, processed meat was positively associated with the prevalence of advanced adenomas in the rectum, but not with the prevalence of advanced adenomas in the proximal colon. And, poultry intake was not associated with the consumption and prevalence of colorectal polyps. The researchers underscored the need for more studies on these associations.[11]

Still, Some Researchers Believe That Interventions Need to Be Devised to Reduce the Intake of Red and Processed Meat and Increase the Levels of Physical Activity

In a qualitative study published in the journal *BMC Cancer*, researchers based in the UK wanted to determine the dietary and physical activity interventions that patients preferred to reduce their consumption of red and processed meat and increase their physical activity. The initial cohort consisted of twenty-eight patients, between the ages of sixty and seventy-four, who had been colonoscopy diagnosed with an intermediate or high-risk adenoma. To learn more, the researchers held four focus groups with most of the patients and some of their partners. During the focus groups, the participants discussed the experience of having polyps and their changing behaviors. In general, the participants noted that they had not associated the removal of their polyps with colorectal cancer, and they did not remember being given any information or advice concerning this relationship. Most expressed interest in learning more about polyps and their association with more serious illnesses. The participants noted that they followed different diets and adhered to varying levels of physical activity, and the participants who made changes tended to be satisfied with their results. Still, many people were reluctant to make changes. The researchers concluded that there were clearly practical, intellectual, and emotional issues associated with developing interventions to change dietary and physical activity behaviors in the participants of the focus groups. Specifically, more attention needs to be paid to tailoring interventions to the needs of individuals, sharing more information about the relationship between colon polyps and colorectal cancer, and focusing on motivating people to change behaviors. While current colonoscopy services tend to reassure patients that their polyps have been removed, there is little discussion about "the significance of a polyp, a precursor to colon cancer." Further, "without a full understanding of the role of high risk polyps in the aetiology of colorectal cancer, the motivation to change entrenched behaviours (such as inadequate physical activity and a diet that includes high levels of red and processed meat) may be lacking."[12]

Vitamins C and E May Offer No Benefits in the Prevention of Colon Polyps

In a double-blind randomized trial published in the journal *Cancer Research*, researchers from Canada examined the effects vitamins C and E had on the rate of recurrence of colorectal polyps. The initial cohort consisted of 200 patients who were believed to be free of polyps after the removal of at least one colon polyp. All of the patients participated in a brief dietary inquiry about their intake of bran cereals, whole wheat breads, fruit, green vegetables, fish, poultry, prepared meats, beef, and pork. This information was collected along with input about current smoking status, usual bowel habits, and history of previous polyps. The subjects received either a supplement of ascorbic acid (vitamin C) and α-tocopherol (vitamin E) or a placebo. By chance, the subjects who received vitamins were a year younger than those on placebos. Most other characteristics did not differ significantly. However, the subjects assigned to take the vitamin supplements reported the regular use of vitamin C supplementation prior to participation in the study significantly more often than those who were assigned placebos. They also noted that they used vitamin E supplements almost twice as often as the subjects on placebos, but this difference was not significant. After approximately two years of supplementation, the 137 subjects who completed the study had a second colonoscopy. Polyps were observed in 41.4 percent of the seventy subjects on vitamin supplementation and in 50.7 percent of the sixty-seven subjects on placebos. Thus, those taking the vitamin supplements had fewer polyps than those on placebos, but this difference was "small." Still, the researchers commented that "the study had insufficient power to rule out the possibility that the small difference in the observed polyp recurrence rates was a chance finding." They emphasized that "a larger study would be required to ensure that an effect of this size was not a chance finding."[13]

Calcium and Vitamin D Supplementation May Raise the Risk of Serrated Polyps

In a randomized, multicenter, double-blind, placebo-controlled trial published in the journal *Gut*, researchers located in several cities in the United States but based in Chapel Hill, North Carolina, and Lebanon, New Hampshire examined the effect of calcium and vitamin D supplementation on the incidence of serrated polyps. At baseline, the cohort consisted of 2,259 patients between the ages of forty-five and seventy-five who had been diagnosed with one or more adenomatous polyps and were due to have a follow-up test in three to five years. Sixty-three percent of the patients were male, and 88 percent were Caucasian. The patients were randomly placed in groups to receive daily calcium carbonate tablets (1,200 mg), daily vitamin D tablets (1,000 IU), both daily calcium and vitamin D tablets, or neither calcium nor vitamin tablets; these treatments were designed to continue until the subjects' next colonoscopy. At baseline, the groups had similar characteristics. During the treatment phase, the researchers observed no effect of either calcium or vitamin D supplementation on the cases of serrated polyps. However, six to twelve years after the trial began, the researchers found an increased risk of serrated polyps among patients taking calcium supplementation alone and among those taking the combination of calcium and vitamin D supplementation. Further, there was evidence that among women and current smokers, calcium was associated with a higher risk of serrated polyps. No association was found between vitamin D supplementation alone and serrated polyps. Nor was an association seen among dietary calcium and serrated polyps. The researchers concluded that "these possible risks must be weighed against the benefits of calcium and vitamin D supplementation."[14]

Cigarette Smoking and Alcohol Consumption Are Risk Factors for Serrated Colon Polyps

In a systematic review and meta-analysis published in the journal *Gastroenterology*, researchers from Northern Ireland investigated the association between lifestyle factors and the risk for serrated colon polyps. The researchers identified forty-three studies on the association between serrated colon polyps and seven different lifestyle factors: smoking, alcohol, body fatness, diet, physical activity, medication, and hormone replacement therapy. Some of the papers reported on multiple risk factors; there were twenty-nine papers on smoking, fourteen on alcohol consumption, twenty on "body fatness," eight on physical activity, twelve on patient medication, and fifteen on dietary factors. When they compared the highest and lowest categories of exposure, the researchers found that several factors increased the risk of serrated colon polyps—tobacco smoking, alcohol intake, body mass index, and the high intake of fat or meat. In contrast, they learned that certain factors significantly decreased the risk of serrated colon polyps. These included the use of nonsteroidal anti-inflammatory drugs or aspirin, as well as the higher intake of folate, calcium, or fiber. The researchers concluded that the risk of serrated colon polyps could be reduced with the implementation of lifestyle changes.[15]

Birthplace Does Not Appear to Be a Determinant of Colorectal Adenomas

In a retrospective study published in the *World Journal of Gastroenterology*, researchers from Australia investigated the association between places of birth and risk of colorectal adenomas in the practice of a single gastroenterologist at a tertiary referral hospital. A total of 623 patients (48 percent male and 67 percent were over the age of fifty years) were recruited and categorized according to birthplace, language spoken, and details of the colonoscopy, including indications, completion rates, complications, and results (prevalence and histopathology of polyps). The researchers determined that 42 percent of the patients were from Australia or New Zealand, 20 percent were from Europe, 15 percent were from Asia, 11 percent were from the Middle East or Africa, 9 percent were from South America, and 3 percent were Pacific Islanders. Twenty-five percent were smokers, 25 percent had elevated levels of cholesterol (hypercholesterolemia), 20 percent had diabetes mellitus, 16 percent were on aspirin, and 7 percent were on nonsteroidal anti-inflammatory drugs. A total of twenty-one colorectal cancers and 635 polyps were identified. The researchers found that the prevalence of polyps varied according to birthplace: Europe 45.1 percent, Australia and New Zealand 39.5 percent, Pacific Islands 33.3 percent, Asia 30.3 percent, Middle East and Africa 26.9 percent, and South America 24.5 percent. However, after correcting for age and male sex, further analyses revealed that birthplace was not an independent predictor of developing polyps, including adenomas and advanced adenomas. Still, it was observed that Asian-born patients had adenomas and advanced adenomas that were detected at younger ages than those born in Australia and New Zealand. According to the researchers, their findings demonstrate that birthplace "should not influence the recommendations for colorectal cancer screening." Far more important than birthplace are the previously identified risk factors such as older age and male sex.[16]

REFERENCES AND FURTHER READING

Baillie, Lesley, Maurice B. Loughrey, and Helen G. Coleman. "Lifestyle Risk Factors for Serrated Colorectal Polyps: A Systematic Review and Meta-Analysis." *Gastroenterology* 152 (2017): 92–104.

Carr, Prudence R., Bernd Holleczek, Christa Stegmaier et al. "Meat Intake and Risk of Colorectal Polyps: Results from a Large Population-Based Screening Study in Germany." *American Journal of Clinical Nutrition* 105 (2017): 1453–1461.

Crockett, Seth D., Elizabeth L. Barry, Leila A. Mott et al. "Calcium and Vitamin D Supplementation and Increased Risk of Serrated Polyps: Results from a Randomized Clinical Trial." *Gut* 68, no. 3 (March 2019): 475–486.

Dowswell, George, Angela Ryan, Aliki Taylor et al. "Designing an Intervention to Help People with Colorectal Adenomas Reduce Their Intake of Red and Processed Meat and Increase Their Levels of Physical Activity: A Qualitative Study." *BMC Cancer* 12 (2012): 255.

Figueiredo, Jane C., Seth D. Crookett, Dale C. Snover et al. "Smoking-Associated Risks of Conventional Adenomas and Serrated Polyps in the Colorectum." *Cancer Causes & Control* 26 (2015): 377–386.

Fliss-Isakov, Naomi, Revital Kariv, Muriel Webb et al. "Mediterranean Dietary Components Are Inversely Associated with Advanced Colorectal Polyps: A Case-Control Study." *World Journal of Gastroenterology* 24, no. 24 (June 29, 2018): 2617–2627.

Fliss-Isakov, Naomi, Shira Zelber-Sagi, Muriel Webb et al. "Smoking Habits Are Strong Associated with Colorectal Polyps in a Population-Based Case Control Study." *Journal of Clinical Gastroenterology* 52, no. 9 (October 2018): 805–811.

Huang, Hsin-En, Yi-Ching Yang, Jin-Shang Wu et al. "The Relationship Between Different Glycemic Statuses and Colon Polyps in a Taiwanese Population." *Journal of Gastroenterology* 49 (2014): 1145–1151.

Kim, Hong-Bae, Yong-Jae Lee, Jae-Yong Shim, and Hye-Ree Lee. "The Association Between Coronary Calcification and Adenomatous Polyps of Colon in Korean Adults." *Clinics and Research in Hepatology and Gastroenterology* 38 (2014): 649–654.

McKeown-Eyssen, Gail, Catherine Holloway, Vartouhi Jazmaji et al. "A Randomized Trial of Vitamins C and E in the Prevention of Recurrence of Colorectal Polyps." *Cancer Research* 48 (August 15, 1988): 4701–4705.

Salimian, Sina, Maryam Habbi, Mojtaba Sehat, and Abbas Hajian."Obesity and Incidence of Polorectal Polyps: A Case-Control Study." *Annals of Medicine & Surgery* 85 (2023): 306–310.

Song, Mingyang, I-Min Lee, JoAnn E. Manson et al. "No Association Between Vitamin D Supplementation and Risk of Colorectal Adenomas or Serrated Polyps in a Randomized Trial." *Clinical Gastroenterology and Hepatology* 19, no. 1 (January 2021): 128–135.

Sonnenberg, Amnon, Kevin O. Turner, and Robert M. Genta. "Increased Risk for Colon Polyps in Patients with Reflux Disease." *Digestive Diseases and Sciences* 63 (2018): 228–233.

Sun, Manchun, Manyi Sun, Li Zhang et al. "Colorectal Polyp Risk Is Linked to an Elevated Level of Homocysteine." *Bioscience Reports* 38, no. 2 (April 2018): BSR20171699.

Tantamango, Y. M., S. F. Knutsen, L. Beeson et al. "Association Between Dietary Fiber and Incident Cases of Colon Polyps: The Adventist Health Study." *Gastrointestinal Cancer Research* 4 (2011): 161–167.

Tran, Fiona and Jenn Hian Koo. "Birthplace Is Not a Determinant of Colorectal Adenomas." *World Journal of Gastroenterology* 20, no. 26 (July 14, 2014): 8606–8611.

CROHN'S DISEASE

INTRODUCTION

A type of inflammatory bowel disease, Crohn's disease causes inflammation or swelling in any part of the digestive tract, from the mouth to the anus. This inflammation may spread to all tissue layers of the affected areas. Approximately 80 percent of patients have involvement of the small intestine. An autoimmune disease, Crohn's disease is a lifelong condition for which there is no known prevention or cure. Still, with proper treatment(s), many people live active and productive lives with Crohn's or ulcerative colitis, the other somewhat common inflammatory bowel disease.

People with Crohn's disease may suffer from a good deal of debilitating pain, and there is the potential for life-threatening complications. Still, there are a number of treatments and therapies that may reduce the signs and symptoms, even resulting in long-term reductions in inflammation and remissions.

While the exact cause of Crohn's disease is unknown, heredity clearly plays a role. Crohn's disease is more common in people who have family members, particularly first-degree relatives, with this disease. Some contend that a virus or bacteria may be triggers. In an attempt to stop the invading virus or bacteria, the body may attack its own cells.

There are a few different types of Crohn's disease. About 50 percent of patients have ileocolitis, which is the inflammation of the lower small intestine and the first portion of the large intestine. Colitis is inflammation of the lining of the large intestine; ileitis is the swelling and inflammation at the end of the small intestine; and gastroduodenal is the inflammation and irritation of the stomach and the first section of the small intestine. With another types of Crohn's disease, jejunitis, there are patchy areas of inflammation in the middle part of the small intestine, and perianal disease is inflammation around the anus, which may cause fistulas and abscesses.

According to the Crohn's & Colitis Foundation, Crohn's disease was first described in 1932 by three physicians—Burrill Crohn, Leon Ginzberg, and Gordon D. Oppenheimer. At the time, diseases of the small intestine were believed to be intestinal tuberculosis. The three physicians collected data from fourteen patients with the symptoms of abdominal cramps, diarrhea, fever, and weight loss, and demonstrated that the symptoms were not caused by tuberculosis or any other known disease. Although first called regional ileitis, the illness was later named Crohn's disease.[1]

SYMPTOMS, RISKS, AND COMPLICATIONS

There are a host of different symptoms associated with Crohn's disease. These include abdominal pain, diarrhea, fatigue, weight loss, and rectal bleeding. Some may have fever, mouth sores, or pain in the mouth or gums, reduced appetite, and pain or drainage near the anus. People with Crohn's disease may also have non-gastrointestinal symptoms. These include inflammation of the skin, eyes, heart, pancreas, and joints; inflammation of the liver or bile ducts; kidney stones; anemia' and delayed growth or sexual development in children.

While Crohn's disease may occur at any age, it is more likely to develop when people are relatively young. Most people with Crohn's are diagnosed before they are in their early thirties. Caucasians have the highest risk for Crohn's, especially Jewish people of Eastern European descent (Ashkenazi Jewish). Still, the incidence is growing among Blacks who live in North America and the UK, people from the Middle East and migrants to the United States. People who smoke cigarettes have a higher risk and an increased risk for more severe cases of this disease. There is some limited evidence that people who have had an appendectomy may have an increased risk. And, people who live in urban areas of developed countries have a higher risk than those in rural areas of less-developed countries.

People with Crohn's disease are frequently forced to deal with complications. A somewhat common problem is a bowel obstruction or stricture, which is caused by the scarring and narrowing of the bowel. This may require a surgical procedure to widen the stricture or remove the diseased portion of the bowel. Ulcers or open sores are another complication. These may appear in any portion of the digestive tract. When ulcers extend completely through the intestinal wall, they are known as fistulas. Fistulas may develop between the intestine and the skin or between the intestine and another organ. They are most often seen near and around the anus. When fistulas are inside the abdomen, they may result in infections and abscesses with collections of pus. These must be treated immediately. People with Crohn's disease have an increased risk for a skin condition known as hidradenitis suppurativa, in which there are deep nodules, tunnels, and abscesses in the armpits, groin, under the breasts, and in the genital area. And, they have an increased risk for osteoporosis, arthritis, and gallbladder and liver disease. Certain Crohn's medications that block functions of the immune system slightly increase the risk of lymphoma, skin cancers, and infections. People with Crohn's may well be prescribed corticosteroids, which increase the risk of osteoporosis, bone fractures, cataracts, glaucoma, diabetes, and high blood pressure. And, it is known that Crohn's disease increases the risk of blood clots in veins and arteries. Because of all these digestive problems, people with Crohn's disease have an increased risk for malnutrition, and people with inflammatory bowel disease have an increased risk for colorectal cancer and should begin screening years before the usual recommendations.

PREVALENCE

While the global incidence of Crohn's disease is around six to eight million people, in the United States about three-quarters of a million people have this disease.[2]

DIAGNOSIS AND TREATMENT OPTIONS

Most people who are diagnosed with Crohn's disease see their medical provider for ongoing problems with chronic diarrhea, abdominal cramps, and/or unexplained weight loss. Most likely, these patients will be referred to a gastroenterologist for further testing. Testing will begin with blood tests to look for any abnormalities and a stool test to check for infections, bacteria, or parasites. The provider will order imaging tests that view the digestive tract. These may include a CT scan, which uses X-rays to show the degree of inflammation, or a MRI scan with enterography, which uses large magnets and radio waves to create images of areas inside the body. Endoscopy testing enables the gastroenterologist to pass slender tubes inside the digestive tract. With an upper endoscopy, the tube is passed from the mouth into the esophagus, stomach, and upper portion of the small intestine. With a colonoscopy, the tube is passed from the anus to the rectum, to the large intestine, and to the end of the small bowel ileum. With a capsule endoscopy, a small plastic capsule with a light and a camera is swallowed and passed through the digestive tract.

Treatment for Crohn's disease depends on the location and severity of the disease. It usually begins with medication that reduces inflammation and calms the immune response. These include anti-inflammatory medications, steroids, immunomodulators, and biologic therapies. Pain medications may be used, as well as antidiarrheal medications and antibiotics. Pills known as Janus kinase inhibitors reduce the immune response and treat Crohn's. Upadacitinib (Rinvoq), a pill, is the only one currently approved for Crohn's disease by the US Food and Drug Administration. Biologic medications may also be used, such as infliximab (Remicade) or adalimumab (Humira), especially for the treatment of moderate to severe Crohn's disease. Sometimes, surgery is needed to treat the complications associated with Crohn's disease. These include surgeries to repair intestinal perforations (holes), fistulas, strictures, and blockages.

RESEARCH FINDINGS

Consumption of Unprocessed/Minimally Processed Food Is Associated with a Reduced Risk of Crohn's Disease

In a study published in the journal *Clinical Gastroenterology and Hepatology*, researchers from numerous locations but based in France evaluated the association between the degree of food processing and the risk of Crohn's disease and ulcerative colitis. The researchers used data from the European Prospective Investigation into Cancer and Nutrition Cohort, which included 413,590 participants from eight European countries; 68.8 percent were women and the mean baseline age was 51.7 years. Dietary data were collected at baseline from validated country-specific dietary questionnaires. During a mean follow-up period of 13.2 years, there were 179 incident cases of Crohn's disease and 431 incident cases of ulcerative colitis. The researchers learned that the prevalence of Crohn's disease was lower in people consuming higher proportions of unprocessed or minimally processed foods, particularly fruits and vegetables. (There was no association between unprocessed and minimally processed food intake and ulcerative colitis.) The highest mean proportion of unprocessed food was seen in the UK and the lowest was in Italy. The researchers concluded that there is "a beneficial impact of giving preference to the consumption of nonprocessed/minimally processed food with regard to CD [Crohn's disease] risk, particularly in persons who are at high risk for this disease such as first-degree relatives of CD patients."[3]

A High-Fiber Diet Appears to Benefit People with Crohn's Disease

In a systematic review and meta-analysis published in the journal *Nutrients*, researchers from Spain wanted to learn if the intake of a high-fiber diet benefited people with Crohn's disease. The researchers identified eleven studies with a total of 5,010 subjects that met their criteria; 2,389 of the subjects in these studies had Crohn's disease. The remainder of the subjects had ulcerative colitis or were healthy. Forty-four percent were men, and 56 percent were women. The subjects ranged in age from thirteen to seventy-seven years. All of the studies were written in English and were either randomized controlled trials or observational in design. Six of the studies included both people with Crohn's disease and ulcerative colitis, and five included only people with Crohn's disease. The researchers learned that a diet with higher amounts of fiber, with or without the administration of routine therapies, improved Crohn's disease remission rates. The researchers commented that a high-fiber diet was not only safe for people with Crohn's disease, but it was also an effective means to deal with the illness. And, they concluded that "a high fiber diet should be an adjuvant treatment in conjunction with other therapeutic strategies to maintain remission."[4]

Exercise Appears to Decrease the Risk of Future Active Disease in People with Crohn's Disease in Remission

In a prospective study published in the journal *Inflammatory Bowel Diseases*, researchers from Chapel Hill, North Carolina, examined the association between exercise and risk reduction for future active disease in patients with Crohn's disease and ulcerative colitis. Using data from the Crohn's and Colitis Foundation of America, the researchers identified 1,308 patients with Crohn's disease and 549 with ulcerative or indeterminate colitis; all of these patients were in remission. After six months, 227 patients (17.4 percent) with Crohn's disease and 135 patients (24.6 percent) with ulcerative or indeterminate colitis developed active disease. The median age for those in the Crohn's group was forty-five years and forty-three years for the second group. The majority of the participants were women. Crohn's disease patients in the less active category were significantly older than those in the highest category of exercise, and more women were in the less active category. The less active Crohn's disease patients were more likely to be smokers, had previous bowel surgery, and were taking steroids. And the median age for disease duration was twelve years for Crohn's and nine years for ulcerative and indeterminant colitis. The researchers learned that a higher exercise level was associated with a decreased risk of active disease for Crohn's disease and ulcerative and indeterminant colitis. However, the difference for Crohn's disease was significant while the difference for ulcerative and indeterminant colitis was not. Among the Crohn's disease patients, 20 percent of those in the low exercise category experienced relapse or developed active disease at six months, compared with 15 percent of those in the high-exercise category, and this was statistically significant. Still, there was an exception. For patients using steroids, those who exercised more had an increased risk of active disease; for those not using steroids, those who exercised more had a decreased risk of active disease. The researchers concluded that their findings "highlighted the need for assessment of exercise status as a potential environmental factor in disease activity." Further, if their findings are replicated, "exercise could be prescribed to prolong and possibly promote remission in patients with IBD."[5]

A Diet Low in Red and Processed Meats Does Not Appear to Reduce the Rate of Crohn's Disease Flares

In a randomized, controlled trial published in the journal *Gastroenterology*, researchers from Philadelphia, Pennsylvania, and Chapel Hill, North Carolina, wanted to learn if eating a low red and processed meat diet would reduce the rate of Crohn's disease flares. The researchers obtained data from the Crohn's and Colitis Foundation Partners Study, which has since been renamed IBD Partners, an internet-based cohort of more than 15,600 participants with inflammatory bowel disease. The researchers initially recruited 118 subjects for the high-meat arm and ninety-five for the low-meat arm; all of the participants were in remission. The participants were more likely to be females who were diagnosed at a relatively young age. They tended to be from the northeastern section of the United States and less often from western states. The primary outcome, symptomatic relapse of Crohn's disease, occurred in 62 percent of the participants during the course of the study, whereas 42 percent and 35 percent had a moderate to severe symptomatic recurrence, respectively. The researchers determined that there were no statistically significant differences in relapse time between the people on the two diets. According to the researchers, this suggests "that reduction of red and processed meats does not reduce the risk of symptomatic CD relapse in patients with quiescent disease."[6]

People with Crohn's Disease Tend to Have Low Levels of Serum Vitamin D

In a systematic review and meta-analysis published in the journal *Nutrition*, researchers from Iran evaluated the relationship between Crohn's disease and vitamin D status. They located a total of sixty-three studies that met their criteria. There were 129,808 patients and 3,711 controls with ages ranging from eleven to forty-nine years. The majority of the studies were from the United States, Denmark, Canada, and Ireland. Different cut-off points were used to define vitamin D deficiency. The studies tended to have matched cases and controls in terms of age and sex. A few studies considered ethnicity, body mass index, weight, and smoking as additional matching variables. When compared to healthy controls, the researchers found that people with Crohn's disease had significantly lower levels of serum vitamin D. In fact, more than half of the patients with Crohn's disease had a vitamin D deficiency. And, those patients with lower concentrations of vitamin D had greater disease activity than those with sufficient concentrations. "Only a minority of recently diagnosed patients had optimal vitamin D levels."[7]

Upadacitinib Reduced the Symptoms of Crohn's Disease within the First Week of Induction Therapy

In a post-hoc analysis of pooled data from two phase three, multicenter, double-blind twelve-week induction trials and one-week maintenance trial published in *Clinical Gastroenterology and Hepatology*, researchers from many locations but based in New York City evaluated the rapidity of symptomatic improvement in patients with Crohn's disease. The initial cohort consisted of 1,021 patients; 674 received 45 mg per day of upadacitinib and 347 took a placebo. The patients in both groups had similar demographic characteristics. For the first fifteen days of treatment, daily diary data were used to analyze improvements in very soft/liquid stool frequency and abdominal pain. Clinical outcomes were assessed at every study visit. The researchers learned that when compared to the patients taking the placebo, the patients taking upadacitinib had a reduction in daily symptoms beginning on day five or six. And, the improvement continued until day fifteen. These improvements occurred irrespective of the prior treatments the patients had received. The researchers concluded that patients with Crohn's disease "may benefit from a convenient therapy that provides quick improvement and early symptoms resolution without the consequences of excessive or prolonged corticosteroid use."[8]

Some Researchers Described Their "Real-World" Experience with Upadacitinib

In an article published in the journal *Digestive Diseases and Sciences*, researchers from Chicago, Illinois outlined their professional experience treating patients with upadacitinib. They described twelve patients with Crohn's disease who were treated at their tertiary center, the University of Chicago Medicine Inflammatory Bowel Disease Center. Nine of the patients (75 percent) were women, and all of the patients were white. Forty-two percent were ever-smokers. The median age at upadacitinib initiation was 40.5 years, and median disease duration prior to medication initiation was 18.2 years. Five patients (41.7 percent) had a history of a Crohn's disease-related hospitalization in the year prior to upadacitinib, and all had failed at least three biologics. Forty-two percent of the patients had been taking ustekinumab (Stelara) prior to taking upadacitinib. For all except one patient, upadacitinib was initially dosed at 15 mg daily; that patient was started on 30 mg per day, but was then lowered to 15 mg per day. Median treatment duration was 5.2 months. Three of the twelve patients reported subjective improvements in their Crohn's disease symptoms, and the researchers found that objective testing demonstrated improvement in five of the patients. Seven patients reported adverse events, such as abdominal pain, fatigue, fever, nausea/vomiting, and headache. The researchers concluded that in their cohort of medically refractory patients with Crohn's disease, "treatment with upadacitinib resulted in subjective and objective response in twenty-five percent and forty-two percent of patients, respectively."[9]

Osteopathic Soft-Tissue Techniques May Improve the Quality of Life of People with Crohn's Disease

In a thirty-day, single-blind, randomized, controlled trial published in the journal *Medicine*, researchers from Spain evaluated the use of osteopathic soft-tissue techniques in patients with Crohn's disease. The cohort consisted of thirty people with Crohn's disease; all of them were diagnosed with Crohn's disease at least one year before the trial began. Sixteen people (eight women and eight men) were placed in the experimental group, and fourteen people (twelve women and two men) were placed in the control group. The mean age for the experimental group was 40.14 years, and the mean age for the control group was 42.56 years. At baseline, the groups were similar in pain levels, anxiety, and depression. Every ten days, those in the experimental group received a forty-five-minute session conducted by a physiotherapist with extensive experience in manual therapy; the members of the control group attended evaluation sessions but did not receive the manual therapy. All of the participants were advised against changing their daily routines; they were assessed at baseline and when the trial ended. The researchers determined that although the treatments significantly improved the quality of life of people with Crohn's disease, they did not reduce their pain. Still, the quality of life improvements were seen in people in both the active and remission phases of the disease. The researchers acknowledged "that patients with higher scores of self-reported pain display lower improvements in QoL [quality of life]."[10]

Cannabis May Have a Limited Usefulness for People with Crohn's Disease

In a prospective trial published in *Clinical Gastroenterology and Hepatology*, researchers from the Gastroenterology Institute at the Meir Medical Center in Israel examined the use of cannabis (marijuana) for people with Crohn's disease. The cohort consisted of twenty-one patients with a mean age of forty years; there were thirteen men. These patients had already failed to respond to at least one of several treatments, such as steroids, immunomodulators, or antitumor necrosis factor-a agents. The patients were assigned to smoke cannabis containing 115 mg THC (Δ9-tetrahydrocannabinol) or placebo cigarettes that contained cannabis flowers from which the THC had been removed. Disease activity and laboratory tests were reviewed during the eight weeks of the trial and two weeks of follow-up. They were evaluated at baseline and at weeks two, eight, and ten. A side-effect questionnaire asked about changes in the ability to concentrate, work, sleep, abdominal pain, appetite, general well-being, and general satisfaction with the treatment. The researchers determined that five of the eleven subjects in the cannabis group achieved a complete remission, as did one of the ten in the placebo group. A clinical response was seen in ten of the eleven subjects in the cannabis group and four of the ten in the placebo group. Three of the patients in the cannabis group were weaned from steroid dependency. Subjects using cannabis reported improved appetite and sleep, with no significant side effects. Yet, four patients in the placebo group (but none in the cannabis group) deteriorated and needed a "rescue intervention" during the study period. (The exact nature of that intervention was not specified.) The researchers observed that the patients in the cannabis group experienced a significant increase in their quality of life, something not seen in the placebo group.

Unfortunately, the benefits were short-lived. The patients relapsed two weeks after the cannabis treatment was stopped. Still, the researchers concluded that "cannabis provided a significantly higher rate of clinical response without any alarming side effects."[11]

In a trial published in *Inflammatory Bowel Diseases*, researchers from Germany evaluated the benefits and adverse effects of cannabis use in patients with inflammatory bowel diseases. The cohort consisted of 319 consecutive patients with inflammatory bowel diseases who were seen at the University of Calgary. They completed a questionnaire on their motives for using cannabis, as well as their patterns of use and any benefits or adverse responses. Subjects who used cannabis specifically for the treatment of their inflammatory bowel disease were compared to non-users. The researchers learned that cannabis had been used by 17.6 percent (fifty-six) of the patients to relieve their symptoms; almost all of these patients (96.4 percent) smoked the cannabis. Forty-two (75 percent) of the cannabis-using patients used it to treat their Crohn's disease. Meanwhile, 263 patients (82.5 percent) said that they never used cannabis to relieve their inflammatory bowel disease symptoms. The patients noted that their healthcare providers did not recommend treatment with cannabis, primarily because of a lack of research on its efficacy for inflammatory bowel diseases. Although the benefits came with frequent side effects, the patients reported that the cannabis relieved their abdominal pain (83.9 percent), abdominal cramping (76.8 percent), joint pain (48.2 percent), and diarrhea (28.6 percent). Patients with Crohn's disease who used cannabis for more than six months were likely to require surgery. Apparently, most patients indicated that they would continue to use cannabis and would recommend cannabis to other patients. The researchers concluded that their findings indicated that cannabis may not be as useful as some patients believe. "Maybe, this is due to cannabis use masking symptoms in the presence of ongoing inflammation." And, the use of cannabis may ultimately lead to poorer outcomes.[12]

Acupuncture with Moxibustion May Provide Some Symptom Relief for People with Crohn's Disease

In a systematic review and meta-analysis published in the *Journal of Pharmacopuncture*, researchers from Korea assessed the use of acupuncture and moxibustion for the symptoms associated with Crohn's disease. They identified twelve randomized controlled trials with 650 participants that met their criteria for inclusion. The different studies used various combinations of treatments. Three of the studies had an overall low risk of bias, while three had a high risk and six had "some concerns." The researchers learned that for patients with mild to moderate Crohn's disease, there was a significant difference between those who received acupuncture and moxibustion and those who received sham acupuncture and sham moxibustion. However, the results for acupuncture alone were inconclusive. The researchers underscored the need for more research. "More studies to expand to the body of knowledge in this field is urgently required."[13]

People with Crohn's Disease See Themselves as Having Substantial Disease Burden

In a study published in the journal *Crohn's and Colitis 360*, researchers from the UK, Indianapolis, Indiana, Belgium, and Canada wanted to learn more about how people with

Crohn's disease perceived their disease burden. The researchers developed a qualitative semi-structured interview guide and conducted two rounds of face-to-face interviews that were audio-recorded and transcribed. The first round of interviews had sixteen adults, with a mean age of 50.3 years, and eight adolescents with a mean age of 15.6 years. Sixteen of the patients were white, and eighteen had moderate or severe Crohn's disease. The most frequently reported symptoms were abdominal pain/cramps, urgent bowel movements, diarrhea, frequent bowel movements, blood in the bowel movements, rectal bleeding, bloating, nausea, and vomiting. The frequency of symptoms varied from subject to subject. Other reported non-gastrointestinal symptoms included fatigue/tiredness, weakness, perianal discharge, leg pain, back pain, dizziness, joint pain, hair loss, skin and eye problems, and shortness of breath. The patients noted that Crohn's disease affected their physical functioning, daily activities, emotional well-being, social functioning, work/education, and relationships. For example, since their symptoms could be unpredictable, it was sometimes difficult to make plans they might not be able to keep. Adolescents seemed particularly dismayed by the impact their Crohn's disease had on friendships. Most noted that to prevent certain symptoms, they had to change their diets, and they avoided certain foods. No major difference in disease was seen between the adults and adolescents. In the second round of interviews, there were six adults with a mean age of 51.5 years; there were two males and four females. Five of the patients were white, and one was Hispanic. Most had a graduate-level education. Patients had been diagnosed with Crohn's disease for a mean of 7.1 years. Three of the patients had moderate disease, and three had severe. All six patients had taken biological therapy, and three had been prescribed corticosteroids. Five of the patients noted that they could consider themselves in remission even if some but not all of their symptoms stopped. The researchers commented that "further exploration of patient perceptions of CD remission and their perceptions of treatment expectations would help align patient and healthcare professional treatment outcome goals and aid the evaluation of treatment success in patient-focused drug development."[14]

Adolescents with Crohn's Disease May Experience Nutritional Problems

In a prospective, cross-sectional study published in the journal *BMC Gastroenterology*, researchers from Brazil examined the association between Crohn's disease and nutritional status in adolescents. Their cohort consisted of twenty-two patients with mild to moderate active Crohn's disease, twenty-nine patients with inactive Crohn's disease, and thirty-five controls, who were first-degree relatives of and in the same age bracket as the Crohn's disease patients. All of the participants were between the ages of 13.2 and 19.4 years. Data were collected on weight, height, and body mass index, as well as information the consumption of macronutrients and micronutrients. Before their medical consultations, seven-day food diaries were completed. When compared to the controls, the patients had a poorer quality of diet, particularly in caloric intake, dietary protein intake, dietary fiber intake, and micronutrient intake. For example, caloric intake was lower than recommended in 50 percent of the patients with active Crohn's disease, in 3.5 percent of those with inactive Crohn's disease, and in 5.7 percent of the controls. And, the prevalence of micronutrient deficiency was higher among the patients with Crohn's disease than among those in the control group, and the deficiencies were greater among those with active Crohn's disease than among those with inactive Crohn's disease. The researchers concluded that adolescents with mild to moderately active Crohn's disease "are at risk for nutritional deficits, which makes it important to conduct nutritional assessments as part of the routine evaluation of such patients, in order to plan nutritional support as part of the overall treatment strategy in this population."[15]

REFERENCES AND FURTHER READING

Albenberg, Lindsey, Colleen M. Brensinger, Qufei Wu et al. "A Diet Low in Red and Processed Meat Does Not Reduce Rate of Crohn's Disease Flares." *Gastroenterology* 157 (2019): 128–136.

Bae, Joon Hyun, Seo Young Kang, Si Eun You et al. "The Effects of Acupuncture on Crohn's Disease: A Systematic Review and Meta-Analysis." *Journal of Pharmacopuncture* 26, no. 3 (2023): 211–226.

Colombel, Jean-Frédéric, Tadakazu Hisamatsu, Raja Atreya et al. "Upadacitinib Reduces Crohn's Disease Symptoms Within the First Week of Induction Therapy." *Clinical Gastroenterology and Hepatology* 22, no. 8 (August 22): 1668–1677.

Costa, Camila Ortiz Prospero Cavalcante, Flair José Carrilho et al. "A Snapshot of the Nutritional Status of Crohn's Disease Among Adolescents in Brazil: A Prospective Cross-Sectional Study." *BMC Gastroenterology* 15 (2015): 172.

Espi-López, Gemma V., Marta Inglés, Isabel Soliva-Cazabán, and Pilar Serra-Añó. "Effect of the Soft-Tissue Techniques in the Quality of Life in Patients in Crohn's Disease." *Medicine* 97, no. 51 (2018): e13811.

Jones, Patricia D., Michael D. Kappelman, Christopher F. Martin et al. "Exercise Decreases Risk of Future. Active Disease in Patients with Inflammatory Bowel Disease in Remission." *Inflammatory Bowel Diseases* 2, no. 5 (May 2015): 1063–1071.

Kitchen, Helen, Mallory Farrar, Tamara Al-zubeidi et al. "Patient's Perspective on Disease Burden, Remission Definition, and Symptoms Associated with Treatment Seeking: A Qualitative Study in Adult and Adolescent Patients with Crohn's Disease." *Crohn's and Colitis 360* 2, no. 2 (April 2020): otaa033.

Meyer, Antoine, Catherine Dong, Corinne Casagrande et al. "Food Processing and Risk of Crohn's Disease and Ulcerative Colitis: A European Prospective Cohort Study." *Clinical Gastroenterology and Hepatology* 21 (2023): 1607–1616.

Naftali, Timna, Lihi Bar-Lev Schleider, Iris Dotan et al. "Cannabis Induces a Clinical Response in Patients with Crohn's Disease: A Prospective Placebo-Controlled Study." *Clinical Gastroenterology and Hepatology* 11 (2013): 1276–1280.

Sadeghian, Mehdi, Parvane Saneei, Fereydoun Siassi, Ahmad Esmaillzadeh. "Vitamin D Status in Relationship To Crohn's Disease: Meta-Analysis of Observational Studies." *Nutrition* 32 (2016): 505–514.

Serrano Fernandez, Victor, Marta Seldas Palomino, José Alberto Laredo-Aguilera et al. "High-Fiber Diet and Crohn's Disease: Systematic Review and Meta-Analysis." *Nutrients* 15 (2023): 3114.

Storr, Martin, Shane Devlin, Gilaad G. Kaplan et al. "Cannabis Use Provides Symptoms Relief in Patients with Inflammatory Bowel Disease But Is Associated with Worse Disease Prognosis in Patients with Crohn's Disease." *Inflammatory Bowel Diseases* 20, no. 3 (March 2014): 472–480.

Traboulsi, Cindy, Fares Ayoub, Alexa Silfen et al. "Upadacitinib Is Safe and Effective for Crohn's Disease: Real-World Data from a Tertiary Center." *Digestive Diseases and Sciences* 68 (2023): 385–388.

DIVERTICULITIS

INTRODUCTION

Diverticulosis is the development of small, irregular bulging pouches in the wall of the large intestine. When these pouches become inflamed, the condition is termed diverticulitis. Normally, the wall of the large intestine or colon is smooth. An irregular bulging pouch in the colon wall is called a diverticulum. Multiple pouches are termed diverticula.

After the age of fifty, diverticula are a common occurrence. Usually found in the lower part of the colon in people of European descent and in the upper part of the colon in people of Asian descent, diverticula often do not cause any problems. Still, when diverticulosis becomes diverticulitis, the condition may become painfully problematic for some people, a situation that has the potential to trigger a medical emergency requiring immediate hospitalization and sometimes surgery.

There are two main types of diverticulitis—acute and chronic. Acute diverticulitis begins suddenly and improves quickly with treatment. People who have recurring episodes of diverticulitis have the chronic form. There are also complicated and uncomplicated forms of diverticulitis. Most of the time, diverticulitis is uncomplicated; there is inflammation and an infection, but they heal relatively quickly. Diverticulitis becomes complicated when it causes additional problems, such as the rupturing of a diverticulum.

Although diverticular disease has become more prevalent in the twentieth and twenty-first centuries, it was first described in the late 1700s by a French surgeon named Alexis Littre. By the very late 1800s, inflammation of the diverticula was termed diverticulitis.[1]

SYMPTOMS, RISKS, AND COMPLICATIONS

The most frequent symptom of diverticulitis is pain, primarily in the lower left abdomen. The pain tends to be sudden and intense, but it may be mild and worsen over time. Inflammation of the diverticula may also cause fever, nausea, mild to severe rectal bleeding, and changes in bowel habits, such as diarrhea or constipation.

Risks associated with developing diverticulitis include aging, obesity, smoking, a low-fiber diet, a high red meat diet, a lack of exercise, a heavy intake of alcohol, a low intake of vitamin D, and certain medications, such as steroids, opioids, nonsteroidal anti-inflammatory drugs (NSAIDs), and naproxen sodium. While many cases of diverticulitis seem to occur by chance, there does appear to be a genetic component in people of European or Asian descent. People with weakened immune systems or autoimmune disorders have an increased risk of repeated bouts with diverticulitis.

About 15 percent of people with diverticulitis develop complications. Among the potential complications are abscesses (pockets of pus), blockages of the colon, a fistula or irregular passageway from the bowel to another organ of the body, tears in the colon, allowing waste to spill out into the abdomen, causing a serious medical problem known as peritonitis, and bleeding from ruptured blood vessels, called diverticular hemorrhage, which may lead to anemia.

PREVALENCE

Although diverticulosis is common, diverticulitis is an uncommon complication. It affects about 4 percent of people with diverticulosis. Once a person has had an attack of diverticulitis, there is about a 20 percent chance that that person will have another attack.

Diverticulosis becomes more common as people age. In the United States, more than one-third of adults between the ages of fifty and fifty-nine and two-thirds of those over the age of eighty have these bulges. Most of these people will never have any problems, but, of course, some will develop diverticulitis.

DIAGNOSIS AND TREATMENT OPTIONS

Generally, healthcare providers begin by ordering blood and urine tests. Then, an abdominal CT or computerized tomography scan may be used to see the extent of inflammation and any related complications. Six to eight weeks after the resolution of the symptoms, a colonoscopy, in which a healthcare provider inserts a long, thin lighted tube (endoscope) inside the anus and rectum into the colon, is used to obtain a better view of the colon and to rule out a colon malignancy. (A colonoscopy is never done to diagnose diverticulitis. If done too soon, it may perforate the colon and spread infection.)

Mild diverticulitis is treated with rest, changes in diet, and possibly antibiotics. Severe diverticulitis may require hospitalization and intravenous antibiotics. Some cases of diverticulitis necessitate surgery. Treatment for diverticulitis frequently begins with several days of consuming a liquid diet and avoiding solid foods. This enables the colon to rest, recover, and heal. Acetaminophen may be used for pain relief, and antibiotics or antispasmodics are sometimes prescribed. (Other common pain relievers, which may upset the gastrointestinal tract, should be avoided.) If conservative treatment does not work, a patient may require hospitalization for intravenous antibiotics, antiviral, and/or pain medications or blood transfusions. Surgery may be needed to treat an abscess, persistent bleeding, a perforation, or a fistula. In rare instances, a problematic section of the bowel has to be removed; this is termed a partial colectomy. Sometimes, this requires a temporary colostomy or the creation of a temporary opening for the colon through the abdomen. People with a colostomy need to use colostomy bags to collect fecal matter.

RESEARCH FINDINGS

Antibiotics May Not Provide Any Benefit for People with Acute Uncomplicated Diverticulitis

In a multicenter, randomized trial published in the *British Journal of Surgery*, researchers from ten surgical departments in Sweden and one in Iceland investigated the usefulness of treating people with antibiotics for acute uncomplicated cases of diverticulitis. The researchers recruited 623 patients with computed tomography-verified acute uncomplicated left-sided diverticulitis; 314 patients were treated with intravenous antibiotics and 309 were treated with intravenous fluids without antibiotics. The patients in the two groups were demographically similar in age, sex, BMI, comorbidities, body temperature, white blood cell count, and levels of C-reactive protein (a measure of inflammation). At the time of admission, all of the patients had a history of acute abdominal pain and fever. Three patients in the antibiotic group and six in the no antibiotics group had complications such as perforation or abscess formation. The median hospital stay for all of the patients was three days. During hospitalization, the patients in both groups had rapid improvements in abdominal pain and tenderness and body temperature. Forty-one patients were lost to follow-up. Of the remaining patients, recurrent diverticulitis occurred in ninety-three patients, with no significant difference between the groups. No differences between the groups were also observed for frequency of surgery, abdominal pain, and changes in bowel habits. The researchers commented that the antibiotic treatment did not prevent complications, accelerate recovery, or prevent recurrence. In fact, "the recommendations of antibiotic therapy are based on tradition and expert opinion, and not on evidence derived from controlled trials." The researchers concluded that "antibiotic therapy does not prevent surgical complications or recurrence, and does not shorten hospital stay. Antibiotics should be reserved mainly for patients with complicated diverticulitis."[2]

In a retrospective, case-control study published in the journal *Colorectal Disease*, researchers from the Netherlands evaluated the need for antibiotics in mild colonic diverticulitis. The cohort consisted of 272 patients with mild colonic diverticulitis who were admitted to one of two hospitals. A total of 191 patients were treated without antibiotics and 81 were treated with antibiotics. At baseline, both groups were comparable with respect to age, sex, comorbidity, and use of nonsteroidal anti-inflammatory drugs, steroids, and aspirin. All of the patients had ultrasound or imaging-confirmed diverticulitis. Treatment failure did not differ between the groups. During follow-up, twelve patients (15 percent) in the antibiotic group had a recurrence, one of whom required emergency surgery. Five patients needed management by an elective resection and primary anastomosis (connection during surgery). Fourteen patients (7 percent) in the non-antibiotic group had one or more recurrences requiring hospitalization. One of these required an acute resection. Seven patients had complications requiring elective surgery. All had a resection and primary anastomosis. Although the association was not statistically significant, treatment with antibiotics resulted in a higher risk of recurrence. The researchers noted that even though "the mandatory use of antibiotics in mild diverticulitis has been a long-standing surgical dogma," it appears to be safe to omit antibiotics in patients with mild cases of diverticulitis.

While antibiotic use may be useful in those patients with elevated temperatures or obvious infections, "current evidence supports the notion that antibiotics can be omitted in selected patients with mild colonic diverticulitis."[3]

Antibiotics Do Not Appear to Reduce the Length of Hospital Stays in Patients with Uncomplicated Diverticulitis

In a double-blind, randomized, controlled trial published in the journal *Clinical Gastroenterology and Hepatology*, researchers from New Zealand and Australia investigated the ability of antibiotic therapy to reduce the length of hospital stays in people with uncomplicated diverticulitis. The initial cohort consisted of 180 patients who were hospitalized for uncomplicated acute diverticulitis, a diagnosis that was confirmed by CT. For seven days, eighty-five patients were assigned to receive antibiotics and ninety-five took placebos. The researchers collected demographic, clinical, and laboratory data and answers to questionnaires every twelve hours for the first forty-eight hours and then daily until discharge. The researchers found that there was no significant difference in the median time of hospital stay between the two groups, and there was no significant difference in adverse events, readmission to the hospital within one week, and readmission to the hospital within thirty days. The researchers concluded that their findings "provided arguably the strongest evidence to date in support of omitting antibiotics in selected patients presenting with uncomplicated acute diverticulitis."[4]

The Combination of a Traditional Herb, Daiobotanpito, and Antibiotics May Be Useful for Acute Diverticulitis

In a retrospective, nonrandomized, open-label trial published in the journal *Evidence-Based Complementary and Alternative Medicine*, researchers from Japan evaluated the use of a combination of daiobotanpito and antibiotics to treat acute diverticulitis. The initial cohort consisted of thirty-four patients with acute diverticulitis. The eleven patients in the first group received daiobotanpito and intravenous antibiotics, and the twenty-three patients in the second group received only intravenous antibiotics. Both groups were comparable in patient demographics and clinical characteristics, such as previous episodes of diverticulitis and the duration of symptoms before admission. The researchers determined that when evaluating the duration of fever, abdominal pain, and antibiotics administration, the patients treated with the combination therapy had significantly better outcomes than those treated only with intravenous antibiotics, and there were no adverse effects in either group. The first group had a trend toward a one-day shorter hospital stay, though the trend did not reach statistical significance. There was a complete resolution of symptoms in both groups. The researchers concluded that the patients benefited from the addition of daiobotanpito to the treatment, and it may be advisable to add this herb to the treatment plan.[5]

Dietary Intake Appears to Play a Role in the Prevention of Diverticular Disease Complications

In a systematic review published in the journal *Nutrients*, researchers from Italy examined the association between dietary habits and the development of diverticular disease complications. The researchers identified eight articles that met their criteria, but none of them was considered to be high quality. Three studies used the same cohort of male patients, which included approximately 47,000 men, and two studies were based on a female cohort including a total of 740,094 patients. In the majority of the studies, dietary assessment was obtained from study participants using a validated semi-quantitative food frequency questionnaire, assessing the consumption of 131 to 148 foods and beverages. Still, the researchers determined that a high intake of fiber was associated with a decreased risk of diverticulitis or hospitalization due to diverticular disease, with protective effects for fruit and cereal fiber but not for vegetable fiber. Conversely, high red meat consumption and a Western diet pattern were associated with a higher risk of diverticulitis. Alcohol consumption seemed to be associated with diverticular bleeding, but not recurrent diverticulitis or diverticular complications. The researchers emphasized the need for more studies on dietary intake and diverticular disease. "Further high quality studies are needed to better define these associations."[6]

In a prospective study published in the journal *Gut*, researchers from the UK examined the association between dietary intake of fiber and the incidence of diverticular disease. The cohort consisted of 690,075 women from the Million Women Study; these women did not have a known history of diverticular disease. At baseline, their mean age was sixty years, and their mean total dietary fiber intake was 13.8 g per day, of which 42 percent came from cereals, 22 percent from fruits, 19 percent from vegetables, and 15 percent from potatoes. During six years of follow-up, 17,325 women were admitted to the hospital or died from diverticular disease. Dietary fiber intake was assessed using a forty-item food questionnaire and measured one year later in 4,265 randomly selected women. Compared with women in the lowest fifth of dietary fiber intake, those in the highest fifth of dietary fiber intake were from higher socioeconomic groups, slightly taller and leaner, much less likely to smoke, less likely to consume red or processed meats, and had a higher intake of total energy. There were forty-eight cases of diverticular disease per 10,000 women-years in the lowest fifth of dietary fiber intake and thirty-five cases per 10,000 women-years in the highest fifth. The researchers noted that "there was a strong and highly significant association between total fibre intake and diverticular disease incidence." Fiber clearly seemed to prevent some cases of diverticular disease.[7]

In a major prospective cohort study published in the *European Journal of Nutrition*, researchers from Sweden assessed the association between intake of dietary fiber from fruits and vegetables and hospitalization for diverticular disease. The researchers used data obtained from the Swedish Mammography Cohort, which included 66,651 women, and the Cohort of Swedish Men, which included 48,850 men. Fiber consumption was determined from food frequency questionnaires. Participants in the two cohorts noted their average consumption of ninety-six foods and beverages over the previous year; the participants chose from eight predefined frequency categories ranging from never to three or more times per day. The amount of fiber intake from cereals, fruits, and vegetables, respectively, was estimated in grams per day for each participant, and the participants were divided into four quartiles. The lowest quartile had those who ate the least fiber and the highest quartile had those who ate the most. During 287,789 person-years of follow-up, 505 women in the Swedish Mammography Cohort were diagnosed with diverticular disease, and during

337,919 years of follow-up, 255 men in the Cohort of Swedish Men were diagnosed with this disease. The researchers learned that compared to the women with the lowest intake of fiber, the women with the highest intake of fiber had a 25 percent decreased risk for hospitalization for diverticular disease. At the same time, when compared to the men with the lowest intake of fiber, the men with the highest intake of fiber had a 39 percent decreased risk of diverticular disease. When compared with women and men with the lowest intake of fruits and vegetables, women and men with the highest intake had about a 30 percent decreased risk of diverticular disease. The researchers commented that a higher intake of dietary fiber, especially fruits and vegetables, reduces the risk of hospitalization for diverticular disease, "while intake of cereals does not influence the risk."[8]

But Another Study Found That Constipation and a Low-Fiber Diet Were Not Associated with Asymptomatic Diverticulosis

In a cross-sectional study published in the journal *Clinical Gastroenterology and Hepatology*, researchers from several cities in the United States but based in Chapel Hill, North Carolina, noted that diverticulitis is often said to be a result of constipation caused by a low-fiber diet. That is why the researchers decided to evaluate the relationship between constipation, low dietary fiber, and the risk of asymptomatic diverticulosis. The cohort consisted of 539 people with diverticulosis and 1569 who did not have diverticulosis. Participants with diverticulosis were older and more likely to be male and white. They had a higher BMI and used tobacco, aspirin, and alcohol more often than the controls. All of the participants were assessed for their diets, levels of physical activity, and bowel habits, and they all had a colonoscopy. The researchers determined that the subjects with less frequent bowel movements (less than seven per week) had a lower risk of diverticulosis than those with regular bowel movements (seven per week). And, those reporting hard stools also had reduced odds. There was no association between diverticulosis and straining or incomplete bowel movements. The researchers noted that they found no difference between the cases and controls in mean dietary fiber intake and reported supplemental fiber intake, and they found no relationship between dietary fiber intake and diverticulosis. And, when they further broke down fiber intake to beans, grains, fruits, and vegetables, they also found no association between dietary fiber intake and the presence of diverticulosis. The researchers commented that their results appear to contradict many of the current beliefs associated with diverticulosis. And, they concluded that "because of the significant health burden of symptomatic diverticulitis, it is time to take a fresh look at risk factors and alternative hypotheses for asymptomatic diverticulosis."[9]

People with Diverticular Disease May Include Nuts, Corn, and Popcorn in Their Diets

In a study published in *JAMA: Journal of the American Medical Association*, researchers from Seattle, Washington, Boston, Massachusetts, and Canada explained that people with diverticular disease are often told not to consume nuts, corn, and popcorn. The researchers wanted to learn if these foods are actually associated with diverticulitis and diverticular bleeding. To conduct their research, the researchers used the database from the Health Professionals Follow-Up Study, a cohort of men who were followed via self-administered medical and dietary questionnaires. At baseline, there were 47,228 men between the ages of forty and seventy-five years who were free of diverticulitis or its complications, cancer, and inflammatory bowel disease. During eighteen years of follow-up, there were 801 incident cases of diverticulitis and 383 incident cases of diverticular bleeding. Twenty-seven percent of the subjects reported eating nuts at least twice per week. Fifteen percent ate corn and popcorn at least twice per week. Consumption of less than one serving per month of nuts, corn, and popcorn was noted in 25 percent, 12 percent, and 36 percent of the men, respectively. Subjects in the highest category of nut consumption tended to be older and to consume more alcohol but were slightly more active than those in the lowest category. Compared to men with the lowest intake of corn, men with the highest intake generally consumed more total fiber and red meat but less alcohol. Men who ate popcorn at least twice per week were, in general, younger and more likely to use analgesics and to be non-smokers than those who ate popcorn less than once per month. The researchers found that nut, corn, and popcorn consumption were not associated with an increased risk of complicated diverticular disease. On the contrary, they observed an inverse association between nut and popcorn consumption and the risk of diverticulitis. And there was no association between corn consumption and diverticulitis, and no significant association between the consumption of nuts, corn, and popcorn and diverticular bleeding. The researchers concluded that their findings "refute the pervasive but unproven belief that these foods invoke diverticular complications, and suggest that the recommendation to avoid these food in diverticular disease should be reconsidered."[10]

People with Diverticulosis with Lower Levels of Serum Vitamin D Have a Higher Risk of Developing Diverticulitis, but High Doses of Vitamin D Supplementation May Not Prevent Diverticular Related Hospitalization

In a trial published in *Clinical Gastroenterology and Hepatology*, researchers from Boston, Massachusetts, and Seattle, Washington, examined the association between pre-diagnostic levels of serum vitamin D and diverticulitis. The researchers used data obtained from the Partners Healthcare Research Patient Data Registry (RPDR). (At the time of the study, Partners Healthcare was an integrated academic healthcare system that provided care for over 1.8 million patients in the greater Boston area.) The researchers identified 9,116 patients with uncomplicated diverticulosis and 922 patients who developed diverticulitis that required hospitalization. Compared to the patients with uncomplicated diverticulosis, the patients with diverticulitis were older, more likely to be female and less likely to have obesity or coronary artery disease. The researchers learned that patients with uncomplicated diverticulosis had significantly higher mean pre-diagnostic levels of serum vitamin D than patients with diverticulitis that required hospitalization. And patients with more serious cases of diverticulitis had lower levels of vitamin D than patients with less serious cases, but these differences usually did not reach significance. Compared to patients in the lowest quartile of serum vitamin D, patients in the highest quartile had a substantially lower risk of developing diverticulitis requiring hospitalization. The risk of diverticulitis dropped dramatically as the levels of serum vitamin D rose. The researchers concluded that their study as well as other studies "highlight the potential importance of vitamin D in the maintenance of colonic health."[11]

In a post-hoc analysis of a community-based randomized double-blind placebo-controlled trial published in the journal *Clinical Nutrition*, researchers from New Zealand and Boston, Massachusetts assessed the efficacy of vitamin D supplementation on diverticular disease hospitalization. The initial cohort consisted of 5,110 community-dwelling participants in Auckland, New Zealand. Fifty-eight percent were male, and the mean age was sixty-six years. During the two years before the trial, forty-three subjects (0.8 percent) had a diverticular disease hospitalization. The participants were randomly assigned to take a monthly capsule of either 100,000 IU vitamin D or a placebo. During a median of 3.3 years of follow-up, there were seventy-four participants who were hospitalized for diverticular disease. The researchers found no difference in the risk of diverticular disease hospitalization between the vitamin D supplement group and the placebo group. Even such a high dose of vitamin D was unable to reduce the risk of hospitalization. The researchers concluded that "monthly 100,000 IU vitamin D3 supplementation does not reduce the risk of diverticular disease hospitalization in the general population." Still, the researchers emphasized the need for more research on the topic.[12]

Smoking May Increase Complications in Diverticular Disease

In a trial published in the *British Journal of Surgery*, researchers from the UK examined the relationship between smoking and the severity of diverticular disease. The cohort consisted of eighty patients with diverticular disease. The forty-five patients in the first group had diverticular disease complications requiring hospitalization or surgery during an eighteen-month period; the thirty-five patients in the second group had asymptomatic diverticular disease or minor symptoms. There was no difference in age or sex between the two groups. Both groups were predominately Caucasian, with twice as many women as men. The mean age was 69.1 years. Only thirty-three patients were retired. Concurrent medical conditions were present with the same frequency in the more elderly patients in both groups. Medication use, especially nitrates, calcium channel blockers, aspirin, nonsteroidal anti-inflammatory drugs, and beta blockers, was equally prevalent in both groups. Twenty-eight of the patients in the first group were diagnosed as a result of an urgent hospital admission. An emergency operation was performed on twenty patients. Two patients died from diverticular disease in the first group; there were no deaths in the second group. The researchers were unable to detect differences in epidemiological factors, concurrent and past medical and surgical conditions, or chronic medication use between the two groups. However, the proportion of smokers in the first group was significantly greater than in the second group. Smoking appeared to be the only independent factor predisposing people to significant complications of diverticular disease. The researchers concluded that "in patients with diverticular disease, smoking is associated with an increased risk of complications."[13]

People with Diverticular Disease Seem to Benefit from Maintaining a Lower BMI and Being More Physically Active

In a systematic review and meta-analysis of prospective studies published in the *European Journal of Nutrition*, researchers from the UK, Norway, and Germany examined the relationship between BMI, physical activity, and the risk of diverticular disease. The researchers located six cohort studies of BMI and diverticular disease, with 28,915 cases and 1,636,777 participants, and five cohort studies of physical activity and diverticular disease risk, with 2,080 cases and 147,869 participants. The studies on BMI were from Europe, the United States, and Australia; the studies on physical activity were from Europe and the United States. The researchers learned that as BMI increased, so did the risk of diverticular disease. For each 5-unit increase in BMI, there was a 28 percent increase in the relative risk of diverticular disease, a 31 percent increase in the relative risk of diverticulitis, and a 20 percent reduction in the relative risk of diverticular disease complications. Likewise, as people became more physically active, they lowered their risk of diverticular disease. There was a 24 percent reduction in the risk of diverticular disease for the highest versus the lowest level of physical activity and a 26 percent reduction in the risk of diverticulitis for the highest versus the lowest level of vigorous physical activity. The researchers concluded that their findings suggested, "excess weight and low physical activity are risk factors for diverticular disease." These findings have important public health implications. "They add diverticular disease to the list of conditions that appear to be associated with adiposity and low physical activity."[14]

There Also Appears to Be an Association between Cardiorespiratory Fitness, BMI, and Diverticulitis in Older Adults

In a cross-sectional trial published in the online journal *PLoS ONE*, researchers from Ames, Iowa, investigated the association between cardiorespiratory fitness, BMI, and diverticulitis in older adults. The cohort consisted of 476 older adults, with a mean age of seventy-one years; 61 percent were female. The subjects had no history of myocardial infarction, stroke, cancer, inflammatory bowel disease, or diabetes. Diverticulitis cases were reported in the medical history questionnaire. Thirty-five (7.4 percent) of the participants had diverticulitis. The researchers learned that the participants who had better cardiorespiratory fitness and lower BMI were less likely to have diverticulitis. According to the researchers, this suggested that there were "potential additive benefits to the combination of high CRF [cardiorespiratory fitness] and lower BMI in relation to the prevalence of diverticulitis in older adults." While the mechanism in which CRF affects diverticulitis is not known, higher levels of BMI are a known risk factor for this disease. And, the researchers concluded that "higher CRF combined with lower BMI is more strongly associated with a lower prevalence of diverticulitis."[15]

REFERENCES AND FURTHER READING

Aune, Dagfinn, Abhijit Sen, Michael F. Leitzmann et al. "Body Mass Index and Physical Activity and the Risk of Diverticular Disease: A Systematic Review and Meta-Analysis of Prospective." *European Journal of Nutrition* 56 (2017): 2423–2438.

Carabotti, Marilia, Francesca Falangone, Rosario Cuomo, and Bruno Annibale. "Role of Dietary Habits in the Prevention of Diverticular Disease Complications: A Systematic Review." *Nutrients* 13 (2021): 1288.

Chabok, A., L. Påhlman, F. Hjern et al. "Randomized Clinical Trial of Antibiotics in Active Uncomplicated Diverticulitis." *British Journal of Surgery* 99, no. 4 (April 2012): 532–539.

Crowe, Francesca, Angela Balkwill, Benjamin J. Cairns et al. "Source of Dietary Fibre and Diverticular Disease Incidence: A Prospective Study of UK Women." *Gut* 63 (2014): 1450–1456.

de Korte, N., J. P. Kuyvenhoven, D. L. van der Peet et al. "Mild Colonic Diverticulitis Can Be Treated Without Antibiotics: A Case-Control Study." *Colorectal Disease* 14, no. 3 (March 2012): 325–330.

Jaung, Rebekah, Sherry Nisbet, Martijn Pieter Gosselink et al. "Antibiotics Do Not Reduce Length of Hospital Stay for Uncomplicated Diverticulitis in a Pragmatic Double-Blind Randomized Trial." *Clinical Gastroenterology and Hepatology* 19 (2021): 503–510.

Maguire, Lillias H., Mingyang Song, Lisa E. Strate et al. "Higher Serum Levels of Vitamin D are Associated with Reduced Risk of Diverticulitis." *Clinical Gastroenterology and Hepatology* 11, no. 12 (December 2013): 1631–1635.

Mahmood, Mahmood W., Mirna Abraham-Nordling, Niclas Håkansson et al. "High Intake of Dietary Fibre from Fruit and Vegetables Reduces the Risk of Hospitalisation for Diverticular Disease." *European Journal of Nutrition* 58 (2019): 2393–2400.

Matrana, Marc R. and David A. Margolin. "Epidemiology and Pathophysiology of Diverticular Disease." *Clinics in Colon and Rectal Surgery* 22, no. 3 (2009): 141–146.

Ogawa, Keiko, Koji Nishijima, Funio Futagami et al. "Effectiveness of Traditional Japanese Herbal (Kampo) Medicine, Daiobotanpito, in Combination with Antibiotic Therapy in the Treatment of Acute Diverticulitis: A Preliminary Study." *Evidence-Based Complementary and Alternative Medicine* 2013 (2013): 305414.

Papagrigoriadis, S., L. Macey, N. Bourantas, and J. A. Rennie. "Smoking May Be Associated with Complications in Diverticular Disease." *British Journal of Surgery* 86 (1999): 923–926.

Perry, Anne F., Robert S. Sandler, Dennis J. Ahnen et al. "Constipation and a Low-Fiber Diet Are Not Associated with Diverticulosis." *Clinical Gastroenterology and Hepatology* 11 (2013): 1622–1627.

Song, B. K., J. M. Saavedra, E. C. Lefferts et al. "Associations Between Cardiorespiratory Fitness and Diverticulitis in Older Adults." *PLoS One* 17, no. 9 (2022): e0275433.

Strate, Lisa L., Yan L. Liu, Sapna Syngal et al. "Nut, Corn and Popcorn Consumption and the Incidence of Diverticular Disease." *JAMA: Journal of the American Medical Association* 300, no. 8 (August 27, 2008): 907–914.

Wu, Z., J. Broad, J. Sluyter et al. "Effect of Monthly Vitamin D on Diverticular Disease Hospitalization: Post-Hoc Analysis of a Randomized Controlled Trial." *Clinical Nutrition* 40 (2021): 839–843.

DYSPEPSIA

INTRODUCTION

Also known as indigestion, dyspepsia is discomfort in the upper abdomen. This discomfort may be an occasional occurrence or an integral component of an individual's daily life. Whether it is an infrequent annoyance or a near-constant life disruptor, dyspepsia is a gastrointestinal problem that is all too often hard to treat effectively.

There are two main types of dyspepsia—organic and functional. With organic dyspepsia, medical providers are able to determine a specific cause. When that cause is corrected, the dyspepsia may well be cured. With functional dyspepsia, there are no obvious physical or mechanical reasons for the symptoms. Currently, functional dyspepsia has two main subtypes—postprandial distress syndrome and epigastric pain syndrome. Postprandial distress syndrome is defined as meal- or food-induced dyspepsia, while epigastric pain syndrome is characterized by the presence of epigastric pain and/or burning. Many people with functional dyspepsia have both types.

Still, people with dyspepsia often also show frequent overlap with other gastrointestinal problems, such as irritable bowel syndrome, abnormal gastric emptying (gastroparesis), postprandial fullness, epigastric pain, nausea, vomiting, and gastroesophageal reflux disease, as well as non-GI diseases, such as anxiety, depression, insomnia, fibromyalgia, chronic fatigue syndrome, interstitial cystitis, and overactive bladder. People with these overlapping medical problems tend to have more frequent and more severe symptoms and a poorer health-related quality of life.

In an article in the *American Journal of Gastroenterology*, researchers from the UK analyzed the annual inpatient and outpatient records of hospitals and dispensaries in Philadelphia, New York, and Boston for the years 1750 to 1920. They determined that dyspepsia was first recorded in hospital statistics at the end of the eighteenth century. After that, the numbers "increased markedly." Throughout the nineteenth and twentieth centuries, it was a common diagnosis.[1]

SYMPTOMS, RISKS, AND COMPLICATIONS

There are a number of symptoms associated with dyspepsia. These include a feeling of nausea and/or fullness soon after eating a relatively small amount of food. (People with dyspepsia often have difficulty eating average-sized meals and may be advised to eat more frequent, smaller meals, which may be difficult to coordinate.) All too often, the eating-related symptoms trigger an unintentional loss of weight, which may be problematic for someone who is already somewhat thin. There may be mild to severe pain and/or a burning sensation between the bottom of the breastbone and the bellybutton. Many people also have bloating in the upper abdomen and/or acid reflux. Other less frequent symptoms include belching, vomiting, and/or heartburn—a pain in the center of the chest that may radiate into the neck or back.

There are a number of known medical problems that increase the risks for developing dyspepsia. These include inflammation of the stomach (gastritis), impaired stomach emptying (gastroparesis), biliary disease, food allergies, Helicobacter pylori, peptic ulcers, celiac disease, gallstones, constipation, pancreas inflammation (pancreatitis), stomach cancer, intestinal blockage, reduced blood flow in the intestine (intestinal ischemia), diabetes, thyroid disease, and pregnancy. Other easier-to-control risks associated with dyspepsia include overeating or eating too quickly, consuming fatty, greasy, or spicey foods, drinking excess amounts of alcohol, eating or drinking foods with higher amounts of caffeine, drinking carbonated beverages, eating chocolate, smoking, experiencing anxiety, and taking certain antibiotics, pain relievers, and iron supplements.

There are still other factors that increase the risk of dyspepsia. These include having a history of anxiety and/or depression, physical and/or emotional abuse, a past Helicobacter pylori infection, the use of nonsteroidal anti-inflammatory drugs (NSAIDs), and having been assigned female at birth.

PREVALENCE

Dyspepsia is an extremely common medical disorder. In fact, dyspepsia is the most common upper gastrointestinal disorder. An article in the *Journal of Neurogastroenterology and Motility* estimated that the organic form of dyspepsia affects about 5–7 percent of the population, and the functional form of dyspepsia is present in between 11.5 and 14.7 percent of the population.[2] Another article in the journal *Lancet Gastroenterology & Hepatology* noted that dyspepsia affects up to 30 percent of the population in the United States, Canada, and the UK, with 70 percent of the affected people having functional dyspepsia.[3] Many cases of dyspepsia are probably not reported. As a result, these statistics probably underrepresent the actual prevalence.

DIAGNOSIS AND TREATMENT OPTIONS

People with suspected dyspepsia will probably be sent for a number of tests. These may include a variety of blood tests, an upper endoscopy, breath tests, and gastric emptying studies. In some cases, these tests will yield an abnormal finding, such as peptic ulcer disease or medication-induced dyspepsia (as from NSAIDs). These people will be diagnosed with organic dyspepsia. In a large number of cases, no abnormal finding will be found. These people will be diagnosed with functional dyspepsia.

There are a number of different treatments for dyspepsia. With organic dyspepsia, treating the specific cause may well cure the dyspepsia. Thus, if the dyspepsia is caused by celiac disease, adhering to a strict gluten-free diet may bring relief. (See the entry on celiac disease.) Or, if the dyspepsia is associated with constipation, finding a constipation-relieving treatment or treatments may help resolve both the dyspepsia and the constipation. Similarly, if the dyspepsia symptoms are a result of a Helicobacter pylori infection, treating the infection with a course of antibiotics and a proton pump inhibitor may well result in the improvement of symptoms. There are many treatment options for those with functional dyspepsia. No one treatment works for everyone. Among the treatment options are acid-reducing medications such as proton pump inhibitors and H2 receptor blockers, as well as prokinetic agents that improve the motility of the digestive system. The medication buspirone, which is used for anxiety, is believed to make it easier for food to pass into the stomach. When the dyspepsia symptoms are associated with the nervous system, also known as the "brain-gut connection," some people may benefit from a low-dose tricyclic antidepressant, such as amitriptyline, desipramine, or imipramine. These medications may even help the stomach relax during digestion. Still another common treatment is a fixed combination of peppermint and caraway oil. It is a frequently used phytotherapy that stimulates motility while calming the digestive system. While these treatments have helped some individuals, many others receive little relief and may try alternatives such as acupuncture, cognitive behavioral therapy, biofeedback, and psychotherapy. Some people try eliminating certain foods from their diet and/or exercising more and/or losing weight. As has been noted, eating smaller, more frequent meals has brought relief to large numbers of sufferers.

Perhaps the most notable complication of dyspepsia is the toll it takes on the quality of life of countless numbers of people. While people with the organic form of dyspepsia may find permanent relief, people with functional dyspepsia tend to be less fortunate. In all probability, they will spend a good deal of time and energy searching for a combination of treatments that relieve their symptoms. And it is believed that only about 20 percent of these people find a permanent solution. According to an article published in the *Journal of Neurogastroenterology and Motility*, treating functional dyspepsia is "difficult and does not currently produce satisfactory results."[4]

RESEARCH FINDINGS

Proton Pump Inhibitors Seem to Be Useful for Functional Dyspepsia

In a systematic review and meta-analysis published in the journal *Clinical Gastroenterology and Hepatology*, researchers from China evaluated the usefulness of proton pump inhibitors for functional dyspepsia. They identified seven randomized, double-blind, placebo-controlled trials with 3,725 subjects that met their criteria. Six were published as full articles and one was in abstract form. Four studies compared omeprazole with a placebo and three compared lansoprazole with a placebo. Six trials recruited patients who had symptoms for at least one or three months, and one trial did not provide any information about the patients' history of functional dyspepsia. In all of the trials, an endoscopy was performed on patients before they were recruited. In five trials, patients with a history of peptic ulcer disease were excluded. In six trials, gastroesophageal reflux disease was considered a reason for exclusion. The mean patient age was 43.1 years, and 37 percent were male. The duration of medical therapy ranged from two to eight weeks. The researchers found that proton pump inhibitors provided a modest but statistically significant degree of relief to people with functional dyspepsia, especially in those subjects with "ulcer-like and reflux-like" symptoms. On the other hand, "no significant difference in the efficacy was observed between PPIs and placebo in patients with dysmotility-like and unspecified dyspepsia."[5]

More Research Is Needed to Determine If Prokinetic Medications Are Useful for Functional Dyspepsia

In a systematic review and meta-analysis published in the *American Journal of Gastroenterology*, researchers from Canada and Thailand wanted to determine if prokinetic medications would be useful for the symptoms associated with functional dyspepsia. They located twenty-nine randomized controlled trials from twenty-six articles involving 10,044 participants that met their criteria. There were 5,949 patients and 4,095 controls. The researchers learned that the percentage of symptom improvement was 40 percent among those taking prokinetic medicines and 26.1 percent among those taking placebos. But five trials with 1,774 subjects failed to show any differences in the quality of life scores between the prokinetic medications and the placebos. Pooled data from seventeen separate studies with 3,811 participants found that adverse events occurred in 29.3 percent of patients on prokinetic medication and 30.8 percent on a placebo. The most common adverse events were diarrhea, abdominal discomfort, and nausea. Unfortunately, the researchers determined that the quality of the evidence was low. For example, there were problems with trial design, unexplained heterogeneity, and possible publication bias. The researchers underscored the need for "high quality RCTs [randomized controlled trials] with large sample sizes of FD [functional dyspepsia] patients . . . to verify the efficacy of prokinetics."[6]

Some Psychotropic Drugs May Be Useful for Functional Dyspepsia

In a systematic review and meta-analysis published in the journal *Gut*, researchers from the UK, Belgium, Canada, and Australia evaluated the usefulness of psychotropic medications for treating functional dyspepsia. The researchers located thirteen randomized controlled trials with 1,241 patients that met their criteria; 673 of the patients received active therapy and 568 took a placebo. Ten of the trials were believed to be at low risk for bias. The proportion of female patients recruited by the trials ranged from 56 percent to 85.3 percent. Six trials excluded people with coexistent mood disorders. Subgroup analyses determined that only two types of psychotropic drugs helped people with functional dyspepsia—antipsychotics and tricyclic antidepressants (TCADs). Further, a significant treatment effect was only found in trials that were held in tertiary or specialized care centers, though that was the type of care in most of the trials. When the researchers only included trials that excluded people with mood disorders, none of the psychotropic drugs had a significant effect on functional dyspepsia. At the same time, when they only included the ten trials with the low risk of bias, the psychotropic drugs were beneficial. The researchers concluded that "overall, psychotropic drugs are more effective than placebo for the treatment of FD [functional dyspepsia]. However, this beneficial effect was limited to antipsychotic drugs, such as sulpiride and levosulpiride, and TCADs, such as amitriptyline and imipramine."[7]

People with Functional Dyspepsia May Also Have GERD and/or Irritable Bowel Syndrome

In a cross-sectional study published in the *Journal of Gastroenterology and Hepatology*, researchers from Japan asked Japanese workers who visited a clinic for a routine health check-up to complete a self-reported questionnaire. (Japanese law required employers to conduct annual health screenings for all employees.) People who had a history of gastrointestinal surgery, peptic ulcer disease, Crohn's disease, and ulcerative colitis were excluded, as were subjects who submitted incomplete questionnaires. The questionnaire included demographic characteristics as well as questions about symptoms associated with gastrointestinal reflux disease (GERD), functional dyspepsia, and irritable bowel syndrome (IBS). A total of 2,680 subjects were included in the analyses. GERD was found in 207 patients, functional dyspepsia in 269 patients, and IBS in 381 patients. The researchers classified the remaining 2,012 subjects as the control group. The percentage of women among the GERD, functional dyspepsia, IBS, and control groups was 30.4 percent, 43.1 percent, 51.4 percent, and 32.9 percent, respectively. When compared to the controls, functional dyspepsia and IBS, but not GERD, were significantly female predominant. Overlaps were found in 160 (6 percent) of the subjects, and an overlap of functional dyspepsia and IBS was the most common, affecting 2.3 percent of all subjects. Overlaps were found in ninety-seven (46.9 percent) of the subjects with GERD, 128 (47.6 percent) of the subjects with functional dyspepsia, and 131 (34.4 percent) of the subjects with IBS. The researchers concluded that overlaps in GERD, functional dyspepsia, and IBS were a common occurrence, and they "worsened the HR-QOL [health-related quality of life] in Japanese adults."[8]

Certain Factors Increase the Risk of Developing Functional Dyspepsia in Children

In a cross-sectional trial published in the journal *BMC Gastroenterology*, researchers from China assessed the risk factors associated with the development of functional dyspepsia in children. The cohort consisted of 6,976 children who ranged in age from seven to seventeen years, with a mean age of 14.3 years; 3,497 were female. They were students at eight primary and secondary schools. The vast majority (85.7 percent) had been breastfed, and 39.8 percent lived independent of their parents. The researchers learned that 209 of the children (3 percent) had functional dyspepsia. These children had a mean age of 15.3 years, and 117 were female. When the researchers compared the children with functional dyspepsia to those without this disorder, they found several notable differences. For example, the children with dyspepsia were older and more likely to live independently of their parents. They never ate breakfast and ate cold and pickled foods. Nevertheless, the researchers commented that "scientific evidence for studying the efficacy of dietary and other related factors in FD are still lacking." That is why, "further well-designed studies are still needed to establish dietary risk factors related to FD."[9]

There Is a High Frequency of Overlap between Functional Dyspepsia, Overactive Bladder, and Irritable Bowel Syndrome

In a web-based cross-sectional trial published in *Neurogastroenterology & Motility*, researchers from Japan investigated the association between functional dyspepsia, overactive bladder, and irritable bowel syndrome. The cohort consisted of 5,330 people who completed web-based surveys with questions about functional dyspepsia, overactive bladder, and irritable bowel syndrome; there were 2,187 men and 3,143 women. Functional dyspepsia, overactive bladder, and irritable bowel syndrome were diagnosed in 438 (8.2 percent), 497 (9.3 percent), and 728 (13.7 percent) of the subjects, respectively. Among the subjects with either functional dyspepsia or overactive bladder, 10.7 percent had both of these disorders. And the overlap between functional dyspepsia and irritable bowel syndrome was 11.2 percent. The researchers noted that their findings confirmed that overactive bladder is "a significant co-morbidity" not only in functional dyspepsia but also in irritable bowel syndrome.[10]

Acupuncture May Be Useful for Postprandial Distress, a Subtype, and Symptom of Functional Dyspepsia

In a five-center, randomized clinical trial published in the journal *Annals of Internal Medicine*, researchers from China tested the usefulness of acupuncture for postprandial distress, a subtype and symptom of functional dyspepsia. The initial cohort consisted of 278 subjects; over a four-week period of time, they were randomly assigned to twelve twenty-minute sessions of acupuncture or sham acupuncture. Five acupuncturists performed both the real and sham acupuncture; patients in the acupuncture group received acupuncture at eight acupoints and one optional point. Evaluations were conducted at the end of week four, and during follow-ups at weeks eight, twelve, and sixteen. Researchers were looking for improvements in postprandial fullness, upper abdominal bloating, and early satiation. A total of fifty patients dropped out of the study; twenty-one in the acupuncture group and twenty-nine in the sham group. After four weeks, the estimated elimination of the three symptoms was 27.8 percent in the acupuncture group and 17.3 percent in the sham group, a difference of 10.5 percentage points. During the follow-ups, the acupuncture group continued to have better results than the sham acupuncture group. The researchers concluded that there is a need for "future research on the long-term effect of acupuncture that incorporates objective outcomes and daily measurement of symptoms."[11]

Buspirone May Be Somewhat Helpful for Some People with Functional Dyspepsia

In a randomized, double-blind, placebo-controlled, crossover trial published in the journal *Clinical Gastroenterology and Hepatology*, researchers from Belgium evaluated the ability of the medication buspirone to help with the symptoms of functional dyspepsia. The cohort consisted of seventeen patients, with a mean age of 38.5 years; there were thirteen women. The trial included two treatment periods of four weeks each, separated by a two-week washout period. In the first part of the trial, seven patients were given buspirone, 10 mg, three times per day, and ten were given a placebo, fifteen minutes before meals. In the second half of the trial, ten patients took buspirone and seven took placebos. At baseline and at the end of the trial, the researchers assessed meal-related symptoms and their severity, gastric sensitivity, accommodation, and emptying. The researchers learned that buspirone significantly reduced the overall severity of dyspepsia symptoms and the individual symptoms of postprandial fullness, early satiation, and upper abdominal bloating. The placebo appeared to have no significant effect. But, buspirone did not significantly alter solid emptying, and it slowed liquid gastric emptying. The researchers underscored the need for future studies with larger sample sizes.[12]

Certain Foods Appear to Exacerbate the Symptoms of Functional Dyspepsia

In a trial published in the *Scandinavian Journal of Gastroenterology*, researchers from Turkey wanted to determine what foods exacerbate the symptoms of functional dyspepsia. The cohort consisted of 168 adults with functional dyspepsia, sixty-four males and 104 females between the ages of eighteen and seventy-six years, and 135 healthy control subjects, fifty-seven males and seventy-eight females. All of the patients received a standardized work-up, including an upper gastrointestinal endoscopy, abdominal ultrasonography, and laboratory tests. The subjects completed a two-part questionnaire that had forty-seven questions and a short-form frequency questionnaire that was designed for functional gastrointestinal disorders. The questionnaire asked about nutritional habits, meal frequency and content, snacking frequency and content, fluid consumption habits, night eating habits, sleeping habits, and symptom-triggering foods. The researchers learned that the patients had slightly higher BMIs than the controls. While 68.5 percent of the patients ate three meals per day, 70.4 percent of the controls ate three meals. About one-third of the people in both groups did not eat any snacks, but the remainder tended to eat one or two snacks. Night snacking was uncommon. And the researchers determined that certain foods, specifically fried and fatty foods, hot spices, and carbonated drinks triggered the symptoms of functional dyspepsia. Other foods that probably contributed to the symptoms include legumes, cracked wheat and rice, and onions. "Removing these foods during the course of treatment might help alleviate the symptoms."[13]

People with Functional Dyspepsia Should Reduce Their Intake of Fat

In an article published in the journal *Advanced Biomedical Research*, researchers from Iran examined studies on the effects of fat intake in people with dyspepsia symptoms. They wanted to learn if actual research studies supported the belief that the intake of fatty foods resulted in more symptoms of fullness, bloating, and nausea in people with functional dyspepsia. The researchers located nineteen studies that met their criteria. These studies yielded a number of important findings. Thus, people with functional dyspepsia frequently report an intolerance to high-fat foods. It makes them feel full very quickly, and they easily become bloated. "The assessments have shown that fullness and bloating, which are caused by the high-fat meal, occur 30 minutes after fat ingestion." And they concluded that "studies show that fatty foods are associated with the occurrence of dyspeptic symptoms, and lower fat intake may alleviate symptoms in patients."[14]

There May Be an Association between Functional Dyspepsia and Vitamin D

In a case-control trial published in the journal *Annals of Medicine & Surgery*, researchers from India examined the relationship between functional dyspepsia and levels of vitamin D. The cohort consisted of 150 patients with functional dyspepsia and 150 controls. The patients attended an outpatient department of a tertiary academic hospital in eastern India from May 2021 to September 2022. The healthy controls were at the hospital for a different reason and had no history of self-reported chronic illness. The patients tended to be older than the controls, but the controls had higher BMI levels. Further, the controls had more people with obesity. The researchers learned that the patients had significantly lower levels of vitamin D than the controls. According to the researchers, this difference may be in part explained by the restrictive diets that people with dyspepsia tend to follow "to relieve unpleasant sensations in [the] gastrointestinal region." The researchers concluded that people with functional dyspepsia may well need vitamin D supplementation.[15]

Dyspepsia Does Not Appear to Shorten Lifespan

In a longitudinal ten-year follow-up study published in the *American Journal of Gastroenterology*, researchers from the UK and Canada wanted to learn if a diagnosis of dyspepsia had any influence on mortality. Data on mortality and the cause of death at ten years were obtained from the Office of National Statistics (in the UK). Baseline demographic data, lifestyle factors, gastrointestinal symptoms, and quality of life were recorded. Symptom data were available for 8,323 of the 8,407 people between the ages of forty and forty-nine years, 53.2 percent female, who were originally enrolled. A notable 3,169 (38.1 percent) had dyspepsia at baseline. Ten years later, 137 people (1.65 percent) had died. But the likelihood of death was no higher in those with dyspepsia than in those without this disorder. The researchers found "no association between symptom status at baseline and risk of death from cancer, including GI tract cancers, other diseases of the GI tract, ischemic heart disease, respiratory disease or central nervous system disorders." Although dyspepsia is associated with "considerable morbidity," it is "unlikely to impact adversely on survival in the general population."[16]

People with Dyspepsia Are Probably More Likely to Have Anxiety and Depression

In a systematic review published in the *Journal of Gastrointestinal and Liver Diseases*, researchers from Indonesia examined the relationship between functional dyspepsia and anxiety and depression. The researchers located thirteen studies with 14,076 subjects that met their criteria. The studies recruited adults ranging in age from seventeen to sixty-five years. All of the studies were considered to have a low risk of bias, and almost all of the studies found that people with functional dyspepsia had significantly higher levels of anxiety and depression than healthy controls. In fact, one study found that when the subjects were treated with anxiolytic medications or antidepressants, the symptoms of functional dyspepsia improved significantly. And, a randomized controlled trial found that acotiamide, a drug used for treating postprandial distress syndrome that is not sold in the United States, improved anxiety symptoms in people with functional dyspepsia. However, another study found that although the mean scores of anxiety and depression were higher among people with functional dyspepsia than controls, the difference was not statistically significant. Yet, the researchers determined that people with functional dyspepsia and psychological distress had more severe digestive symptoms, longer recovery times, increased healthcare costs, and more healthcare-seeking behavior. The researchers concluded that "identifying psychological factors in FD patients is essential to help clinicians determine the best choice of treatment and improve the prognosis and quality of life of the patients."[17]

Psychological Interventions May or May Not Help Deal with the Symptoms of Functional Dyspepsia

In a systematic review and meta-analysis published in the journal *Frontiers in Psychology*, researchers from China examined the ability of psychological interventions to help with the symptoms associated with functional dyspepsia. They located fourteen randomized controlled trials with 1,434 patients that met their criteria. There were 717 people in the intervention groups and 717 in the control groups. The psychological interventions included psychotherapy, psychodrama, cognitive behavioral therapy, relaxation therapy, and hypnosis. The people in the control groups received supportive therapy or no psychological interventions.

The sample sizes ranged from 30 to 348; follow-up periods ranged from two weeks to fourteen months. The overall quality of evidence for all assessed outcomes was rated as low or moderate. The researchers determined that the psychological interventions had "a significant beneficial effect" on symptom improvement. And this improvement continued during follow-up. But this effect was primarily seen as a result of psychotherapy "with fewer trials for other psychological interventions."[18]

Internet-Delivered Cognitive Behavioral Therapy May Be Useful for Adolescents with Functional Dyspepsia

In a trial published in the journal *Behavior Therapy*, researchers based in Stockholm, Sweden, evaluated the ability of internet-delivered cognitive behavioral therapy to ease the symptoms of functional dyspepsia or functional abdominal pain in adolescents. The cohort consisted of thirty-one adolescents between the ages of thirteen and seventeen. Sixty-five percent were female. All of the teens participated in a ten-week program together with one of their parents. The program focused primarily on the situations and behaviors that triggered abdominal symptoms. For example, in the second module, the teens mapped their gastrointestinal-specific behaviors, and in the fourth module, the teens were taught to "provoke" symptoms. The goal was to teach them to deal with their symptoms and prevent their symptoms from interfering with their activities. On average, the adolescents completed 7.2 modules or 72 percent of the program. Parents had five modules to help them "reduce unhelpful parental behaviors." On average, the parents completed four modules or 80 percent. Assessments were conducted at pretreatment, posttreatment, and at a six-month follow-up. The researchers noted that their findings determined that the intervention was "feasible and acceptable" and "potentially efficacious in reducing pain intensity, GI symptoms, avoidant behavior, fear of symptoms, and quality of life." Moreover, six months after the program ended "the improvements were sustained or significantly further increased across outcomes."[19]

REFERENCES AND FURTHER READING

Azizz, I., O. S. Palsson, H. Törnblom et al. "Epidemiology, Clinical Characteristics, and Associations for Symptom-Based Rome IV Functional Dyspepsia in Adults in the USA< Canada, and the UK: A Cross-Sectional Population-Based Study." *Lancet Gastroenterology & Hepatology* 3, no. 4 (2018): 252–262.

Baron, Jeremy Hugh and Amnon Sonnenberg. "Early History of Dyspepsia and Peptic Ulcer in the United States." *American Journal of Gastroenterology* 104, no. 12 (December 2009): 2893–2896.

Bonnert, Marianne, Ola Olen, Maria Lalouni et al. "Internet-Delivered Exposure-Based Cognitive-Behavioral Therapy for Adolescents with Functional Abdominal Pain or Functional Dyspepsia: A Feasibility Study." *Behavior Therapy* 50 (2019): 177–188.

Das, D. S., G. K. Saharia, M. K. Pnigrahi, and D. Sahoo. "Association of Vitamin D and Functional Dyspepsia: A Case-Control Study." *Annals of Medicine & Surgery* 85 (2023): 4667–4673.

Esterita, T., S. Dewi, F. G. Suryatenggara, and G. Glenardi. "Association of Functional Dyspepsia with Depression and Anxiety: A Systematic Review." *Journal of Gastrointestinal and Liver Diseases* 30, no. 2 (June 18, 2021): 259–266.

Ford, Alexander C., David Forman, Alastair G. Bailey et al. "Effect of Dyspepsia on Survival: A Longitudinal 10-Year Follow-Up Study." *American Journal of Gastroenterology* 107, no. 6 (June 2012): 912–921.

Ford, Alexander C., Pavit Luthra, Jan Tack et al. "Efficacy of Psychotropic Drugs in Functional Dyspepsia: Systematic Review and Meta-Analysis." *Gut* 66 (2017): 411–420.

Fujiwara, Yasuhiro and Tetsuo Arakawa. "Overlap; in Patients with Dyspepsia/Functional Dyspepsia." *Journal of Neurogastroenterology and Motility* 20, no. 4 (October 2014): 447–457.

Göktas, Zeynep, Seyfettin Köklü, Derya Dikmen et al. "Nutritional Habits in Functional Dyspepsia and Its Subgroups: A Comparative Study." *Scandinavian Journal of Gastroenterology* 51, no. 8 (2016): 903–907.

Kaji, Makiko, Yasuhiro Fujiwara, Masatsugu Shiba et al. "Prevalence of Overlaps Between GERD, FD and IBS and Impact on Health-Related Quality of Life." *Journal of Gastroenterology and Hepatology* 25, no. 6 (June 2010): 1151–1156.

Khodarahmi, Mahdieh and Leila Azadbakht. "Dietary Fat Intake and Functional Dyspepsia." *Advanced Biomedical Research* 5, no. 1 (2016): 76.

Matsuzaki, J., H. Suzuki, Y. Fukushima et al. "High Frequency of Overlap Between Functional Dyspepsia and Overactive Bladder." *Neurogastroenterology & Motility* 24, no. 9 (September 2012): 8221–8227.

Pittayanon, R., Y. Yuan, N. P. Bollegala et al. "Prokinetics for Functional Dyspepsia: A Systematic Review and Meta-Analysis of Randomized Controlled Trials." *American Journal of Gastroenterology* 114, no. 2 (2019): 233–243.

Tack, Jan, Peter Janssen, Tatsuhiro Masaoka et al. "Efficacy of Buspirone, A Fundus-Relaxing Drug, in Patients with Functional Dyspepsia." *Clinical Gastroenterology and Hepatology* 10, no. 11 (November 2012): 1239–1245.

Wang, Wei Hong, Jia Qing Huang, Ge Fan Zheng et al. "Effects of Proton-Pump Inhibitors on Functional Dyspepsia: A Meta-Analysis of Randomized Placebo-Controlled Trials." *Clinical Gastroenterology and Hepatology* 5, no. 2 (February 2007): 178–185.

Wei, Z., X. Xing, X. Tantai et al. "The Effects of Psychological Interventions on Symptoms and Psychology of Functional Dyspepsia: A Systematic Review and Meta-Analysis." *Frontiers in Psychology* 13 (April 2022): 827220.

Wei, Z., X. Yang, X. Xing et al. "Risk Factors Associated with Functional Dyspepsia in Chinese Children: A Cross-sectional Study." *BMC Gastroenterology* 21 (2021): 218.

Yang, Jing-Wen, Li-Qiong Wang, Xuan Zou et al. "Effect of Acupuncture for Postprandial Distress Syndrome: A Randomized Clinical Trial." *Annals of Internal Medicine* 172, no. 12 (June 16, 2020): 777–785.

FOOD POISONING

INTRODUCTION

Food poisoning or foodborne illness occurs when a person eats or drinks a food or beverage that is contaminated; the food or drink is infected with a toxic organism, such as a bacterium, fungus, parasite, or virus. When a toxic substance is consumed, the body attempts to remove it forcefully by vomiting, diarrhea, or both. It is not uncommon to also develop a fever. These are the body's attempts to restore itself to good health.

Food may become contaminated during any stage of the food production process—from harvesting to transportation to storage to cooking to preparation to serving. Contamination may occur when food is not fresh, not washed well, not handled in a safe manner, not cooked for a sufficient amount of time at the correct temperature, not served in a safe and proper way, or not refrigerated or frozen in a timely manner.

Responses to the toxin vary according to the type of toxin. In some cases, people begin feeling ill within minutes or hours. In other cases, it may take days or even weeks.

Though there are more than 250 specific types of food poisoning, there are several common types. Perhaps the most well known is Salmonella, which is most often found in raw eggs and undercooked poultry. But, it has also been found in other foods such as meats, milk and other dairy products, salads, cream-filled baked goods, and sandwich fillings. Campylobacter is a bacterial infection that causes severe upper gastrointestinal upset and may continue for weeks. Common causes are undercooked poultry, meats, or eggs, poorly processed meats, contaminated vegetables, and raw milk or water. It may also spread via cross-contamination. E. coli may be found in meat, unpasteurized milk or juice, soft cheeses from unpasteurized milk, fresh fruits and vegetables, contaminated water, and feces of infected people. Listeria is contained in hot dogs, luncheon meats, unpasteurized milk, soft cheeses from unpasteurized milk, refrigerated smoked fish, refrigerated patés or meat spreads, and fresh fruits and vegetables. Norovirus may be in shellfish, fresh fruits and vegetables, ready-to-eat foods such as salads and sandwiches handled by people with the virus, and food or water contaminated with vomit or feces of a person with the virus. And, Shigella bacteria are found in uncooked vegetables, shellfish, and cream or mayonnaise-based salads. It may cause blood or mucus in diarrhea, which is why it is sometimes termed bacillary dysentery. Staphylococcus may produce a toxin that causes the sudden onset of nausea and vomiting. It usually occurs when food handlers contaminate the food, especially dairy, meat, eggs, and salads.

The infections associated with food poisoning may spread from one person to another through tiny amounts of vomit or stool that linger on surfaces or fingers and then transfer to another person's food or mouth. That is why meticulous handwashing must be practiced whenever food poisoning is suspected.

While anyone may become ill with food poisoning, some people are at greater risk than others. These include children, pregnant women, the elderly, or anyone who may have a weakened immune system, and people who are generally in poorer health. Healthier people may experience such mild symptoms that they are unaware they are dealing with a toxic food or drink. Still, just about everyone knows a strong, healthy, younger person who has suffered a debilitating case of food poisoning.

Since the earliest of times, people have had to deal with food poisoning. In fact, researchers believe that there were cases during the Stone Age. It has been suggested that the first documented case may be traced back to 323 BC when Alexander the Great is believed to have died from typhoid fever, which was caused by salmonella typhi.[1]

SYMPTOMS, RISKS, AND COMPLICATIONS

The most common symptoms of food poisoning include nausea, vomiting, diarrhea with or without bloody stools, stomach pain, stomach cramps, headache, weakness, and fever. Other less common symptoms include blurred or double vision, loss of movement in limbs, swallowing problems, weakness, tingling or numbness of the skin, and changes in the sound of the voice.

Several improper food handling practices increase the risk of food poisoning. These include poor handwashing, especially after using the bathroom. People who handle food must be extra vigilant with handwashing. Inadequately cleaned counters and utensils are also problematic. Counters must be thoroughly cleaned, and utensils are best cleaned in a dishwasher. And, incorrectly stored food is another notable risk factor. Food left out at room temperature too long may become spoiled, as may food stored too long in the refrigerator. It is even possible for the temperature in the refrigerator to be too warm to completely and adequately cool and preserve the freshness of the food, especially if the refrigerator is malfunctioning.

The most frequent complication associated with food poisoning is severe dehydration or a potentially dangerous loss of water, salt, and minerals. Both vomiting and diarrhea may cause dehydration. People dealing with food poisoning often have a difficult time staying hydrated, especially if they have ongoing nausea and vomiting. Without adequate hydration, they may need to be hospitalized and receive intravenous fluids. Without such an intervention, a person's condition may further deteriorate and result in organ damage and even death. But, there are other food poisoning complications. Thus, the salmonella and campylobacter bacteria may cause joint damage and chronic arthritis. The campylobacter bacteria may cause a neurological disorder called Guillain-Barré syndrome. Listeria is particularly harmful for a developing fetus; it may cause neurological damage and death. And E. coli may result in hemolytic uremic syndrome and kidney failure. That is exactly what occurred in a 2024 outbreak at scores of different McDonald's restaurants in the United States. Apparently, they had been sent tainted food from a supplier.

PREVALENCE

In the United States, and in fact throughout the world, food poisoning is an incredibly frequent occurrence. It has been estimated that in the United States about one in every six people is annually sickened. That means that each year, about forty-eight million people become ill, 128,000 are hospitalized, and 3,000 die.[2] In all probability, many of these cases are preventable.

DIAGNOSIS AND TREATMENT OPTIONS

If a healthcare provider suspects food poisoning, he or she will ask about food or drink that has recently been consumed. This discussion will generally point to a few highly probable possibilities. Did the patient eat uncooked or poorly cooked food? Attend an outside picnic in hot weather? Was the food left outside for more than a few hours? Did last night's dinner have food that was used beyond the expiration date? And, what about the raw fish in the sushi? Wasn't it placed a little too close to the fresh cantaloupe slices? In any case, to check for specific bacteria or parasites, the healthcare provider may well order blood and/or stool tests.

Outside the hospital setting, food poisoning treatment tends to focus on trying to stay hydrated. In many cases, a form of hydration that has balanced electrolytes is advised. These are sold in pharmacies and in many food stores. One example is Pedialyte, which may be used by children and adults. Some types of food poisoning need to be treated with antibiotics, but antidiarrheal medicines are usually not advised, other than an over-the-counter medicine such as Pepto Bismol (bismuth subsalicylate).

While the body is healing, it may be best to refrain from eating a normal diet. Instead, consume foods such as fruit juice, ice pops, and gelatin. When it is time to reintroduce food, eat small amounts of bland foods, such as broth and crackers or unbuttered toast. The water and sodium in the broth are good for rehydration, and the crackers and toast add a small amount of nutrition. Certain foods may worsen the symptoms associated with food poisoning. These include high-fiber foods, dairy, spicy foods, and high-fat foods. Avoid these for at least several days.

It is important to note that the vast number of food poisoning cases are short-lived—no more than a few days. That is how long it takes for the body to purge itself of the infection. And, though those few days may be miserable, complications are rare. However, if larger amounts of toxin have been consumed, if a person has a weakened immune system, or if the ingested toxin needs a specific treatment, such as an antibiotic, it may require a healthcare provider visit and more time. Fortunately, truly serious cases of food poisoning are uncommon.

RESEARCH FINDINGS

In the United States, Leafy Greens Are a Source of Foodborne Illness

In a study published in the *Journal of Food Protection*, researchers from Columbus, Ohio, analyzed the extent to which leafy greens are a source of foodborne illness in the United States. In this study, the researchers combined results from three outbreak-based models with illness incidence and economic costs. From this data, they determined that up to 9.18 percent of foodborne illnesses in the United States are linked to leafy greens. That means that every year in the United States, as many as 2,307,558 cases of food poisoning are caused by leafy greens, such as iceberg and romaine lettuce. Among the most prevalent toxins were norovirus, Shiga toxin-producing *E. coli*, *Salmonella*, and *Campylobacter*. And, according to these researchers, the annual economic costs of these illnesses are estimated to be up to $5.278 billion, "emphasizing the significant burden on healthcare and productivity due to the consumption of contaminated leafy greens."[3]

In the United States, the Annual Costs of Foodborne Illness Are High

In a study published in the *Journal of Food Protection*, a researcher from Columbus, Ohio, who was also a researcher in the previous study, discussed the financial costs associated with all foodborne illness cases. Since the study was published more than a decade ago, it should be assumed that these numbers have increased markedly. According to this researcher, it may be conservatively estimated that the average cost of each foodborne illness is $1,149, which leads to an overall annual economic burden of $55.5 billion. Another less conservative figure put the costs at $93.2 billion. Whatever the actual costs, they are extraordinarily high. Still, as might be expected, the costs vary from location to location. The reasons for this variation, according to this researcher, include differences in the incidence of illness, differences in medical and productivity costs, and differences in welfare losses caused by death and lost quality of life. Thus, using a conservative model, the researcher found that the average cost per case in West Virginia was $888 and $1,766 in the District of Columbia. A less conservative model found the average cost per case to be $1,505 in Kentucky and $2,591 in Maryland.[4] Again, these costs are probably considerably lower than they are now. In the intervening years, they may have risen by many billions of dollars.

A Foodborne Illness Outbreak in a Restaurant May Take a Huge Financial Toll

In a study published in the journal *Public Health Reports*, researchers from Baltimore, Maryland, wanted to estimate the costs restaurants may face from an outbreak of foodborne illness. So, they developed a computational simulation model which included various scenarios depending on the outbreak size, the pathogen, the type of restaurant, the amount of lost revenue, and the costs of lawsuits, legal fees, and insurance premium increases. From the calculations, the researchers estimated that the cost of a single foodborne illness outbreak ranged from $3,968 to $1.9 million for a fast food restaurant, $2.1 million for a fast-casual restaurant, $8,030 to $2.2 million for a casual dining restaurant, and $8,273 to $2.6 million for a fine dining restaurant. These costs varied from one in which there were a minimum of problems, such as five people involved with no lost revenue, lawsuits, or legal fees, to a large problematic situation such as a 250-person outbreak with high lost revenues and high amounts of lawsuits and legal fees. The most expensive outbreaks were caused by Listeria and the least expensive ones were from Bacillus cereus. These costs represented ten to 5,790 percent of a restaurant's annual marketing costs and 0.3 to 101 percent of annual profits and revenues. The largest costs were from lawsuits and legal fees, outbreak size, and lost revenue. The researchers commented that their findings might help restaurant owners determine how much they should invest in order to improve their infection-control measures. And, the researchers concluded that "a single foodborne illness outbreak can incur substantial costs, enough to compose a large portion of a restaurant's annual profits. Many of these costs outweigh the costs of various infection prevention and control measures that are available to restaurants."[5]

Additional Training Appears to Improve the Amount of Information and Knowledge but Not the Safety Practices of the Food Handlers in Restaurants

In a study published in the journal *Nutrition Research and Practice*, researchers from Korea wanted to determine if additional training would improve the knowledge and safety practices of the people who handle food in restaurants. Twelve restaurants participated in this study; they were divided into two groups—seven small franchise restaurants received training and five Korean-style restaurants did not. Questionnaires and trained panelists evaluated employee knowledge and practices before and after the training program. Before the training, the level of knowledge between the groups was similar. The ratio of males to females was about one to two, and 41.5 percent of the intervention group and 53.1 percent of the control group had graduated from high school. The majority listed their work experience as either one year or less or more than four years. The researchers determined that the level of knowledge about food safety improved significantly more in the intervention group than the control group. However, employee practices and sanitation performance did not improve. As a result, the researchers concluded that there, "more job-specific and hand-on training materials for restaurant employees should be developed and more continuous implementation of the food safety training and integration of employees appraisal with the outcome of safety training were needed."[6]

Parents in Palestine Have a Basic Knowledge about Food Safety Practices, but Could Use More Education

In a cross-sectional trial published in the journal *BMC Public Health*, researchers from Palestine evaluated the knowledges, attitudes, and practices related to food poisoning among parents of the children in Nablus, Palestine. During 2015, data were collected using structured questionnaire interviews in primary healthcare centers in Nablus. Slightly over 400 parents were interviewed; almost all of them were mothers. The mean age of the subjects was 29.62 years, and more than half of them lived in the city. Almost 80 percent were unemployed, and they reported that they, as mothers, were responsible for food preparation. The vast majority appeared to have basic knowledge about foodborne illness. For example, when asked about higher-risk foods for food poisoning, they knew that eating raw or half-cooked food, such as raw vegetables, poorly cooked eggs, and raw milk, was potentially dangerous. Further, they generally knew the importance of washing fruits and vegetables and refrigeration. And, about two-thirds were aware that food handlers without clinical symptoms could still contaminate food. But, only 49 percent correctly agreed that some toxins that cause food poisoning are resistant to heating. Overall, the researchers found that the subjects with higher levels of education and those who lived in cities had significantly more knowledge about foodborne illness and food safety. The researchers determined that the subjects generally had a good deal of knowledge, a good attitude, and good hygienic practices. And, there was a significant positive association between their knowledge and practice. Those who knew more about foodborne illness and food poisoning had better food handling and preparation practices. The researchers concluded that "educational programmes or campaigns should start with parental awareness regarding the direct hazards to their family health from food poisoning, as by realising their susceptibility to food poisoning, their motivation to change becomes stronger and beneficial, as parents are more likely to change their behaviours as long as it benefits their children."[7]

Students of Dietetics and Food Handlers Need to Improve Some of Their Actions and Attitudes to Prevent Food Poisoning

In a cross-sectional trial published in the *Journal of Pharmacy and BioAllied Sciences*, researchers from Malaysia analyzed the food-related knowledge, attitudes, and practices of students of dietetics and food handlers in a public university in Malaysia. A self-administered questionnaire was distributed to 106 students and food handlers; it had four sections—sociodemographic, knowledge, attitude, and practice. Data were collected from February 17, 2016, to February 26, 2016. The cohort included fifty-three students of dietetics and fifty-three food handlers. Both groups had more females than males. The subjects ranged in age from eighteen to fifty-one years, with a mean age of 27.14 years. The researchers learned that the subjects generally had good knowledge about safe food practices, but they had a "poor attitude" about food poisoning. The scores for the students tended to be better than those for the food handlers. Thus, 98.1 percent of the students and 52.8 percent of the food handlers identified salmonella as a cause of food poisoning, and 94.3 percent of the students and 52.8 percent of the food handlers were aware that raw eggs could cause food poisoning. And, all of the students and 90 percent of the food handlers knew that vomiting and diarrhea were symptoms of food poisoning. But, only about half of all of the subjects realized that slices of honeydew, baked potato, leftover turkey, and chocolate cake kept overnight on the counter and eaten may cause food poisoning. It was very concerning to realize that only 52.8 percent of the students and 86.8 percent of the food handlers always washed their hands with soap and water after using the bathroom. Clearly, both of these groups should be more aware of the need to wash their hands for food safety. On the other hand, almost everyone washed fresh fruits and vegetables before eating. The researchers concluded that their findings may help to develop "effective methods to promote better understanding about FP [food poisoning] and improving their knowledge and awareness."[8]

Students in Saudi Arabia Also Need to Learn More about Foodborne Illness

In a cross-sectional trial published in the *International Journal of Food Science*, a researcher based in Saudi Arabia noted that awareness about foodborne pathogens may help reduce the incidence of foodborne illnesses. That is why he wanted to determine the level of knowledge that students had about this public health problem. The cohort consisted of 399 university students from four major cities in Saudi Arabia—Abha, Dammam, Jeddah, and Riyadh. A little more than half of the students were female. About one-quarter were younger than twenty years, with the majority between the ages of twenty and thirty years. More than three-quarters were enrolled in a bachelor's level program. The subjects were questioned about five major microbial pathogens—Salmonella, Campylobacter, Staphylococcus, Listeria, and E. coli. Using questionnaires, data were collected through interviews with trained personnel. Each questionnaire took about ten to twenty minutes to complete. The researcher learned that only 34.5 percent of the students knew about these pathogens. Awareness varied according to the pathogen, and the differences seemed to be related to age, sex, education, and field of study. So, as might be expected, computer science students knew less about these pathogens than students in the health sciences. Female students were more knowledgeable than the males. Still, the researcher commented that the students had a generally poor knowledge about foodborne illnesses. The researcher noted "that there is a need for health education programs for students, especially those emphasizing foodborne pathogens." Further, "there is a need to conduct food safety education programs for university students to improve their level of awareness about foodborne pathogens."[9]

Emergency Room Physicians Should Learn More about Illness from Foodborne Disease

In a descriptive, cross-sectional trial published in the journal *Cureus*, researchers from Qatar and Egypt noted that in Qatar, foodborne illnesses are among the top ten events reported to the Ministry of Public Health. And, efforts to increase the surveillance of these illnesses may not be accomplished without the involvement of emergency departments. That is why the researchers wanted to learn if the emergency department physicians knew a sufficient amount about collecting stool samples from people who may have a foodborne illness. The data were gathered in the emergency department of Hamad General Hospital in Qatar in 2018. Sixty-five physicians completed a four-part questionnaire, a response rate just under 30 percent. Less than half of the physicians were specialists; almost two-thirds graduated between 2000 and 2013, with the earliest graduate from 1983 and the latest being in 2017. Almost all had worked at the hospital for one or more years. Eighty-four percent noted that they had seen a patient with acute diarrhea in the emergency department during the previous month. Eighty percent said that a stool culture is needed for patients reporting acute bloody diarrhea and a fever. Seventy-five percent identified specific pathogens, such as salmonella, as pathogens of diseases. But, for various reasons, such as the fact that it would not alter disease management, 72 percent who had a patient with acute diarrhea did not order a stool culture, and 62 percent who ordered a stool culture did not learn the results. At the same time, when taking a history of a patient with acute diarrhea, all of the physicians asked about travel history, 93.6 percent asked about sick contacts, and "a large percentage" asked about associated symptoms such as abdominal pain, fever, and bloody stools. The researchers concluded that there were clearly "several gaps regarding the knowledge and practice of emergency physicians toward the surveillance of foodborne disease."[10]

Street Food Vendors in Bangladesh Have Inadequate Food Safety Knowledge and Hygiene Practices

In a cross-sectional study published in the journal *Scientific Reports*, researchers from Bangladesh, Abilene, Texas, and Sweden evaluated the food safety knowledge and hygiene practices of street food vendors in Dhaka, Bangladesh, the capital city of the country. The cohort consisted of 350 subjects in seven areas of Dhaka. Trained data collectors gathered data during in-person interviews with street vendors using a pretested questionnaire. Most of the questions had yes, no, or don't know answers. The survey questions consisted of thirteen items that measured information on handwashing, eight items on gloves, nineteen questions about foodborne illnesses, and ten items on the types of health problems that can affect food safety. Ninety-eight percent of the vendors were male, with 48 percent having a secondary education and a notable 85 percent having no food safety training. They were primarily young adults between the ages of twenty-five and thirty-four years. Slightly more than half worked as chefs, 7.3 percent were cleaners, 23.3 percent were cutters, and 8.2 percent were food servers. For about three out of four of the vendors, selling food on the street was their primary job. Although about 89 percent of the vendors practiced some degree of handwashing, only 5.6 percent wore gloves when handling raw foods. An even smaller number wore gloves when cleaning tables, preparing foods, or handling garbage. Yet, 90 percent reported having some experience with foodborne illnesses and knew the signs and symptoms of these diseases. Although 45 percent said that they would stop working immediately if they became ill, almost one-fifth noted that they would continue working. The researchers found an association between educational levels and work experience with handwashing practices, use of gloves, and knowledge about foodborne illnesses. Why is this important? Because, according to the researchers, "numerous studies have consistently identified food handlers as the main contributors to foodborne diseases by using improper handling practices." Their findings may be useful "to develop intervention efforts [such a training programs in food safety practices] in street foods and prevent foodborne disease."[11]

Older Consumers Do Not Necessarily Have Adequate Knowledge about Foodborne Illnesses

In a systematic review and meta-analysis published in the journal *Food Control*, researchers from Canada noted that people over the age of sixty years, who tend to have weakened immune systems and may well have chronic medical problems, are at increased risk for foodborne illnesses. That is why it is important for them to be well-versed on this topic. The researchers located fifty-seven relevant studies published between 1996 and 2018. Most of the studies were journal articles that used a cross-sectional design and were published in the United States, and most reported on food safety behaviors and knowledge outcomes.

The researchers were primarily interested in information on people who prepare food for themselves and others in the household, as well as people who live independently but receive meals from outside, such as a meal delivery service. The researchers learned that the subjects tended to refrigerate their food in a timely manner. On the other hand, there was a good deal of variability in handwashing, both before and after preparing food and when rinsing raw meat and storing it in the refrigerator. In general, the subjects did not monitor the temperature of their refrigerators. But, they tended to be careful about defrosting foods in the refrigerator and not at room temperature, as well as checking the "use-by" and "best-before" dates on the label. However, the subjects were not sufficiently aware of the pathogen Listeria and the safe operating temperatures of refrigerators. And, they all too often ate undercooked eggs. The researchers noted that future studies should investigate whether older adults are eating foods with a high risk of foodborne illnesses, such as seafood, deli meat, unpasteurized milk, and soft cheeses, and the frequency with which they consume these foods. In addition, there need to be "interventions and education campaigns [that] focus on increasing knowledge of Listeria and improving food safety refrigeration practices."[12]

Certain Practices Increase the Risk of Foodborne Illness in the Home Setting

In a study published in the journal *Foods*, researchers from Italy examined certain at-home practices that placed people at increased risk for food poisoning. The researchers recruited fourteen households who lived in the Italian provinces of Padua, Bologna, and Venice.

Families with more vulnerable members, such as pregnant women, children, and people over the age of sixty years, were included. In the home settings of the families, the researchers observed the everyday practices of the family members in October and November 2019, primarily at the activities associated with lunch and dinner, with an average duration of two hours per visit. Each family was visited by two observers who gathered the data. The first observer focused on recording the actions related to the handling, cooking, and storage of food. The second observer examined the organization and management of domestic space, work tools, and family dynamics. In addition, photos were taken of specific sources of risk in the kitchen, such as the arrangement of work surfaces, products, and areas outside and inside refrigerators, freezers, cabinets, and drawers. A total of twenty-eight diaries, fourteen kitchen maps, fourteen photographic sets of domestic refrigerators, and many photographs of potential risk situations were collected. The researchers learned that thirteen of the fourteen families had inappropriate handwashing and handling of food; eleven had inappropriate washing of utensils, work surfaces, and food. Eleven families used towels and sponges improperly and had objects unrelated to the preparation of food, such as keys, wallets, bags, books, and games in the kitchen. Seven families had food stored in unsuitable containers or materials, and five families had problematic conservation practices, such as placing food in the wrong section of the refrigerator, and they overcooked food, which may cause chemical food hazards such as the development of carcinogenic substances. Three families did not manage their children and pets properly; the pets were allowed to eat from the plates of the children. And one family's food preparation was contaminated by detergent, which probably contained chemicals. The researchers noted that all of these problems facilitate food-related microbiological risks in the kitchen, and they commented that family members tend to rely on their senses, such as sight and smell, to determine if food is safe to eat. The family members expressed particular concern about chemicals in foods, such as dyes, preservatives, and pesticides. As a result, they preferred to buy from neighbors, friends, and traditional shops and markets closer to home. The researchers concluded that their findings "suggest that the adoption of appropriate food practices is not always related to risk knowledge." And, "the most frequently found inadequacies are those related to microbiological risks."[13]

Food Provided through a School Lunch Program May Make Children Ill

In an article published in the *Journal of Food Protection*, researchers from several locations in the United States but based in Atlanta, Georgia, investigated a food poisoning outbreak that occurred in three North Dakota schools following lunches that contained burritos. The illness included the symptoms of nausea, headache, abdominal cramps, vomiting, and/or diarrhea that began after lunch at the elementary, middle, and high schools in a rural town in North Dakota. The three schools served similar food. Most children ate the same foods because the same six food items were placed on every child's lunch tray. Five hundred and four students and staff experienced these symptoms as quickly as thirty-five minutes after lunch, and the median duration of the illness was 6.2 hours. At the elementary school, the fire department was called to hose down the school playground, which was filled with the children's vomit. Thirty-eight children were sent to the local hospital emergency department. No one was hospitalized or died. Since the various burritos had different fillings, the researchers determined that the source must be the actual burritos. No definitive answers were obtained from plant inspections, tracebacks, and laboratory tests. Still, more than 2 million pounds of burritos were recalled or withheld from distribution. The researchers commented that "the short incubation period and the symptoms of the illness suggest that a preformed toxin or other short-acting agent that targets the stomach or upper intestine is the etiologic agent." Apparently, the burritos had been shipped before an appropriate cooling period which "may have provided an environment that allowed the causative agent to flourish."[14]

Parents Sometimes Pack Lunches That May Easily Become Sources of Food Contamination

In a trial published in the journal *Pediatrics*, researchers from Texas wanted to learn if the temperature of the foods packed in lunches for children was kept sufficiently cold. As a result, they decided to measure the lunches of preschool children who attended child care centers. All of the parents of children ages three to five who were in full-time child care at nine central Texas centers were invited to take part in the trial. Two of the centers were small and the others were far larger. Two hundred and thirty-five parent/child dyads volunteered to participate. Over the course of the three-day study, there were a total of 705 lunches. About 91 percent were packed in thermally insulated plastic bags. Although three centers used refrigerators, teachers often failed to place the lunches in them and left the lunches at room temperature. The temperature of food packed by the parents for their child's lunch was individually measured 1½ hours before being served to the children. All of the lunches contained at least one perishable item. Yet, about 39 percent of the lunches had no ice packs. Slightly more than 45 percent had a single ice pack. In some cases, frozen teething rings and drink boxes were used as ice packs. Almost all of the lunches were found to be at unsafe temperatures. Even when multiple ice packs were used, more than 90 percent of the lunch items were at unsafe temperatures. When measured, 97.4 percent of the meats, 99 percent of the dairy, and 98.5 percent of the vegetables were not at acceptable temperatures. Of the 1631 perishable food items that the researchers tabulated, only twenty-two were at an acceptable temperature range. The researchers concluded that there is an obvious need for further training on how to pack children's lunches. "Education of parents and the public must focus on proper methods of packing lunches that allow the food to remain in the food safety zone."[15]

REFERENCES AND FURTHER READING

Al-Mohaithef, Mohammed. "Awareness of Foodborne Pathogens Among Students: A Cross-Sectional Study in the Kingdom of Saudi Arabia *International Journal of Food Science* 2021 (May 2021): 9971748.

Bartsch, Sarah M., Lindsey Asti, Sindiso Nyathi et al. "Estimated Cost to a Restaurant of a Foodborne Illness Outbreak." *Public Health Reports* 133, no. 3 (2018): 274–286.

Chehab, M. A., M. Nour, G. Bryant et al. "Knowledge and Practice of Emergency Physicians Regarding Food-borne Disease Surveillance at Hamad General Hospital in Qatar." *Cureus* 11, no. 6 (2019): e4934.

Islam, S., N. Tanjia, A. K. Mitra et al. "Inadequate Food Safety Knowledge and Hygiene Practices Among Street Food Vendors in Dhaka, Bangladesh." *Scientific Reports* 14 (2024): 17349.

Menini, AL, G. Mascarello, M. Giarette et al. The Critical Role of Consumers in the Prevention of Foodborne Diseases: An Ethnographic Study of Italian Families." *Foods* 11 (2022): 1006.

Mohd Yusof, A. M., N. A. A. Rahman, and M. Haque. "Knowledge, Attitude, and Practice Toward Food Poisoning Among Food Handlers and Dietetic Students in a Public University in Malaysia." *Journal of Pharmacy & BioAllied Sciences* 10, no. 4 (October–December 2018): 232–239.

Park, Sung-Hee, Tong-Kyung, and Hye-Ja Chang. "Evaluation of the Food Safety Training for Food Handlers in Restaurant Operations." *Nutrition Research and Practice* 4, no. 1 (2010): 58–68.

Scharff, Robert I. "States Estimates for the Annual Cost of Foodborne Illness." *Journal of Food Protection* 78, no. 6 (2015): 1064–1071.

Steinberg, Ellen B., Alden Henderson, Adam Karpati et al. "Mysterious Outbreaks of Gastrointestinal Illness Associated with Burritos Supplied through School Lunch Programs." *Journal of Food Protection* 69, no. 7 (July 2006): 1690–1698.

Thaivalappil, A., I. Young, C. Paco et al. "Food Safety and the Older Consumer: A Systematic Review and Meta-Analysis of Their Knowledge and Practices at Home." *Food Control* 107 (2020): 106782.

Yang, X. and R. Scharff. "Foodborne Illnesses from Leafy Greens in the United States: Attribution, Burden, and Cost." *Journal of Food Protection* 87 (2024): 100275.

Zyoud, S. J. Shalabi, K. Imran et al. "Knowledge, Attitude and Practices Among Parents Regarding Food Poisoning: A Cross-Sectional Study from Palestine." *BMC Public Health* 19 (2019): 586.

GALLSTONES

INTRODUCTION

Gallstones are hardened pieces of cholesterol, mucin, and calcium salts of bilirubinate or palmitate. They may appear in the gallbladder, a condition known as cholelithiasis, or in the bile ducts, a condition known as choledocholithiasis. (Chole means bile and lithiasis means stone forming.) While they are often present and do not cause any problems, gallstones may become lodged in the biliary tract and block the flow of bile, a condition which may be extremely painful and potentially dangerous.

There are three types of gallstones; stones made of cholesterol are the most common type. Black pigment stones are made of calcium bilirubinate and are a result of the destruction of blood. Brown pigment stones usually occur when there is a bacterial infection or parasitic infestation of the biliary system. Gallstones range in size from as small as a grain of sand to as large as a golf ball. Some people develop just one gallstone. But, people tend to develop more than one.

The major problem with gallstones is that they grow. While they may begin quite tiny, every time bile washes over them, they slowly and steadily grow. Eventually, gallstones may be large enough to stop the flow of bile, especially if they get caught in a narrow space, such as a bile duct or the neck of the gallbladder.

Although it is impossible to be certain when gallstones first appeared, it is known that they probably date to prehistoric times. It has been shown that people in ancient societies, such as Egypt and Greece, had gallstones. In an article published in the *International Journal of Paleopathology*, researchers from Colombia and Italy noted that gallstones were found in archeological mummies from Colombia.[1]

SYMPTOMS, RISKS, AND COMPLICATIONS

Unless they become lodged and create a blockage, gallstones usually do not cause symptoms. But, a host of different symptoms is associated with larger gallstones that are blocking bile ducts, a medical problem known as a gallstone attack or a gallbladder attack. The two most common symptoms are sudden, severe, right upper abdominal pain, termed biliary colic, and nausea. Other symptoms may include sweating, fever, fast heart rate, drop in blood pressure, fever, chills, indigestion, pain in the right shoulder, pain in the back between the shoulder blades, abdominal swelling and tenderness, intolerance of fatty foods, yellow tint to the eyes and skin (jaundice), and dark-colored urine and light-colored stool. These attacks tend to occur after a meal, especially a fatty meal. Biliary colic may last for only a few minutes or may continue for hours. The episode is over when the stone moves or the pressure somehow eases.

While everyone is theoretically at risk for gallstones, they are more common in women between the ages of twenty and fifty years, when estrogen may increase the amount of cholesterol in the blood, and in people assigned female at birth. The risk for men increases after the age of sixty. A few conditions and lifestyle factors increase the risk. These include obesity, Crohn's disease, leading a sedentary lifestyle, being pregnant, eating a high-fat diet, eating a high-cholesterol diet, eating a low-fiber diet, rapid weight loss, diabetes, excessive amounts of cholesterol and/or bilirubin in the blood, and the failure of the bile ducts and/or gallbladder to work properly. Taking hormone replacement therapy drugs, especially estrogen, may raise the levels of cholesterol, thereby increasing the risk in some people, though that does not appear to be the case for the hormones from oral contraceptives. Even fasting may be problematic. It decreases the functioning of the gallbladder, which may cause the bile to become overconcentrated with cholesterol. And, there is probably a genetic link; in fact, Native Americans and people of Mexican descent, who tend to have higher levels of cholesterol, have an increased risk.

It is known that when certain people eat a rich, fatty meal, they may easily have a gallstone attack. As the gallbladder squeezes the bile needed to help digest the meal, stones may become trapped. Once a person has had his or her first gallstone attack, he or she is at increased risk for subsequent attacks. Eventually, a gallstone may stay in place; when that occurs, it quickly becomes an emergency situation. Bile that is unable to flow backs up into the bile ducts and organs, causing acute inflammation and fostering the growth of bacteria. Potential complications include cholecystitis (inflammation of the gallbladder), pancreatitis (inflammation of the pancreas), cholangitis (inflammation of the bile duct), hepatitis (inflammation of the liver), jaundice (bilirubin in the blood), and septicemia (infection of the blood).

PREVALENCE

At least 10 percent of the population of the United States has gallstones. Up to 75 percent of them are females and people assigned female at birth. But, only 20 percent of those diagnosed with gallstones will have symptoms or require treatment. While people throughout the world have gallstones, it is known that rates vary in different countries. Thus, the Swedes and Chileans have high rates of gallstones, and the Japanese have low rates. The prevalence rates are extremely low in some African societies.[2]

DIAGNOSIS AND TREATMENT OPTIONS

People who appear to be having gallstone symptoms may have blood tests to look for inflammation, infection, and jaundice, and imaging tests to locate a blockage in the biliary tract. The imaging tests will probably begin with a transabdominal ultrasound, which may easily locate gallstones in and near the gallbladder. This is considered the most useful test to detect gallstones. When that test is inconclusive, other imaging tests, such as an endoscopic ultrasound, may be ordered. During this test, which is conducted as part of an upper endoscopy, a medical provider views the stomach lining and gallbladder. In certain patients, a cholescintigraphy (HIDA scan) may be used to rule out cholecystitis. The HIDA scan uses an injectable chemical called a radioactive tracer to take images.

Most often, problematic gallstones require a cholecystectomy or the surgical removal of the gallbladder. Today, it is a common laparoscopic procedure. Most people never again need treatments for gallstones. After the gallbladder is removed, bile flows unimpeded from the liver to the small intestine. Some people do develop a type of chronic diarrhea. This is caused by bile flowing continuously in the intestines, and it is treatable with bile acid binders. If surgery is not advised, a cholecystostomy may be performed. In this procedure, a catheter is placed in the gallbladder to drain the stones. There are medications for gallstones, such as ursodiol and chenodiol. But, they are only useful for very small stones, and it may take a long time for them to work. On occasion, they may be used to prevent the formation of gallstones. Thus, someone who plans to lose weight very quickly may be prescribed one of these medications to prevent the formation of gallstones.

RESEARCH FINDINGS

A "Healthy" Dietary Intake May Lower the Risk of Gallstones

In a hospital-based, case-control study published in the *International Journal of Preventive Medicine*, researchers from Iran evaluated the association between dietary intake and gallstones. The cohort consisted of 110 patients with gallstones confirmed by ultrasonography. The 230 control subjects were patients admitted to other wards of the hospital for medical problems such as traumas and orthopedic conditions; they were matched based on age and sex. The average age for the gallstone group and controls was 57.66 and 56.00 years, respectively. The researchers used a semi-quantitative food frequency questionnaire to evaluate the frequency of food consumption during the previous year. Food items on the questionnaire were categorized into twenty-eight food groups. The researchers characterized a healthy dietary pattern to contain higher amounts of vegetable oils, vegetables, fruits, fish, legumes, and nuts and a low consumption of hydrogenated fats and salt. And, they described an unhealthy dietary pattern to have higher amounts of artificial juice, processed meats, refined grains, sweets and desserts, pickles, snacks, and red meats. The researchers determined that people in the highest levels of the healthy diet were significantly less likely to have gallstones. At the same time, the unhealthy diet appeared to increase the incident cases of gallstones. The researchers commented that their study "was among the few studies to evaluate the association of dietary patterns with risk of gallstones conducted among Iranian population."[3]

Higher Dietary Fiber Intake Is Associated with a Lower Risk of Gallstones

In a case-control study published in the journal *BMC Gastroenterology*, researchers from Iran wanted to determine if a higher intake of fiber would reduce the risk of developing gallstones. The cohort consisted of 189 patients with newly diagnosed gallstones and 342 age-matched controls. Dietary intakes were assessed with a 168-item semi-quantitative food frequency questionnaire. The patients with gallstones had a higher mean age, consumed more fat, and were more likely to be female; they were less physically active and consumed less total, soluble, and insoluble dietary fiber. In fact, there was an inverse association between the consumption of total, soluble, and insoluble dietary fiber and the risk of gallstones. People who consumed the most total, soluble, and insoluble fiber had the least risk for gallstones. "Comprehensive assessment of the associations of dietary fiber intake with GSD [gallstone disease] showed that higher intakes of dietary fiber were significantly associated with reduced GSD risk."[4]

Physical Activity May Reduce the Risk of Symptomatic Gallstones

In a prospective study published in the *European Journal of Gastroenterology & Hepatology*, researchers from the UK evaluated the ability of physical activity to reduce the risk of symptomatic gallstones. The initial cohort consisted of 25,639 volunteers, between the ages of forty and seventy-four years, who were recruited into the European Prospective Investigation of Cancer (EPIC), Norfolk. They completed a questionnaire about occupational and recreational physical activity. Participants were then placed in one of four physical activity groups—inactive, moderately inactive, moderately active, and active. The cohort was monitored over fourteen years for symptomatic gallstones. By the time the researchers conducted their analyses, the cohort had 24,255 participants. The researchers determined that after five years, the highest level of physical activity was associated with a 70 percent reduction in the risk of symptomatic gallstones. When compared to the inactive group, the risk of gallstones was significantly lower in the active group; and, the findings were similar in men and women. Even those participants who were moderately active or moderately inactive had lower rates of symptomatic gallstones than the participants in the inactive group. Interestingly, the researchers commented that "if the whole population increased their level of physical activity by one category, seventeen percent of symptomatic gallstone disease could be prevented over a five-year period." The amount of physical activity in the highest category was equivalent to either exercising for one hour a day if employed in a sedentary job or exercising for thirty minutes per day if employed in a standing job or working in a heavy manual job. The researchers concluded that their findings "support public health policy to increase exercise in the population to reduce the incidence of symptomatic gallstones, although high levels of physical activity would be needed."[5]

In a systematic review and meta-analysis published in the *Journal of Clinical Gastroenterology*, researchers from China also assessed the relationship between physical activity and the risk of gallstones. They located a total of sixteen studies that comprised nineteen independent reports with approximately 260,000 participants. Of the sixteen studies, there were five case-control studies and eleven, including an abstract from a conference meeting, cohort studies. Of the nineteen independent reports, nine involved only women, six involved only men, and four had men and women. Nine were conducted in the United States, six were conducted in Europe, three in Asia, and one in Australia. The researchers found that the studies consistently found that increasing levels of physical activity resulted in lower levels of gallstone risk. "Future research should focus on the dose-response relationship between physical activity and gallstone disease risk." And, it needs to address "whether physical activity actually reduces the risk of stone formation or merely reduces the onset of symptoms of the disease."[6]

Both Diet and Physical Activity Seem to Impact the Development of Gallstones

In a population-based, case-control trial published in the *American Journal of Clinical Nutrition*, researchers from Italy and Buffalo, New York, examined the ability of the combination of dietary factors and physical ability to reduce the risk of gallstones. The initial cohort consisted of one hundred newly diagnosed patients with gallstones and 290 randomly selected control subjects who did not have gallstones. The patients and controls lived in Italy, and the gallstones were diagnosed with ultrasonography. Both the patients and controls completed a questionnaire about their usual diet and physical activity during the twelve months before their diagnosis. The researchers learned that, when compared to the controls, the patients with gallstones tended to be older. Their BMIs were higher, and they were more likely to be dealing with diabetes. In addition, the researchers determined that the higher intake of saturated fats and refined sugars may increase the risk of gallstones, while higher intake of monounsaturated fats, fiber from cellulose, and more physical activity may protect against gallstone formation. The researchers concluded that their findings "suggest that a sedentary lifestyle and a diet rich in animal fats and refined sugars and poor in vegetable fats and fibers are significant risk factors for gallstone formation."[7]

There Appears to Be an Association between Hormone Replacement Therapy and Gallstones

In a systematic review and meta-analysis published in the journal *Medicine*, researchers from China reviewed studies on the association between oral contraception, hormone replacement therapy, and gallstones. The researchers located nineteen studies with approximately 556,620 subjects that met their criteria. There were nine case-control studies and ten cohort studies. The age of the subjects ranged from fourteen to eighty years; most of the studies focused on women and oral contraceptives and hormone replacement therapy. Only one study addressed estrogen use in men being treated for prostatic cancer. The researchers found that oral contraceptives appeared to work against the formation of gallstones, while hormone replacement therapy may significantly increase the risk of gallstones. And, the one study of the use of estrogen in men being treated for prostate cancer found that the estrogen promoted the incidence of gallstones. The researchers observed that most of their included studies were high quality, well designed, and did not have publication bias. The researchers commented that they "demonstrated that HRT [hormone replacement therapy] is a risk factor for cholelithiasis, whereas OC [oral contraception] is not."[8]

After Bariatric Surgery, Caucasians and Females Are at Increased Risk for Gallstones

In a systematic review and meta-analysis published in the journal *Lipids in Health and Disease*, researchers from China wanted to determine what factors place people at increased risk for gallstones after bariatric surgery. They located nineteen articles with 20,553 participants that met their criteria; there were 5,169 male patients and 15,384 female patients. After evaluating a host of different factors, the researchers found that race and sex played a crucial role in which people developed gallstones. For Caucasians and females were far more likely to have this response to weight loss surgery. Other factors, such as smoking, preoperative BMI, type of surgical procedure, hypertension, diabetes mellitus, and dyslipidemia did not appear to have any effect—neither positive nor negative. So, they neither provided any protection from gallstones nor increased the risk of gallstones. As a result, women and Caucasians who undergo bariatric surgery may be advised to take a medication that helps prevent the formation of gallstones.[9]

There Seems to Be an Inverse Association between the Consumption of Coffee and Gallstones in Some Women

In a study published in the journal *Clinical Gastroenterology and Hepatology*, researchers from Sweden evaluated the association between the consumption of coffee and the risk of a cholecystectomy. They used data from 30,989 women and 40,936 men from the Swedish Mammography Cohort and the Cohort of Swedish Men. Baseline information on coffee consumption was collected using a food frequency questionnaire. The participants reported their average daily or weekly consumption of coffee. At baseline, the median coffee consumption was 3.1 cups per day in women and 3.4 cups per day in men. Women and men with the highest coffee consumption were younger, had less education, smoked more cigarettes, and consumed less tea. In women, the high coffee consumers were less likely to have used hormone replacement therapy. During a total follow-up period of 905,933 person-years, the researchers identified 1,057 women and 962 men who had a cholecystectomy. The researchers learned that there was a statistically significant inverse association between coffee consumption and risk of cholecystectomy in women who were premenopausal or used hormone replacement therapy. Each two cup per day increase in coffee consumption was associated with a risk reduction of 19 percent. No such association appeared to exist for other women and men. The researchers commented that their findings "were both in line and in contrast with those see in previous studies, reflecting the conflicting evidence on the association between coffee consumption and risk of gallstone disease."[10]

In a prospective study published in the journal *Gastroenterology*, researchers from Boston, Massachusetts, also assessed the association between the drinking of caffeinated coffee and cholecystectomy. Their cohort consisted of 80,898 married women between the ages of thirty-four and fifty-nine years, who had no history of gallstone disease. They were all participants in the original Nurses' Health Study. During twenty years of follow-up, when there were 1,389,936 person-years of follow-up, 7,811 of the women reported having a cholecystectomy. When the researchers compared the women who consumed no caffeinated coffee to those who consumed varying amounts of coffee, the women consuming caffeinated coffee had consistently fewer cholecystectomies. As the consumption of coffee increased, the risk of cholecystectomy decreased in a linear fashion. Moreover, a consistent intake of four cups or more of coffee per day was associated with a 25 percent risk reduction. The researchers commented that "of the few studies that have examined the relationship between coffee consumption and gallstone disease, most, but not all, are compatible with a decreased risk of gallstone disease in person with high coffee intake."[11]

Alcohol Consumption Seems to Reduce the Risk of Gallstones

In a systematic review and meta-analysis published in the *European Journal of Gastroenterology*, researchers from China assessed the ability of alcohol consumption of alcohol to reduce the risk of gallstone disease. The researchers located ten case-control studies from eight articles and eight cohort studies from seven articles that met their criteria. These studies included 415,747 participants. Eleven of the studies were conducted in Europe, two in Asia, three in America, and two in Oceania. Among the eighteen studies, nine included men and women, five included only women, and four had only men. Nine of the studies showed a statistically significant inverse association between alcohol consumption and the risk of gallstone disease; the rest of the studies showed no statistically significant association. Results from a dose-response analysis showed that the risk of gallstone disease reduced by 12 percent for each 10 g per day increment in alcohol consumption. The researchers concluded that "the association between different types of drink and the risk of gallstone disease should be confirmed by well-designed prospective studies."[12]

People Taking Statin Medications for Longer Periods of Time May Reduce Their Risk of Developing Gallstones

In a systematic review and meta-analysis published in the journal *PeerJ*, researchers from Taiwan evaluated the association between the use of statin medications and the risk of gallstones and cholecystectomy. The researchers located eight studies with 590,086 patients that met their criteria; six were case-control studies and two were retrospective cohort studies. Five studies recruited patients who had cholecystectomy because of gallstone disease, and the other three studies included patients with a diagnosis of gallstone disease. The researchers learned that the use of statins was associated with a marginally significant lower risk of gallstone disease. Further analyses determined that shorter use of statins was associated with a higher risk of gallstone disease in both current and former users. Medium-term current statin users had a significantly lower risk of gallstone disease compared to non-users. Long-term use of statins significantly reduced the risk of gallstone disease in current users, but former users had a comparable risk of gallstone disease compared to non-users. The researchers concluded that "long-term and medium-term use of statins without discontinuation lowered the risk of gallstone disease or cholecystectomy."[13]

In a nested, case-control study published in the journal *Pharmaceuticals*, researchers from Korea also examined the association between the use of statin medications and gallstones. The researchers used data from the Korean National Health Service Health Screening Cohort (2002 to 2019). Among the 514,866 participants, 22,636 were diagnosed with gallstones. The people with gallstones were then matched to 90,544 controls for age, sex, income, and residential area. The people in the gallstone group had higher levels of dyslipidemia than those in the control group. As in the previous study, long-term users of statins, defined in this study as more than 545 days, were associated with a lower likelihood of developing gallstones. Conversely, the short-term use of statins, defined as between 180 and 545 days, did not impact the incidence of gallstones. The researchers commented that their findings appear "to support a potential relationship between statin administration and the decrease of incident gallstones in the adult Korean population."[14]

Even Those Who Are Metabolically Healthy but Have Excess Weight and Obesity Are at Increased Risk for Gallstones

In a cross-sectional study published in the journal *Nutrition & Medicine*, researchers from China examined the relationship between excess weight and increased risk for gallstones in people who are otherwise metabolically healthy. The cohort consisted of 125,668 participants between the ages of eighteen and eighty years. There were 70,915 (56.4 percent) males and 54,753 (43.6 percent) females. The mean age was 43.9 years; the mean BMI was 24.7 for males and 22.4 for females. Each participant had a comprehensive health check-up at a hospital in China, and gallstones were diagnosed with an abdominal ultrasonography. Metabolic health was defined as not meeting the criteria for metabolic syndrome. The researchers determined that 5,486 (4.4 percent) of the participants had gallstones, 21,407 (17 percent) were metabolically healthy overweight individuals, and 3,322 (2.6 percent) were metabolically healthy obese individuals. Participants with gallstones tended to be older and were more likely to have metabolic syndrome. The prevalence of gallstones increased with increasing BMI in both those with and without metabolic syndrome. And, the researchers found that overweight people and people with obesity who were metabolically healthy had a higher risk for gallstones, as well as larger and more numerous gallstones than metabolically healthy normal-weight participants. The researchers concluded that their findings "suggested that obesity per se can increase the risk of gallstones even in relatively metabolically healthy adults."[15]

People with Diabetes Mellitus Seem to Have an Increased Risk of Gallstones

In a population-based cohort study published in the journal *Gastroenterology Review*, researchers from Oman, the United States, and the UK evaluated the association between diabetes mellitus and the risk of gallstones. The researchers used data from the National Health and Nutrition Examination Survey database for the years 2017 to 2018. The final analyses included 5,376 subjects with a mean age of 51.3 years. Females were 51.5 percent of the subjects, and the overall mean BMI was 29.8. Non-Hispanic white was the most common race, with 34.9 percent of the subjects. Almost half of the subjects were married, and about a third had taken some college classes or had earned an associate's degree. Among the included subjects, the prevalence of diabetes was 16.2 percent, with a mean age of 50.6 years when diabetes was diagnosed. Only 4.5 percent were taking insulin. The prevalence of gallstones was 11.2 percent with a mean age of 44.4 years at diagnosis, and 11.3 percent already had a cholecystectomy. After adjusting for all available covariates, the researchers learned that people with diabetes had a 46 percent higher risk of developing gallstones. In addition, people taking insulin were more likely to develop gallstones than those not on insulin medication. And, they concluded that diabetes and insulin "are possible risk factors for developing cholelithiasis."[16]

There Seems to Be an Association between Hypertension and Gallstones but Not between Hypertension and Symptomatic Gallstones

In a cross-sectional study published in *BMC Gastroenterology*, researchers from China assessed the association between gallstones and hypertension or elevated levels of blood pressure. Their cohort consisted of 318,403 men and women who had a physical examination; there were 171,276 (53.8 percent) males and 147,127 (46.2 percent) females. Among the subjects in the cohort, 27,463 (8.6 percent) were diagnosed with gallstone disease; 12,452 (3.9 percent) had gallstones and 15,017 (4.7 percent) had a cholecystectomy. Meanwhile, there were 69,372 (21.8 percent) people diagnosed with hypertension, and 22,106 (6.9 percent) with simple systolic hypertension. The researchers learned that hypertension was significantly associated with the risk of gallstone disease, and this association was stronger in women than in men. As the severity of hypertension increased, so did the risk of gallstone disease. However, hypertension was not significantly associated with cholecystectomy. So, it may be assumed that hypertension was associated with asymptomatic gallstone disease. By the time symptoms appeared and surgery became necessary, the association was no longer significant. The researchers concluded that "more attention should be paid to subjects with hypertension, thus to have better screening and provide clues for studying the pathogenesis of gallstone disease."[17]

REFERENCES AND FURTHER READING

Banim, Paul J. R., Robert N. Luben, Nicolas J. Wareham et al. "Physical Activity Reduces the Risk of Symptomatic Gallstones: A Prospective Cohort Study." *European Journal of Gastroenterology* 22 (2010): 983–988.

Cárdenas-Arroyo, Felipe and Maria Cristina Martina. "Two Findings of Gallstones in Archeological Mummies from Colombia." *International Journal of Paleopathology* 24 (2019): 53–59.

Chang, Yu, Hong-Min Lin, Kuan-Yu Chi et al. "Association Between Statis Use and Risk of Gallstone Disease and Cholecystectomy: A Meta-Analysis of 590,086 Patients." *PeerJ* 11 (April 2023): e15149.

Dai, Yu, Bujiangcun Luo, and Weizheng Li. "Incidence and Risk Factors for Cholelithiasis After Bariatric Surgery: A Systematic Review and Meta-Analysis." *Lipids in Health and Disease* 22 (2023): 5.

Kwon, Mi Jung, Jung Woo Lee, Ho Suk Kang et al. "Association Between Gallstones Disease and Statin Use: A Nested Case-Control Study in Korea." *Pharmaceuticals* 16 (2023): 536.

Leitzmann, Michael F., Meir J. Stampfer, Walter C. Willett et al. "Coffee Intake Is Associated with Lower Risk of Symptomatic Gallstone Disease in Women." *Gastroenterology* 123 (2002): 1823–1830.

Misciagna, G., S. Centonze, C. Leoci et al. "Diet, Physical Activity, and Gallstones – A Population-Based, Case-Control Study in Southern Italy." *American Journal of Clinical Nutrition* 69 (1999): 120–126.

Naseri, Kaveh, Saeede Saadati, Hamid Asadzadeh-Aghdaei et al. "Healthy Dietary Pattern Reduces Risk of Gallstones: Results of a Case-Control Study in Iran." *International Journal of Preventive Medicine* 13 (2022): 66.

Nordenvall, Caroline, Viktor Oskarsson, and Alicja Wolk. "Inverse Association Between Coffee Consumption and Risk of Cholecystectomy in Women But Not Men." *Clinical Gastroenterology and Hepatology* 13 (2015): 1096–1102.

Ratheesh, Rani, Michael T. Ulrich, Sherief Ghazy et al. "The Association Between Diabetes and Gallstones: A Nationwide Population-Based Cohort Study." *Gastroenterology Review* 18, no. 3 (2023): 292–299.

Tehrani, A. N., S. Saadati, Z. Yari et al. "Dietary Fiber Intake and Risk of Gallstone: A Case-Control Study." *BMC Gastroenterology* 23 (2023): 119.

Wang, J., X. Duan, B Li, and X. Jiang. "Alcohol Consumption and Risk of Gallstone Disease: A Meta-Analysis." *European Journal of Gastroenterology* 29, no. 4 (2017): e19–e28.

Wang, Siqi, Yuqiong Wang, Jinming Xu, and Yuxin Chen. "Is the Oral Contraception Or Hormone Replacement Therapy a Risk Factor for Cholelithiasis." *Medicine* 96 (2017): 14 (e6556).

Zhang, Junlu, Liangli Chen, Keqing Shen et al. "Association Between Metabolically Healthy Overweight/Obesity and Gallstones in Chinese." *Nutrition & Metabolism* 20 (2023): 20.

Zhang, Yalan, Li Sun, Xin Wang, and Zongtao Chen. "The Association Between Hypertension and the Risk of Gallstone Disease: A Cross-Sectional Study." *BMC Gastroenterology* 22 (2022): 138.

Zhang, Yan-Peng, Ya-Lei Zhao, Yu-Ling Sun et al. "Physical Activity and the Risk off Gallstone Disease: A Systematic Review and Meta-Analysis." *Journal of Clinical Gastroenterology* 51 (2017): 857–868.

GASTRITIS

INTRODUCTION

Gastritis, a condition in which the lining of the stomach (the mucosa) is red and inflamed, may be caused by a number of different factors. The primary causes include infection due to bacteria, viruses, fungi, or parasites and autoimmune disease. Some authorities contend there are also other causes, such as extreme stress, the longtime use of NSAIDs, such as ibuprofen and naproxen sodium, drinking excess amounts of alcohol, smoking, major surgery, burns, traumatic injury, chemotherapy, trauma, critical illness, radiation, celiac disease, HIV/AIDS, inflammatory conditions such as Crohn's disease, and chronic acid reflux.

Sometimes, medical providers combine the cause of gastritis with the name. Examples are stress-induced gastritis, drug-induced gastritis, alcohol-induced gastritis, infectious gastritis, and autoimmune gastritis. Gastritis that appears suddenly is known as acute gastritis; gastritis that appears over a longer period of time is chronic gastritis. Atrophic gastritis occurs when chronic inflammation leads to the loss of glands in the stomach lining that make stomach acid and enzymes.

The term "gastritis" was first used in 1728 by the German physician Georg Ernst Stahl to describe the inflammation of the inner lining of the stomach. Then, it was considered a histological finding; today, it is known as an actual disorder.

SYMPTOMS, RISKS, AND COMPLICATIONS

While symptoms may vary from person to person, the most common symptoms include stomach upset or pain, belching and hiccups, abdominal bleeding, nausea and vomiting, feelings of fullness and/or burning in the stomach, loss of appetite, heartburn, and blood in the vomit or stool. In some cases, people with gastritis have no symptoms.

The risk of gastritis increases with age; older people have higher risks than younger people. And, infection with Helicobacter pylori (H. pylori) infection significantly increases the risk. It may surprise many that gender, education, alcohol consumption, and family history of gastric cancer do not significantly increase the risk of gastritis.

Gastritis that actually eats away at the stomach lining is called erosive gastritis; it may progress to peptic ulcer disease, which may cause bleeding and lead to anemia. Frequent ulcers may cause scarring, which is problematic if they narrow or block the opening to the small intestine. An ulcer that does not heal may eventually result in a hole all the way through the stomach wall. This allows bacteria and acid from the stomach to escape into the abdominal cavity, a serious condition known as peritonitis, which may in turn lead to a serious infection called sepsis. Gastritis that does not cause any erosive changes is termed nonerosive gastritis. Still, over time, this condition may cause the stomach mucosa to atrophy and lose functionality. This may diminish the body's capacity to absorb vitamin B12 in the intestine, as intrinsic factor, a substance that is produced in the stomach, is needed to complete the process. The resulting problem is called pernicious anemia.

PREVALENCE

Gastritis is believed to be very common. Many people with gastritis probably treat themselves with over-the-counter medicine and never discuss their symptoms with a medical provider. Globally, chronic gastritis is seen in more than 50 percent of the population, usually due to Helicobacter pylori (H. pylori) infection in childhood.[1] In the United States, statistics vary widely. However, it is generally thought that the prevalence of atrophic gastritis is as high as 15 percent of the population.[2]

DIAGNOSIS AND TREATMENT OPTIONS

Various tests may be used to detect gastritis. These include upper gastrointestinal X-rays or a barium swallow, upper endoscopy, blood tests, stool samples that look for bacteria and/or blood, and a breath test that detects the H. pylori bacteria in the stomach.

Treatment options depend on the cause of the gastritis. Generally, healthcare providers treat gastritis with antacids and other over-the-counter and prescription medicines, such as proton pump inhibitors, that reduce stomach acid. These should ease symptoms and help heal the stomach lining. If gastritis is caused by bacteria, such as H. pylori, antibiotics and a proton pump inhibitor will be prescribed. If gastritis is caused by an illness or infection, that problem will be treated. In rare instances, gastritis will be treated with surgery.

RESEARCH FINDINGS

There Appears to Be an Association between Gastritis Symptoms and Eating Habits

In a cross-sectional trial published in the journal *Evidence-Based Complementary and Alternative Medicine*, researchers from China examined the relationship between gastritis symptoms and eating habits. The cohort consisted of 526 adult patients with chronic gastritis who were recruited from three different hospitals in Beijing, China; 346 were female and 180 were male. The mean age of the subjects was forty-nine years, with about 44 percent of the subjects between nineteen and forty-four years. Almost half of the subjects had H. pylori, and over half had a normal body mass index. Either alone or with the assistance of trained medical personnel, all of the subjects completed a detailed fifteen to thirty-minute questionnaire which included questions about their eating habits and gastritis symptoms. The subjects reported that their most common symptoms were stomachache, gastric distension, and hiccup/belching. Over half reported that their symptoms were related to dietary factors. More than 40 percent of the female subjects believed that emotional factors affected their symptoms. Problematic eating habits included eating too fast, irregular mealtimes, irregular meal sizes, eating at restaurants, fried foods, sour foods, snacks, salty foods, barbecues, and eating leftover food. Their most popular foods were sweets, spicy foods, and meat. The researchers learned that many of the symptoms associated with gastritis seemed to be related to "unhealthy eating habits and food preferences, among which irregular mealtimes, salty foods, and sweets are the strongest risk factors." The researchers noted that the male subjects should limit their consumption of alcohol, barbecue, and spicy foods and reduce the frequency of eating outside the home. At the same time, the female subjects should control their intake of sweets. The researchers concluded that their findings "provided evidences that eating habits and food preferences were indeed associated with gastrointestinal symptoms."[3]

There May Well Be an Association between Chronic Atrophic Gastritis, Levels of Serum Vitamin B12, and Peripheral Neuropathy

In a trial published in the *World Journal of Gastroenterology*, researchers from China investigated the relationship between chronic atrophic gastritis, vitamin B12, and peripheral neuropathy. The cohort consisted of 593 subjects—295 males and 298 females—diagnosed with chronic gastritis by a gastroscopy and pathological examination. The patients ranged in age from young adults to senior citizens, with an average age of 46.5 years, and their average BMI was 21.16. A variety of tests, such as gastric acid, serum gastrin, serum vitamin B12, and peripheral nerve conduction velocity, were performed. The researchers determined that 162 of the subjects had peripheral neuropathy, and 431 had no evidence of such a disorder. When compared to the subjects without peripheral neuropathy, the subjects with peripheral neuropathy were older, had higher rates of H. pylori infection, and higher rates of chronic atrophic gastritis. Meanwhile, when compared to the subjects with normal levels of vitamin B12, the subjects with vitamin B12 deficiency were older, had higher rates of H. pylori infection, and higher rates of chronic atrophic gastritis. The researchers determined that vitamin B12 deficiency may be a major risk factor for people with chronic atrophic gastritis and peripheral neuropathy. So, they treated some subjects with atrophic gastritis and H. pylori with vitamin B12. And, they found that treating the subjects with vitamin B12 had the potential to significantly improve the symptoms of peripheral neuropathy. The researchers concluded that vitamin B12 deficiency may be a major risk factor for chronic atrophic gastritis patients with peripheral neuropathy, and chronic atrophic gastritis and H. pylori infection may be risk factors for chronic gastritis patients with vitamin B12 deficiency. At the same time, "this study confirmed that treating the primary disease with the supplementation of vitamin B12 can significantly improve peripheral neuropathy symptoms, suggesting that the timely supplementation of vitamin B12 can prevent or improve CAG [chronic atrophic gastritis] in patients with peripheral neuropathy."[4]

People with Atrophic Gastritis May Be Deficient in Vitamin B12

In a study published in the journal *Gut*, researchers from Australia wanted to learn if people with moderate to severe chronic atrophic gastritis were at increased risk for vitamin B12 deficiency. The cohort consisted of nine men and twenty-one women; their mean age at diagnosis was fifty-six years. The mean duration of the follow-up was nine years, but some subjects were studied for up to fourteen years. The researchers learned that the levels of vitamin B12 tended to fluctuate from month to month, but in the majority of patients, there was a general downward trend. Analysis of the lowest levels of vitamin B12 showed that seven subjects were in the pernicious anemia range, eighteen were in the pre-pernicious anemia range, and five were in the normal range. Yet, the degree of gastric atrophy did not correlate with the serum vitamin B12 levels. Subjects with moderate or severe levels of gastric atrophy tended to have similar levels of vitamin B12. While the subjects generally did not complain, they did experience some symptoms associated with vitamin B12 deficiency, such as increasing weakness, loss of memory, depression, and "flatulent dyspepsia." The researchers noted that there are older people "who suffer chronic atrophic gastritis and resulting vitamin B12 deficiency. This causes distressing symptoms which could be relieved by treatment with vitamin B12."[5]

In a case report published in the journal *Case Reports in Hematology*, researchers from Neptune Township, New Jersey, described a case study of a forty-six-year-old Haitian male with no past medical history who presented with chest pain, fatigue, and progressive weakness, which had been ongoing for a month. As a result of these symptoms, he had experienced reductions in appetite and a subsequent 30-pound weight loss. He also reported constipation. After a medical examination and numerous tests, the man was diagnosed with anemia caused by a vitamin B12 deficiency. Following further testing, including an endoscopy and biopsies of the stomach, the man was also diagnosed with atrophic gastritis. After intramuscular vitamin B12 was initiated, the man improved. Following discharge, he was told to continue taking vitamin B12 supplementation. The researchers commented that "this case highlights both a rare cause and presentation of vitamin B12 deficiency."[6]

People with Chronic Autoimmune Gastritis Seem to Have a Tendency for Vitamin D Deficiency

In a trial published in the journal *BMC Gastroenterology*, researchers from Italy evaluated the relationship between chronic autoimmune atrophic gastritis (CAAG) and vitamin D deficiency. The cohort consisted of eighty-seven people with CAAG with a mean age of sixty-four years; seventy-one were female. A control group had 1,232 healthy subjects—276 males and 956 females with a mean age of 62.3 years. All of the people with CAAG had upper gastrointestinal endoscopies and a variety of blood tests, including testing for levels of serum vitamin D. The researchers determined that thirty-seven subjects had mild gastritis, thirty-four had moderate gastritis, and sixteen had severe chronic gastritis. The researchers determined that the vitamin D levels in the CAAG group were significantly lower than the levels in the control group. In fact, vitamin D deficiency was seen in fifty-seven of the eighty-seven CAAG subjects. And, there was a direct relationship between the level of gastritis severity and the degree of vitamin D deficiency. The researchers commented that "the pathogenic mechanism underlying this association has not been fully elucidated, but it is probably due to a decreased absorption of vitamin D."[7]

In a single-institution observational study published in the journal *Digestive and Liver Disease*, researchers from Milan, Italy, described the micronutrient deficiencies seen in their patients with CAAG. The researchers noted that from January 2005 to January 2016, they saw 122 patients with previously or newly diagnosed CAAG. There were 100 females and twenty-two males ranging in age from twenty-five to ninety years, with a median age of sixty-five. Of these, seventy-six had nutritional deficiencies. Twenty-four patients had a single detected deficiency and fifty-two had multiple deficiencies. The most common deficiency was vitamin D. Mild vitamin D deficiency was found in twenty-four patients, moderate deficiency was found in thirty-five patients, and severe deficiency was seen in seventeen patients. And vitamin D deficiency was not only seen in women over the age of sixty but also in "young patients" or twenty-seven out of the seventy-six patients with vitamin D deficiency. According to the researchers, such a high percentage of patients suggests, "the possible pathogenic role of vitamin D deficiency in the onset and development of CAAG."[8]

People with Gastritis May Benefit from Folic Acid Supplementation

In a systematic review and meta-analysis published in the journal *BMC Gastroenterology*, researchers from China investigated the use of folic acid supplementation to halt or even reverse atrophic gastritis and other potentially gastric precancerous conditions (GPC). The researchers located thirteen studies with 1252 subjects that met their criteria. Eleven were clinical randomized controlled trials, one was a conference report, and one was an unpublished research paper. All of the studies were conducted in China, and the subjects were all Chinese. Eleven of the studies were generally deemed to have a low risk of bias. The researchers learned that when the dose of folic acid was between 20 and 30 mg per day and the treatment duration was continued for three to six months, folic acid had a significant therapeutic effect on the pathological changes of GPC. Moreover, five trials found that folic acid had an even better therapeutic effect when the dose was 30 mg per day and the treatment duration was three months. The researchers concluded that their findings "may provide potential evidence for the clinical application of folate in GPC treatment."[9] (Folate is the natural form of vitamin B9; folic acid is the synthetic form. Though they are different entities, the two terms are often used interchangeably.)

There Seems to Be a Link between Atrophic Gastritis and Colorectal Polyps

In a retrospective study also published in *BMC Gastroenterology*, researchers from China investigated the relationship between atrophic gastritis, H. pylori, and colorectal polyps. The cohort consisted of 792 patients who had a gastroscopy and a colonoscopy; there were 381 males and 411 females. They had a mean age of 54.34 years. Colorectal polyps were diagnosed in 385 patients, and a total of 332 patients were diagnosed with atrophic gastritis. The researchers learned that the number of colorectal polyps in the patients with atrophic gastritis was significantly higher than in the non-atrophic gastritis patients, and a significant difference was observed between the two groups in the number of adenomas and the diameter of the polyps. Further, the incidence and number of polyps correlated with the severity of the atrophy. The researchers concluded that "atrophic gastritis was an independent risk factor for colorectal polyps."[10]

A Diet That Supports Higher Levels of Inflammation Increases the Risk of Gastric Diseases Such as Gastritis

In a population-based cohort study published in the journal *Nutrients*, researchers from Korea and Columbia, South Carolina, United States, evaluated the association between the intake of foods that promote inflammation and gastric diseases, such as gastritis. Specifically, the study examined the association between the dietary inflammation index and the development of gastric diseases at baseline and after a mean follow-up of 7.4 years. The cohort consisted of 144,196 subjects from the Korean Genome and Epidemiology Study_Health Examination (KoGES_HEXA). According to the researchers, this study is defined as "a large prospective cohort study that explores the relationship between genetic, environmental, and lifestyle factors in chronic diseases . . . among Koreans." During the follow-up, the researchers learned that there were 1,571 cases of gastritis—412 males and 1,159 females. The researchers found that people with higher dietary inflammation scores were more likely to be older and overweight and have a lower level of education. They were less physically active, experienced menopause, and had a family history of cancer. There was a statistically significant relationship between a higher inflammatory diet and the risk of gastric disease, especially among females and postmenopausal females. The researchers recommended that the diet focus on anti-inflammatory foods such as whole grains, fruits, vegetables, beans, legumes, and fish and other foods that have abundant amounts of folate, flavonoids, and antioxidants.[11]

Green Tea May Protect against H. pylori Infection and Gastritis

In a cross-sectional study published in the *Journal of Epidemiology*, researchers from Japan wanted to determine if green tea was protective against gastritis. The research was conducted in a farming village in Kyushu, Japan, which was famous for its green tea production. At the time of the study, the total population of the village was slightly over four thousand. The initial cohort consisted of 1,207 residents; they answered questionnaires and gave blood samples. After people were eliminated for a variety of different reasons, the cohort consisted of 636 residents between the ages of thirty and sixty years. The researchers learned that the rates of H. pylori infection in males and females were 48.6 percent and 48.8 percent, respectively. The prevalence of chronic atrophic gastritis in males and females was 33.5 percent and 34.5 percent, respectively. The researchers found a positive association between H. pylori infection and the development of chronic atrophic gastritis. And, they determined that people who drank higher amounts of green tea—more than ten cups per day—had lower rates of chronic atrophic gastritis, even after adjustment for H. pylori infection. The researchers concluded that the consumption of green tea may "play a role in the prevention of CAD [chronic atrophic gastritis] in Japan."[12]

Certain Factors Appear to Be Associated with Gastritis Among University Students

In a cross-sectional trial published in the *American Journal of Theoretical and Applied Statistics*, a researcher from Ethiopia studied the prevalence of gastritis among students in the agriculture college at a university. In addition, the researcher assessed the factors associated with gastritis among this population. The cohort consisted of 174 regular students; there were more than twice as many males as females. Of these, seventy-two students reported having a gastric irritation problem and 102 said they had no such problem. Among the seventy-two with gastric irritation, fifty students developed the problem after entering the university. Twenty-two students arrived at the university with gastric irritation. About 44 percent of those students reading four or more hours per day reported gastric irritation, while 38 percent who said they read less than four hours per day had gastric irritation. Interestingly, 91 percent of the students reported eating at the cafeteria. Among those who said they had gastric irritation, 93.1 percent ate at the cafeteria and 6.9 percent did not. The researcher noted that gastric irritation appeared to be significantly related to the consumption of hot drinks like coffee and tea, and it was also significantly related to anxiety and anti-inflammatory drugs like aspirin and ibuprofen. The researcher recommended that the university and others "create awareness and knowledge for students about the causes of gastritis and the way of treating gastritis before it reaches a chronic level."[13]

People with Gastritis May Consume More Starchy Foods and Fewer Sugary Foods

In a trial published in the journal *Clinical Nutrition Research*, researchers from Korea studied the food and nutrient intake of people with chronic gastritis. With the assistance of personal interviews and various tests, the researchers compared the daily food and nutrient intake, antioxidant indicators in the urine, and blood lipids of nineteen people with chronic gastritis to twenty-seven people with a normal gastroscopy. The two groups were similar in age, height, weight, body mass index, and blood pressure. While the subjects in both groups had similar daily intakes of calories, the mean cholesterol intake of the subjects in the gastritis group was significantly lower than the subjects in the normal group. Further, the subjects with gastritis consumed significantly less sugar and significantly more starchy food, such as potatoes and legumes, than the subjects in the normal group. The serum triglyceride levels of the subjects in the gastritis group were significantly higher than the levels of those in the normal group. There were no significant differences in the urinary oxidative biomarkers between the two groups. The researchers concluded that their findings "indicate a possible relationship between a dietary pattern of chronic gastritis patients and a change in serum lipid levels."[14]

Moderate Alcohol Consumption Is Associated with Reduced Rates of Chronic Atrophic Gastritis

In a study published in the *International Journal of Cancer*, researchers from Germany assessed the association between the consumption of alcohol and chronic atrophic gastritis among older adults in Germany. The researchers used data from ESTHER, a large population-based cohort study of older adults in Germany; initially, they had data on 9,953 participants (45 percent male), between the ages of fifty and seventy-four years, with a mean age of sixty-two years. They were recruited by their general practitioners during a general health check-up in Saarland, a state in southwest Germany. The participants completed a questionnaire and provided blood samples. The final analyses included 9,444 participants, with 4,244 males and 5,200 females, with a mean age of 62.1 years. A notable 4,961 participants were infected with H. pylori and 534 were serologically determined to have chronic atrophic gastritis. The researchers learned that the moderate consumption of alcohol, defined as less than 60 g per week and a lifetime total of 51,376 g or less, was associated with significant decreases in the risk of chronic atrophic gastritis. Though the results were not statistically significant, the consumption of higher amounts of alcohol also reduced the risk of chronic atrophic gastritis. The researchers concluded that the inverse relationship between moderate alcohol consumption and chronic atrophic gastritis may be partially explained by the fact that alcohol eliminates H. pylori. "However," according to the researchers, "mechanisms other than H. pylori infection are likely to contribute to the association as well."[15]

There Are Differences between Older and Younger People with Autoimmune Gastritis

In a study published in the journal *Geriatrics & Gerontology International*, researchers from Turkey compared the symptoms and laboratory parameters of autoimmune gastritis in younger and older age groups. The cohort consisted of 355 patients with autoimmune gastritis. Of these, 119 were sixty-five years old or older and 236 were under the age of sixty-five. The older group, which had seventy women, had a mean age of 69.47 years, and the younger group, which had 158 women, had a mean age of 45.79 years. The gastritis diagnosis had been determined on the basis of several test results, including the histopathological findings in the gastric biopsy tissue. The researchers learned that the elderly subjects were more often investigated for vitamin B12 and/or iron deficiency, and they were more likely to have a vitamin B12 deficiency and pernicious anemia. These findings were far less likely to trigger a gastrointestinal investigation in the younger patients. For them, tests were more often ordered when there were actual upper gastrointestinal symptoms. Further, polyautoimmunity was more common in older subjects, and autoimmune thyroiditis and rheumatoid arthritis were the most common. And, the older subjects had higher rates of significantly prolonged gastric emptying time.[16]

Shift Workers Are More Likely to Have Gastritis Than Non-Shift Workers

In a cross-sectional trial published in the *Scandinavian Journal of Work, Environment & Health*, researchers from Korea evaluated the relationship between shift work and gastritis. The researchers collected questionnaire data from a total of 1,254 subjects; 737 were male and 517 were female. There were 964 non-shift workers and 290 shift workers at an electronics company; they were all between the ages of twenty-two and forty years. (Shift work was defined as night work, rotation work, and/or work during irregular hours.) There was a high percentage of females in the shift workers. One of seven specialists performed the endoscopies, and the results were recorded in the subjects' medical records. The researchers learned that except for nausea and vomiting, gastrointestinal complaints were more common in the shift workers. In particular, indigestion was significantly higher among shift workers. There were more endoscopic findings of gastritis among shift workers than daytime workers, but the difference was not significant. Night shift workers were more likely to have gastritis than day shift workers. Age and the consumption of alcohol were also positively associated with gastritis. The researchers concluded that their findings support the belief "that shift work negatively affects the gastrointestinal system."[17]

There May Be an Association between Gastritis and Osteoporosis

In a cross-sectional trial published in the online journal *PLoS ONE*, researchers from Korea and Honolulu, Hawaii investigated the association between atrophic gastritis and osteoporosis in postmenopausal women sixty years of age or older. The cohort consisted of 401 postmenopausal women who had their routine healthcare in Seoul, Korea. The women had dual-energy X-ray absorptiometry to determine bone mineral density of the lumbar spine, total hip, and femoral neck and an upper gastrointestinal series or endoscopy to look for gastritis and other gastrointestinal problems. The researchers learned that the proportion of women with atrophic gastritis was 56.9 percent in the osteoporotic group and 43.1 percent in the non-osteoporotic group. So, gastritis was more likely to occur in women with osteoporosis. The percentage of H. pylori infections was also higher in the osteoporotic group than the non-osteoporotic group, but the difference was not significant. The researchers concluded that "atrophic gastritis is associated with an increased odds of osteoporosis in elderly women after adjusting for anthropometric, laboratory, and social parameters."[18]

There May Not Be an Association between Gastritis and Colorectal Cancer

In a study published in the journal *Cancer Causes & Control*, researchers from Bethesda and Baltimore, Maryland, and Finland evaluated the relationship between atrophic gastritis and incident colorectal cancer. The cohort consisted of 20,928 Finnish male smokers, between the ages of fifty and sixty-nine years, who were participants in the Alpha-Tocopherol, Beta-Carotene Cancer Prevention Study. They all had tests to measure their levels of serum pepsinogen 1 (SPGI). Subjects with low SPGI levels, which puts them at higher risk for atrophic gastritis, were asked to have a gastroscopy. Of these, 1,059 had a gastroscopy, and atrophic gastritis was confirmed in 1,006 subjects (95 percent). During a mean follow-up of 11.3 years, there were 425 incident cases of colorectal cancer. The incidence rates were 1.82, 1.48, and 1.82 per one thousand person-years of follow-up for participants with normal SPGI, low SPGI, and biopsy-confirmed atrophic gastritis, respectively. Thus, compared to the subjects with normal SPGI, there was no increased risk of colorectal cancer among subjects with low SPGI. The researchers concluded that "the factors that predispose [people] to the development of atrophic gastritis may not increase the risk of colorectal cancer through direct effect on gastric homeostasis."[19]

Cigarette Smoking Seems to Promote Atrophic Gastritis in People with Helicobacter Pylori

In a trial published in the journal *Digestive Diseases and Sciences*, researchers from Japan investigated the relationship between atrophic gastritis, aging, cigarette smoking, and H. pylori. The cohort consisted of 327 patients who had upper endoscopies at a hospital in

Hiroshima, Japan. Two hundred and thirty-one of the patients were H. pylori positive and ninety-six were H. pylori negative. The patients were divided into groups according to their smoking history and age. The researchers determined that both H. pylori infection and aging were "important risk factors" for atrophic gastritis, and smoking promoted atrophic gastritis in patients who were H. pylori positive. Apparently, patients who are H. pylori negative have a significantly lower prevalence of atrophic gastritis.[20]

REFERENCES AND FURTHER READING

Choi, Mi-Kyeong, Myung-Hwa Kang, and Mi-Hyun Kim. "Dietary Intake Assessment and Biochemical Characteristics of Blood and Urine in Patients with Chronic Gastritis." *Clinical Nutrition Research* 4 (2015): 90–96.

Gao, Lei, Melanie N. Weck, Christa Stegmaier et al. "Alcohol Consumption and Chronic Atrophic Gastritis: Population-Based Study Among 9,444 Older Adults from Germany." *International Journal of Cancer* 125, no. 12 (December 2009): 2918–2922.

Gebru, Demisew. "Factors Associated with Gastric Disease Among Students of Hawassa University: The Case of College of Agriculture Students." *American Journal of Theoretical and Applied Statistics* 7, no. 6 (2018): 207–214.

Kalkan, Çagdas and Irfan Soykan. "Differences Between Older and Young Patients with Autoimmune Gastritis." *Geriatrics & Gerontology* 17, no. 7 (July 2017): 1090–1095.

Kim, H. W., Y-H Kim, K. Han et al. "Atrophic Gastritis: A Related Factor for Osteoporosis in Elderly Women." *PLoS One* 9, no. 7 (2014): e101852.

Laiyemo, Adeyinka O., Farin Kamangar, Pamela M. Marcus et al. "Atrophic Gastritis and the Risk of Incidental Colorectal Cancer." *Cancer Causes & Control* 21 (2010): 163–170.

Lee, Sangyoon, Chang Ho Chae, Chulyong Park et al. "Relationship of Shift Work with Endoscopic Gastritis Among Workers of an Electronics Company." *Scandinavian Journal of Work, Environment & Health* 46, no. 2 (March 1, 2020): 161–167.

Lei, Jing, Fugang Ren, Wenyuan Li et al. "Use of Folic Acid Supplementation to Halt and Even Reverse the Progression of Gastric Precancerous Conditions: A Meta-Analysis." *BMC Gastroenterology* 22 (2022): 370.

Li, Yuan, Zeqi Su, Ping Li et al. "Association of Symptoms with Eating Habits and Food Preferences in Chronic Gastritis Patients: A Cross-Sectional Study." *Evidence-Based Complementary and Alternative Medicine* 2020 (2020): 5197201.

Massironi, Sara, Federica Cavalcoli, Alessandra Zilli et al. "Relevance of Vitamin D Deficiency in Patients with Chronic Autoimmune Atopic Gastritis: A Prospective Study." *BMC Gastroenterology* 18 (2018): 172

Nakamura, Masaru, Ken Haruma, Tomoari Kamada et al. "Cigarette Smoking Promotes Atrophic Gastritis in Helicobacter Pylori-Positive Subjects." *Digestive Diseases and Sciences* 47, no. 3 (March 2002): 675–681.

Shao-hua, Zhang, Ren Lin-lin, Su Shen et al. "Atrophic Gastritis Rather Than Helicobacter Pylori Infection Can be An Independent Risk Factor of Colorectal Polyps: A Retrospective Study in China." *BMC Gastroenterology* 23 (2023): 213.

Shibata, Kazunori, Masaki Moriyama, Tetsuhito Fukushima et al. "Green Tea Consumption and Chronic Atrophic Gastritis: A Cross-Sectional Study in a Green Tea Production Village." *Journal of Epidemiology* 10, no. 5 (2000): 310–316.

Sreeja, Sundara Raj, Trong-Dat Le, Bang Wool Eom et al. "Association Between the Dietary Inflammation Index and Gastric Disease Risk: Findings from a Korean Population-Based Cohort Study." *Nutrients* 14 (2022): 2662.

Wood, I. J., M. Ralston, B. Ungar, and D. C. Cowling. "Vitamin B12 Deficiency in Chronic Gastritis." *Gut* 5 (1964): 27.

Woodford, Amanda M., Rabbea Chaudhry, Gabriella A. Conte et al. "Chronic Atrophic Gastritis Presenting as Hemolytic Anemia Due to Severe Vitamin B12 Deficiency." *Case Reports in Hematology* 2021 (2021): 9571072.

Yang, Guo-Tao, Hong-Ying Zhao, Yu Kong et al. "Correlation Between Serum Vitamin B12 Level and Peripheral Neuropathy in Atrophic Gastritis." *World Journal of Gastroenterology* 24, no. 12 (March 28, 2018): 1343–1352.

Zilli, Alessandra, Federica Cavalcoli, Clorinda Ciafardini, and Sara Massironi. "Deficiency of Micronutrients in Patients Affected by Chronic Atrophic Autoimmune Gastritis: A Single-Institution Observational Study." *Digestive and Liver Disease* 51 (2019): 505–509.

GASTROENTERITIS

INTRODUCTION

Commonly known as the stomach flu, gastroenteritis is an intestinal infection that triggers watery diarrhea, stomach cramps, nausea and/or vomiting, and, sometimes, fever. Gastroenteritis literally means inflammation in the stomach and intestine. Inflammation makes these organs feel swollen and sore. Highly contagious, it is easily passed from person to person, but it may also be acquired from consuming contaminated food or water or touching a surface that has become contaminated and then touching one's mouth. People who are generally healthy tend to recover fairly quickly. However, infants and young children, the elderly, and those with compromised immune systems may become seriously ill and require hospitalization. And, for some people, a bout with gastroenteritis has the potential to be fatal.

Many viruses may cause gastroenteritis. Worldwide, the most common cause of foodborne gastroenteritis is norovirus, which is known to rapidly sweep through families, schools, and workplaces. It is especially likely to spread among people in confined spaces, such as cruise ships. Meanwhile, the most common cause of viral gastroenteritis in children is rotavirus. Generally, children are infected when they put their fingers on objects contaminated with the virus into their mouths, but the virus may also spread through contaminated food. The infection is most severe in infants and young children. While infected adults may not have symptoms, they are still able to spread rotavirus. Gastroenteritis may also be caused by bacteria, fungi, parasites, large amounts of alcohol, drugs or medications, or chemicals. Thus, campylobacter is an example of bacterial gastroenteritis, and candidiasis is an example of fungal gastroenteritis. Chemotherapy may cause a medication-induced gastroenteritis, and heavy metals may trigger a chemical-related gastroenteritis.

It appears that the term gastroenteritis was first associated with a description of "winter vomiting disease" by Dr. John Zahorsky in 1929. Noroviruses were later identified to be the cause of this illness, named after a diarrhea outbreak among elementary students in Norwalk, Ohio, in 1968.

SYMPTOMS, RISKS, AND COMPLICATIONS

There are several symptoms associated with gastroenteritis. These include watery diarrhea, nausea and/or vomiting, stomach cramps and pain, chills, fatigue, muscle and body aches or headache, and low-grade fever. Following infection, these symptoms usually appear within one to three days. Most often, the symptoms last for a few days. On occasion, they may last up to a few weeks.

Though anyone at any age may become ill with gastroenteritis, certain people have an increased risk. These include young children, older adults, schoolchildren, dormitory residents, and anyone with a weakened immune system. And, people exposed to young children, especially children who are cared for in a group setting, such as a day care program, have an increased risk. Elders living in group settings, such as nursing facilities, also have a higher risk. People with less access to clean water, proper nutrition, sanitation, and healthcare are more vulnerable. Of course, eating raw fish or raw meat may well increase the risk, even in healthy people.

The primary complication of viral gastroenteritis is dehydration—the severe loss of fluids and essential salts and minerals, which may lead to fainting and low blood pressure. This is particularly worrisome for children and the elderly. In some cases, people may need to be hospitalized to replace the lost fluids intravenously. A gastroenteritis illness that continues for longer periods of time may cause damage to the stomach and/or intestines.

PREVALENCE

Gastroenteritis is very common. Just about everyone will deal with at least one bout. Many people deal with multiple bouts. In the majority of cases, gastroenteritis is not serious.

DIAGNOSIS AND TREATMENT OPTIONS

In general, healthcare providers diagnose gastroenteritis from the symptoms reported by their patients. Sometimes, especially when a diagnosis is not obvious, a blood or stool test may be ordered. But, since most cases resolve in a few days, that is not normally necessary. Patients will be advised to remain home and rest. Stay close to a bathroom, and take small sips of water or an oral rehydration solution. Patients who are able to eat should only consume bland foods, such as white rice and bananas. If the symptoms persist for more than a few days, healthcare providers may recommend intravenous fluids and/or medications for nausea and diarrhea.

RESEARCH FINDINGS

Certain Foods and Aspects of Life at Home Appear to Increase the Risk of Gastroenteritis

In a study published in the journal *Epidemiology & Infection*, researchers from Australia wanted to learn if there were certain home-based factors that may increase the risk for people to become ill with gastroenteritis. The data for this study were collected from six hundred Melbourne, Australian families with a total of 2,811 subjects. All of the families had at least four members and included two children between the ages of one and fifteen years. Over a fifteen-month period, family members recorded episodes of highly credible gastroenteritis. A total of 2,669 episodes were recorded by 1,407 subjects. Within a week following an episode, the children or their parents were asked to complete a phone questionnaire concerning the preparation and consumption of the food in the previous week; questionnaires were completed for 2,003 cases by 842 subjects. Of the subjects, 553 had a single highly credible gastroenteritis event during the study period, 182 had two events, sixty-nine had three events, twenty-two had four events, nine had five events, five had six events, one had seven events, and the last one had fourteen events. Before the study concluded, food handling and food storage questionnaires were mailed to all of the families. At random times during the study, nearly all families were asked to complete a control questionnaire, and a second set of control data were generated from the subjects who did not report any cases of gastroenteritis. The researchers learned that the people who became ill with gastroenteritis were more likely to have eaten cold sliced salami, fried rice, fast foods or take-away foods, as well as food at a reception or restaurant and to have had a baby in the house in diapers for at least four hours during the week before having gastroenteritis. At the same time, the people who became ill were less likely to have eaten chicken that was bought cooked, cold sliced ham or sliced chicken, salad of any description, including home-prepared, soft cheeses, raw or cooked eggs, home-cooked chicken or red meat that had been purchased raw but frozen at home before cooking. The researchers noted that food prepared at home from raw ingredients tended to be safer than consuming pre-cooked foods or eating food away from home. While drinking water was not found to be a source of gastroenteritis in this population, alternative sources of infection included pets, swimming pools, and person-to-person contact. The researchers concluded that "the source and type of food eaten were the most strongly associated risk factors for gastroenteritis."[1]

Researchers Determined That Bread Products from a Specific Bakery Caused a Norovirus GII Outbreak in Xiamen City, China

In a case-control study published in the *International Journal of Infectious Diseases*, researchers from China described their investigation of a gastroenteritis outbreak that occurred at a university in China. They explained how they identified the etiological agent of the outbreak, the source of the infection, the mode of transmission, and the risk factors. The researchers noted that eighty-seven, or 1.2 percent of 7,141 students became ill. Sixty-one percent were male, and their median age was twenty years. No cases were identified among faculty or staff members, and there were no cases among family members of the teachers or staff or among the urban residents living around the university. Of the eighty-seven cases, sixty-two experienced vomiting and other common symptoms such as nausea, diarrhea, abdominal pain, fever, headache, and dizziness. No one was hospitalized. The outbreak lasted for twelve days. The researchers learned that sixty-three of the people who became ill had eaten bread products from a specific bakery two days before the onset of illness, and the bread was contaminated with norovirus GII. Although asymptomatic, a food handler from that bakery was found to have the same infectious agent. The researchers concluded that because of the importance of food handlers in the prevention of norovirus infection, "all means should be used to promote health education, hygienic manipulation of food, cleaning, and disinfection."[2]

Certain Foods Are More Likely to Harbor the Infectious Agents Associated with Gastroenteritis

In a retrospective cohort study published in the journal *Emerging Infectious Diseases*, researchers from the UK wanted to learn what foods had the potential to cause campylobacter infections, a source of gastroenteritis. That is why they compared 213 patients with sporadic campylobacter infections with 1,144 patients with negative fecal samples. The subjects with campylobacter had a median age of forty-three years, and those who were negative had a median age of thirty-six years. The population studied included people living in the Cardiff area of the UK who consulted with their general practitioner for gastrointestinal symptoms and subsequently submitted a diagnostic fecal sample for microbiological testing during a one-year period of time. In questionnaires, they were asked about food history, animal contact, foreign travel, leisure activities, medical conditions, and medication use. Interestingly, the researchers learned that those who were not sick were more likely to come from a household that included a child under the age of five years. Not surprisingly, the sick subjects were more likely to report symptoms, particularly fever, muscle aches, and abdominal pain, than the subjects who were not sick. Nearly all of the sick subjects and most of the non-sick subjects had diarrhea, but the sick subjects were more likely to report blood in the stool. The researchers identified several main risk factors for campylobacter infection. Most important was the consumption of chicken during the seven days before the onset of illness. The other risk factors included eating salad vegetables such as tomatoes or cucumbers, eating outside the home during the previous seven days, particularly from a fried chicken outlet, sandwich bar, or other unspecified restaurant, drinking bottled mineral water, and having direct contact with cows or calves. "The association with salad may be explained by cross-contamination of food within the home, but the possibility that natural mineral water is a risk factor for campylobacter infection could have wide public health implications."[3]

Outbreak of Acute Gastroenteritis Associated with Drinking Water

In a matched, case-control study published in *PLOS Global Public Health*, researchers from Kazakhstan, a country in Central Asia, conducted a multiday investigation into the increased rates of gastroenteritis in a rural village in northern Kazakhstan. Included in the cohort were the residents who presented for medical treatment at any healthcare facility for diarrhea, fever, vomiting, or weakness from May 14 to June 15, 2021. Symptom onset peaked on May 27, 2021. Most of the cases were in children, with 44 percent under the age of six years. The attack rate was twenty-seven per 1,000 for the entire village and fifty-three per 1,000 for the old section of the village. Controls were residents matched by age, with two controls for every patient. Using structured questionnaires, the cases and controls were interviewed, and clinical data were obtained from medical records. From this information, the researchers identified 154 cases of acute gastroenteritis, with symptoms such as diarrhea, fever, vomiting, abdominal pain, nausea, weakness, and decreased appetite. One hundred and seven cases were included in the study; they were matched to 219 controls. Disease was mild in thirteen cases and moderate in ninety-four. Of the seventy-nine households with cases, 73 percent had a single case. The others had two or three cases. Seventy-four percent of the cases reported drinking unboiled tap water; only 18 percent of the controls drank the tap water unboiled. This was the only risk factor associated with the illness. The city had two water supply networks, and the cases were clustered in the one in the "old" part of the village. The "new" section of the village's water supply network was completely replaced, but the water supply network in the "old" section had not been renovated for more than thirty years. Meanwhile, the researchers determined that the safety and quality of the water had not been monitored since 2018, which was required by national regulations.

In fact, the researchers found no records of water quality and safety control in the distribution network from 2018 to 2021. District epidemiologists had tested water samples taken from fifteen patient homes four days after the first case was reported and found high levels of bacterial colony-forming units. The researchers determined that "the outbreak was likely due to contaminated drinking water. This conclusion is substantiated by the nearly twenty-fold odds of having the disease among persons who drank unboiled tap water and the decreased odds of having disease among persons who only drank from other sources (specifically water dispensers, bottled soda)."[4]

There May Well Be an Association between Family Food Handling Behaviors and Foodborne Acute Gastroenteritis

In a cross-sectional investigation published in the journal *BMC Public Health*, researchers from Anhui Province, China, analyzed the association between family food handling behaviors and foodborne acute gastroenteritis. The cohort consisted of 1,516 subjects; males comprised 56.5 percent of the subjects, and over 60 percent of the subjects were between the ages of eighteen and fifty years. Almost 57.7 percent of the subjects lived in rural areas and 42.3 percent lived in urban areas. Data on these individuals was collected via a questionnaire survey. For those younger than twelve years, the questions were answered by parents or guardians. During a one-year period of time, 165 of these subjects, or 10.9 percent, reported experiencing the symptoms of foodborne acute gastroenteritis during the previous four weeks. The monthly incidence of foodborne illness was 15.3 percent in females and 7.5 percent in males. Students and children had the highest incidence (13.9 percent) of foodborne acute gastroenteritis, followed by peasant workers (13.1 percent) and peasants (13 percent). But, the differences between these groups did not reach significance. The researchers learned that certain behaviors were more common in people with symptoms. These included not thoroughly heating milk, not thoroughly heating cooked food purchased from outside, not thoroughly heating leftovers stored in the refrigerator, and infrequently storing leftovers in the refrigerator. Other behaviors associated with foodborne acute gastroenteritis included often eating raw seafood, often storing raw and cooked meat in the same container, and infrequently thoroughly cooking green beans. The researchers commented that "most people are not educated in the proper handling of food. Inappropriate food handling occurs in food production, food processing, storage, and consumption." And, they concluded that "inappropriate food handling behaviors in the family environment were associated with foodborne acute gastroenteritis."[5]

In Turkey, Rotavirus-Associated Acute Gastroenteritis Cases Are Very Common in Early Childhood

In a meta-analysis published in the journal *Children*, researchers from Turkey noted that it is generally understood that rotavirus is the most common viral pathogen in childhood gastroenteritis. That is why they wanted to estimate the number of Turkish children who suffer from early childhood rotavirus-associated gastroenteritis. The researchers located thirty-eight prospective, cross-sectional, and cohort studies published in English and Turkish that met their criteria. In these studies, 80,113 Turkish children up to the age of five years were diagnosed with the symptoms of acute gastroenteritis. Stool samples of 13,651 of these children were positive for rotavirus. Thus, the pooled prevalence of rotavirus was 18 percent in these children, 12 percent in children younger than two years, and 5 percent in children between two and five years. The highest prevalence was found in the winter, and the highest incidence was in the winter and spring. The ratio of rotavirus positivity was highest in December and January, while the lowest was in July. Why is this information so important? "Viral gastroenteritis is the most common cause of hospitalization in early childhood," and viral gastroenteritis caused by rotavirus, "occurs at similar frequency in developed and developing countries regardless of cleaning conditions." The researchers concluded that rotaviruses are a significant public health concern in Turkey and elsewhere. "In this context, the World Health Organization recommends that all countries add rotavirus vaccines to their national vaccination programs."[6]

Worldwide, There Appears to Be a High Risk of Human Noroviruses Contamination from Vegetables

In a systematic review and meta-analysis published in the *International Journal of Food Microbiology*, researchers from China wanted to assess the worldwide prevalence of human noroviruses in vegetables. After reviewing articles published between January 1, 1972, and June 1, 2023, they identified twenty-seven studies that met their criteria. The continent with the largest number of studies was Europe, and the highest number of samples was lettuce. Noroviruses were found in 18 percent of vegetables from farms, but only 4 percent from retail stores. The researchers found that the pooled human norovirus prevalence in vegetables was at least 7 percent, and even relatively smaller amounts of contamination may cause serious problems. The researchers concluded that their findings of human norovirus contamination in vegetables "should improve our understanding of the risk to consumers."[7]

Untreated Rainwater Is Probably Not a Source of Gastroenteritis

In a double-blinded, randomized controlled study published in the *American Journal of Public Health*, researchers from Australia examined the ability of untreated rainwater to be a source of gastroenteritis infections. The researchers noted that because of water shortages, people in developed countries have been drinking more untreated rainwater.

The cohort consisted of three hundred households that had a total of 1,352 residents. One hundred and fifty-two of the households had active water treatment units, and 148 households had sham water treatment units. The number of participants per household was 4.59 in the active water treatment group and 4.42 in the sham group. The mean number of children, aged sixteen years or younger, was 2.29 in the active group and 2.25 in the sham group. During the entire twelve-month data collection period, a total of ninety-three households withdrew from the study, forty-five from the active group and forty-eight from the sham group. Still, the researchers found that there were 0.78 episodes of "highly credible gastroenteritis" per person in the active group and 0.76 in the sham group. Highly credible gastroenteritis episodes were experienced by 41.7 percent of the participants in the active group and 38.6 percent in the sham group. The researchers determined that highly credible gastroenteritis rates between the two groups were not significantly different. Thus, the households drinking treated and untreated water had essentially the same rates of highly credible gastroenteritis. And, the researchers concluded that their findings "suggest that consumption of untreated rainwater does not contribute appreciably to community gastroenteritis."[8]

The Severity of Symptoms in Single- versus Multiple-Virus Gastroenteritis Appear to Be Similar

In a study published in the *International Journal of Molecular Sciences*, researchers from Japan and Pittsburgh, Pennsylvania, wanted to learn if cases of gastroenteritis caused by a single virus had different levels of symptom severity than those caused by multiple viruses. The cohort consisted of 1,245 children who had gastroenteritis over a three-year period of time; 2,383 stool samples were collected from these children, who were all patients in a pediatric clinic in Japan. The children had a median age of 2.6 years, and 52 percent were male. At the time of the clinic visits, the children did not have any other disease conditions and they were taking no medications. The stool samples were tested for eleven different viruses. At least one virus was found in 1,706 (71.6 percent) of the specimens, and multiple viruses were found in 565 cases. Norovirus GII was the most common virus, and it was detected during all the seasons. Though clinical symptoms were found to be significantly different in some single versus multiple-virus infections, the disease severity between the two groups was statistically non-significant. "No differences were observed when comparing disease severity in this analysis."[9]

In Children, the Symptoms of Gastroenteritis Tend to Follow a Certain Pattern

In a seven-day, prospective, follow-up study published in the journal *BMC Primary Care*, researchers from the Netherlands examined the course of vomiting, diarrhea, fever, and clinical deterioration in children with cases of gastroenteritis. The cohort consisted of 359 children who were seen in an out-of-hours primary care service. The median age of the children was 1.5 years, and 184 were female. In most of these children, all of the symptoms decreased within five days. Vomiting and fever decreased rapidly, but diarrhea decreased at a slower pace, especially among the children who were six to twelve months old. For them, diarrhea tended to be over seven days after it began. Thirty-one (8.6 percent) of these children developed complicated illness and required referral or hospitalization. Children who deteriorated during follow-up had higher frequencies of vomiting at presentation and had higher frequencies of vomiting and fever during follow-up. The most frequent symptom of dehydration was no urine output for twenty-four hours, and that occurred in forty-five of the children (13.3 percent). The researchers learned that most of the children presented with vomiting, and 20–50 percent were still vomiting two days later. By day five, 10 percent of the children were still vomiting. Diarrhea was the second most common symptom, and fever was the third. The researchers concluded that it is important that clinicians be aware of the normal course of events in average cases of gastroenteritis; they should also be knowledgeable about the signs and symptoms of deterioration. And, they recommended that medical providers "educate parents about the duration of symptoms and what alarm symptoms to monitor as part of this safety netting advice."[10]

Vitamin B6 Had No Effect on the Vomiting Associated with Gastroenteritis

In a double-blind, placebo-controlled trial published in the *Global Journal of Health Science*, researchers from Iran assessed the ability of oral vitamin B6 to help prevent the vomiting associated with gastroenteritis. The cohort consisted of ninety-six children with mild to moderate gastroenteritis who were admitted to a hospital in Tehran, Iran. They ranged in age from six months to twelve years. The children were randomly assigned to one of two groups, each with forty-eight subjects. The groups were matched for age, sex, and symptoms of dehydration. The children in the experimental group were given vitamin B6, and the children in the control group were given a placebo. A physician evaluated the severity of vomiting and dehydration in the children before and after treatment. Forty-one children in the vitamin B6 group and forty in the control group had mild dehydration. Vomiting was managed in twenty-eight children in the vitamin B6 group and in thirty-seven children in the placebo group. According to the researchers, there was no significant difference between the two groups. Thus, the researchers commented, "the prescription of vitamin B6 did not have curable impact on vomiting in children," and they concluded that vitamin B6 has "no useful effect in treatment of pediatric nausea and vomiting following acute gastroenteritis."[11]

REFERENCES AND FURTHER READING

Chen, Y., Y. Wen, J. Song et al. "The Correlation Between Family Food Handling Behaviors and Foodborne Acute Gastroenteritis: A Community-Oriented, Population-Based Survey in Anhui, China." *BMC Public Health* 18 (2018): 1290.

Derakhshanfar, Hojjat, Arash Hadian Amree, Hossein Alimohammadi et al. "Results of Double-Blind Placebo Controlled Trial to Assess the Effect of Vitamin B6 on Managing of Nausea and Vomiting in Pediatrics with Acute Gastroenteritis." *Global Journal of Health Science* 5, no. 6 (2013): 197–201.

Evans, Meirion R., C. Donald Ribeiro, and Roland L. Salmon. "Hazards of Healthy Living: Bottled Water and Salad Vegetables as Risk Factors for Campylobacter Infection." *Emerging Infectious Diseases* 9, no. 10 (October 2003): 1219–1225.

Gao, J., L. Xue, Y. Li et al. "A Systematic Review and Meta-Analysis Indicates a High Risk of Human Noroviruses Contamination in Vegetable Worldwide, with GI Being the Predominant Genogroup." *International Journal of Food Microbiology* 413 (March 2, 2024): 110603.

Guo, Z., J. Huang, G. Shi et al. "A Food-Borne Outbreak of Gastroenteritis Caused by Norovirus GII in a University Located in Xiamen City, China." *International Journal of Infectious Diseases* 28 (2014): 101–106.

Güzel, Mustafa, Orhan Akpmar, and Muhammet Burak Kılıç. "Prevalence of Rotavirus-Associated Acute Gastroenteritis Cases in Early Childhood in Turkey: Meta-Analysis." *Children* 7, no. 10 (October 2020): 159.

Hikita, T., T. Phan, S. Okitsu et al. "A Comparative Study of Acute Gastroenteritis Symptoms in Single-verses-Multiple-Virus Infections." *International Journal of Molecular Sciences* 24 (2023): 8364.

Mitakakis, T. Z., R. Wolfe, M. I. Sinclair et al. "Dietary Intake and Domestic Food Preparation and Handling as Risk Factors for Gastroenteritis: A Case-Control Study." *Epidemiology & Infection* 132 (2004): 601–606.

Orysbayeva, M., B. Zhuman, D. Turegeldiyeva et al. "Outbreak of Acute Gastroenteritis Associated with Drinking Water in Rural Kazakhstan: A Matched Case-Control Study." *PLoS Global Public Health* 2, no. 12 (2022): e0001075.

Rodrigo, Shelly, Martha Sinclair, Andrew Forbes et al. "Drinking Rainwater: A Double-Blinded, Randomized Controlled Study of Water Treatment Filters and Gastroenteritis Incidence." *American Society of Public Health* 101, no. 5 (Mary 2011): 842–847.

Weghorst, Anouk A. H., Irma J. Bonvanie, Gea A. Holtman et al. "Course of Uncomplicated Acute Gastroenteritis in Children Presenting to Out-of-Hours Primary Care." *BMC Primary Care* 23 (2022): 125.

GASTROESOPHAGEAL REFLUX DISEASE (GERD)

INTRODUCTION

Gastroesophageal reflux disease (GERD) occurs when stomach acid repeatedly flows back into the esophagus, the tubal structure that connects the mouth to the stomach. The backflow, known as acid reflux, may irritate the lining of the esophagus. Almost everyone has occasional acid reflux, which is experienced as indigestion, a burning stomach, heartburn, or no symptoms at all. When these problems occur often and produce symptoms, the culprit is probably GERD. It is important to understand that the contents of the stomach are supposed to go only one way—through the intestinal tract. They are not intended to flow back into the esophagus.

When people swallow, a circular band of muscle around the bottom of the esophagus (lower esophageal sphincter or LES) relaxes. This allows food and liquid to flow into the stomach. Then the sphincter closes again. If the sphincter does not relax properly, stomach acid may flow back into the esophagus. This recurrent backwash of acid irritates the lining of the esophagus and may cause it to become inflamed.

Although GERD has probably existed as long as humankind, the modern description of GERD was first outlined by Asher Winkelstein, who was Chief of Gastroenterology at Mount Sinai Hospital in New York City. In June 1934, he presented five cases of a "new" clinical entity he referred to as "peptic esophagitis" to the Eighty-Fifth Annual Session of the American Medical Association in Cleveland. His manuscript on the topic was published in 1935 in *JAMA*.[1]

SYMPTOMS, RISKS, AND COMPLICATIONS

The most common symptoms of GERD include heartburn or a burning sensation in the chest, often after eating, upper abdominal or noncardiac chest pain, trouble swallowing (dysphagia), a sour or bitter taste at the back of the mouth, the regurgitation of food or liquid from the stomach to the mouth, a sense of fullness, and the feeling that there is a lump in the back of the throat. Other more alarming symptoms include difficulty swallowing, pain when swallowing, nausea or vomiting, weight loss, anemia, and bleeding. Sometimes, GERD triggers asthma-like symptoms such as chronic coughing, wheezing, and shortness of breath.

Gastroesophageal reflux (GER) is very common during infancy. The term GERD is used when there are consequences, such as poor weight gain, respiratory problems, or esophagitis (inflammation of the esophagus). Symptoms of GERD in babies or small children include excessive fussiness, difficulty sleeping, refusal to eat, trouble swallowing, irritability or arching of back during or after feeding, weight loss or poor growth, recurring cough or pneumonia, difficulty sleeping, gagging or choking, vomiting episodes, wheezing, hoarseness, and bad breath. In older children and adolescents, symptoms include chronic heartburn, trouble swallowing, recurrent regurgitation, cough, and pneumonia.

There are several conditions that increase the risk of developing GERD in adults. These include obesity, birth defects, such as esophageal atresia, hiatal hernia, pregnancy, older age, connective tissue disorders, such as scleroderma, and delayed stomach emptying. Other factors may aggravate acid reflux. These include smoking, eating larger meals or eating at night, eating fatty or fried foods, drinking alcohol and/or coffee, and taking medications, such as aspirin. Some medications that relax the lower esophageal sphincter increase the risk of acid reflux and GERD. These include benzodiazepines, calcium channel blockers, tricyclic antidepressants, nonsteroidal anti-inflammatory drugs, theophylline (an asthma medication), and hormone treatments for menopause. There are even foods that may relax the esophageal sphincter. These include chocolate, mint, garlic, and onions.

People who deal with frequent bouts of GERD are at increased risk for a number of complications. One of the most common is esophagitis. Esophagitis occurs when stomach acid breaks down tissue in the esophagus, which causes inflammation, bleeding, and sometimes an ulcer or open sore. Esophagitis causes pain and makes it more difficult to swallow. Over time, scar tissue may form, and the esophagus may narrow, which is known as esophageal stricture. GERD increases the possibility for Barrett's esophagus to develop. This condition may lead to a rare cancer that is called esophageal adenocarcinoma. Some people with GERD also develop laryngopharyngeal reflux, which is reflux that travels all the way to the throat. It has the potential to cause swelling, hoarseness, and vocal cord growths, and acid particles may aspirate into the airway.

PREVALENCE

In a systematic review published in the journal *Gut*, researchers from Houston, Texas, the UK, and Australia examined studies on the prevalence of GERD. They found that GERD is one of the most common gastrointestinal disorders, with a prevalence of about 20 percent in Western cultures. The range of GERD prevalence estimates was 18.1 to 27.8 percent in North America, 8.8 to 25.9 percent in Europe, 2.5 to 7.8 percent in East Asia, 8.7 to 33.1 percent in the Middle East, 11.6 percent in Australia, and 23 percent in South America. There is evidence that the prevalence has increased since 1995, particularly in North America and East Asia.[2]

DIAGNOSIS AND TREATMENT OPTIONS

Several tests are used to diagnose GERD. During an upper endoscopy, a physician inserts a thin tube through the mouth into the esophagus and stomach. A camera at the end of the tube enables the physician to view the tissues, and tissue samples or biopsies are taken. An esophageal pH test may be used to measure the acid content of the esophagus. An esophageal manometry uses pressure sensors embedded in a nasogastric tube to measure the muscle activity of the esophagus. It may show which muscles are not working properly. And, it may assess the LES. In very occasional cases, an esophagram, a type of X-ray that takes moving pictures of the esophagus, may be performed. This test may detect a hiatal hernia and the extent of the reflux.

Healthcare providers tend to begin GERD treatment by recommending a number of lifestyle modifications. Since larger meals expand the stomach and put pressure on the LES, smaller, more frequent meals may be advised. Because gravity works against reflux, it is a good idea to eat an early dinner and elevate the head of the bed. Sleeping on the left side places the LES in an air pocket above the contents of the stomach. In contrast, lying on the back or right side lowers the valve. To reduce abdominal pressure, wear loose-fitting clothing and, if appropriate, lose weight. Because both smoking and alcohol weaken the LES, it may be useful to quit smoking and at least reduce drinking. Removing dietary triggers, such as caffeine, chocolate, high-fat foods, carbonated beverages, and peppermint may be helpful.

A number of medications are used to treat GERD. Healthcare providers may begin by recommending antacids, which neutralize stomach acid. As a result, when reflux occurs, it does not harm the esophagus. Antacids work well for occasional acid reflux. Alginates, which are sugars derived from seaweed, float on top of stomach acid, thus creating a barrier between the acid and the esophagus. Alginates may be purchased as a sole ingredient or in combination with antacids. Antacids and alginates are over-the-counter medications. Still, other treatments require a prescription. Histamine receptor antagonists (H2 blockers) block the chemical that signals the body to produce histamine. In so doing, they reduce stomach acid. Proton pump inhibitors are strong acid blockers that promote healing. They are 90 percent effective for reducing acid reflux. And, baclofen is a muscle relaxant, which is frequently prescribed to relieve muscle spasms. It may help reduce the frequency of LES relaxation events, which calms acid reflux.

GERD that does not respond well to medication, or that has complications such as chronic cough or disease of the larynx, may require surgery. The most common surgery for GERD is the Nissen fundoplication. During this procedure, the surgeon wraps the top of the stomach around the lower esophagus. Stitches are used to tighten the junction. A newer procedure, termed magnetic sphincter augmentation, works by augmenting the LES with a series of magnets. The magnets enhance the functioning of the LES while also permitting the passage of food.

RESEARCH FINDINGS

Lifestyle Factors Appear to Be Associated with the Symptoms of GERD

In a trial published in the journal *Digestive Diseases and Sciences*, researchers from Japan wanted to determine which lifestyle factors were associated with GERD. The cohort consisted of 2,853 subjects who participated in a health promotion program in Japan; there were 1,975 men and 878 women with a mean age of 56.8 years and a range in age from twenty-seven to eighty-eight years. GERD symptoms were assessed using the Japanese version of the Carlson-Dent self-administered questionnaire. All of the subjects had an upper gastrointestinal endoscopy as part of their routine examination. The researchers determined that 667 (23.4 percent) of the subjects had GERD. Among the subjects in the GERD group, 232 had asymptomatic erosive reflux disease, ninety-one had symptomatic erosive reflux disease, and 344 had nonerosive reflux disease. In order to assess the influence of lifestyle on the disease, the subjects were asked a series of questions about their lifestyle. These included questions about sleep, exercise, smoking habits, and the intake of alcohol, green tea, and coffee. The researchers learned that the factors associated with GERD included a high BMI, hiatal hernia, and drinking green tea. Sleeping fewer hours and smoking were primarily factors in men, and a lack of exercise was primarily a factor in women. The researchers concluded that their findings "clearly demonstrated that even nonsymptomatic people can suffer from GERD, and that lifestyle and gender differences may very well modulate GERD in individuals."[3]

In a study published in the journal *Gastroenterology Research and Practice*, researchers from China and New York City investigated the relationship between lifestyle factors and the symptoms associated with GERD. The cohort consisted of 37,442 people who had a routine physical examination at a hospital in China; 72.84 percent were men and 27.16 percent were women. In addition to general demographic questions, the subjects were asked about smoking, drinking, diet, and exercise, as well as any symptoms that may be related to GERD. The researchers learned that about 20 percent of the subjects appeared to have GERD. The percentage of men with suspected GERD was significantly higher than the percentage of women with suspected GERD, and the prevalence of GERD was higher in the young and middle-aged than in the elderly. The prevalence of GERD increased with weight gain and in those who smoked, consumed excessive amounts of alcohol, lacked physical activity, and ate larger amounts of oil, meat, fish, salt, cereals, and eggs. In contrast, an adequate intake of fruit and vegetables was correlated with a significantly lower incidence of GERD. The researchers concluded that "suspected GERD or a high risk of GERD is very common in the population of individuals undergoing health examinations." And, "unhealthy lifestyles are closely related to a high incidence of suspected GERD."[4]

In a cross-sectional trial published in the journal *Obesity Research & Clinical Practice*, researchers from Philadelphia, Pennsylvania examined the prevalence and risk factors for GERD in an impoverished area surrounding Temple University in Philadelphia (19140 zip code). The cohort consisted of 503 subjects. Information on demographics, medical history, lifestyle habits, and the symptoms of reflux disease was obtained during in-home interviews, convenience sampling, and targeted mailing. The participating subjects measured their height, weight, and hip and waist circumference. Only people who had lived in this specific zip code for three or more years were eligible to participate. Of the 503 subjects, 129 (25.6 percent) met the criteria for GERD. Many of the subjects had unhealthy levels of waist-to-hip ratios, and the average BMI of all participants was very high, both those with and without GERD reported gaining "considerable" weight since age eighteen. The prevalence of higher alcohol use and eating at fast food restaurants was high for both groups. The researchers found a direct association between waist circumference and GERD. In fact, they determined that "central obesity, rather than overall BMI, is of primary importance in predisposing to GERD." Subjects in the highest quartile of waist circumference had more than double the odds of having GERD. Likewise, people who smoked also had a higher risk. "Active smoking increased the odds ratio considerably compared to non-smokers." So, for this cohort, central obesity and smoking were the two most important risk factors for GERD.[5]

Eating a Predominantly Mediterranean Diet Seems to Decrease the Risk of GERD

In a cross-sectional trial published in the journal *Diseases of the Esophagus*, researchers from Albania and the Netherlands evaluated the relationship between the consumption of a predominately Mediterranean diet and GERD in adult men and women from Albania, a country in southeastern Europe. The cohort consisted of 817 adults who lived in Tirana, the capital of Albania; there were 333 men with a mean age of 51.2 years and 484 women with a mean age of 49.5 years. The subjects were classified as having GERD if, during the past year, they reported heartburn or regurgitation at least once per week and having at least moderate problems from such symptoms. On the other hand, the subjects without such symptoms were classified as non-GERD. The subjects were interviewed about their dietary habits, and a summary score for the Mediterranean and non-Mediterranean diet was calculated for each subject. Demographic data were collected, and a physical examination included the measurement of height and weight. Based on self-reporting, the researchers found the overall prevalence of GERD to be 8.9 percent. Four hundred and forty-five subjects ate a predominately Mediterranean diet and 372 ate a mostly non-Mediterranean diet. Women were more likely than men to eat the Mediterranean diet, and people who smoked were less likely to follow the diet. There was no evidence of a significant relationship between the Mediterranean diet and socioeconomic status, alcohol intake, or physical activity. In both sexes, those who ate the Mediterranean diet were less likely to have GERD. However, "no single component of the Mediterranean dietary score had a significant influence on GERD risk." On the other hand, "when these components were integrated into a single Mediterranean dietary score, there was evidence of a significant protective effect which may be explained by the synergistic and antagonistic interactions between different ingredients of the Mediterranean diet."[6]

There Appears to Be Some Association between GERD and Anxiety and Depression

In a large, retrospective, cross-sectional study published in the *Journal of Neurogastroenterology and Motility*, researchers from Korea collected data from 19,099 subjects who had undergone an upper endoscopy procedure. All of the subjects completed a structured, self-administered questionnaire about their basic demographic characteristics, general health and lifestyle, medical history, and gastrointestinal symptoms. Other factors, such as height, weight, and BMI, were determined. Levels of anxiety and depression were measured with the State-Trait Anxiety Inventory and the Beck Depression Inventory. The researchers determined that 1,574 subjects had reflux symptoms, and 1,368 had endoscopically proven esophageal mucosal erosions/ulcers but did not have any reflux symptoms. The remaining 16,157 subjects were classified as controls. The researchers learned that the subjects with erosive reflux disease had higher state anxiety and depression levels than the subjects in the control group, and the subjects with nonerosive reflux disease had higher levels of state and trait anxiety and depression than the subjects in the control group. Subjects with asymptomatic erosive esophagitis did not have these associations. The researchers concluded that "a multidisciplinary approach to assess and manage these psychological factors is needed for the treatment of GERD."[7]

People Who Smoke and Eat Later Dinners Are at Increased Risk for GERD

In a matched, case-control trial published in the *American Journal of Gastroenterology*, researchers from Japan evaluated the association between smoking, bedtimes, and GERD. The cohort consisted of 147 people with GERD; thirty-eight had a diagnosis of nonerosive GERD and 109 had erosive esophagitis. The subjects with GERD were age and sex matched to 294 people who did not experience GERD symptoms during the previous year. The researchers observed that the subjects who smoked were more likely to have GERD, while there were no differences in BMI and drinking habits between the people with GERD and the controls. In addition, those subjects who ate later dinners or had a significantly shorter "dinner-to-bed time interval" had a significantly increased risk for GERD. The researchers concluded that there is a need to determine if "avoiding going to bed within three hours after eating dinner would reduce or improve GERD symptoms, especially nighttime symptoms."[8]

Baclofen Seems to Relieve the Symptoms of GERD

In a systematic review and meta-analysis, researchers based in China evaluated the usefulness of the medication baclofen for the treatment of GERD. The researchers located nine randomized controlled double-blinded trials with 283 patients with GERD and healthy subjects that met their criteria. Most of the patients were adults in their forties, except for thirty children in their "10s." The treatment duration ranged from twelve hours to four weeks. The trials were conducted in primary and secondary care settings in different countries. The researchers found a statistically significant difference in the reduction of the incidence of GERD between baclofen-treated and placebo-treated patients. Three of the trials provided information on the incidence of transient lower esophageal sphincter relaxation. These trials found that baclofen decreased the rate of this relaxation better than the placebo, and the difference between baclofen and the placebo was statistically significant.[9]

Acupuncture May Be Useful for GERD

In a trial published in the *Chinese Journal of Integrative Medicine*, researchers from China studied the efficacy and safety of treating GERD with acupuncture. The cohort consisted of sixty patients with confirmed cases of GERD. For six weeks, thirty patients (sixteen males and fourteen females between the ages of seventeen and sixty-seven years) were treated with acupuncture and thirty patients (seventeen males and thirteen females between the ages of eighteen and sixty-eight years) were treated with the medications omeprazole and mosapride. Assessments were conducted at baseline, immediately after the treatments ended, and four weeks later. When the treatments ended, the researchers determined that both protocols were equally effective. However, while the patients in the acupuncture group continued to experience relief four weeks later, the patients in the medication group were once again dealing with GERD symptoms. The researchers concluded that acupuncture "is beneficial to the esophageal membrane repairing without evident adverse reaction and after withdrawal relapse."[10]

In a single-center, randomized, controlled four-week trial published in the journal *Integrative Medicine Research*, researchers from Vietnam examined the ability of thread-embedding acupuncture to treat the symptoms of GERD. According to these researchers, thread-embedding acupuncture "involves selecting acupuncture points similar to those used in manual acupuncture and electroacupuncture." Unlike regular acupuncture, which may be administered daily, treatments with thread-embedding acupuncture are given every few weeks. The cohort consisted of sixty-six subjects with GERD; they were no younger than eighteen or older than sixty years. Thirty-three subjects received two sessions of thread-embedding acupuncture and a proton pump inhibitor, and thirty-three subjects were treated with a proton pump inhibitor. The baseline characteristics of the subjects in both groups were similar. One subject in each group was lost to follow-up. The researchers learned that the subjects taking the combination therapy had far better symptom relief than those who only took the proton pump inhibitor. For example, the combination therapy gave faster symptom relief and reduced the severity of the symptoms. A total of five patients experienced adverse events, such as a local hematoma, pain, local swelling, and pruritus. All were mild and resolved within a week without treatment. The researchers concluded that the combination of thread-embedding acupuncture and proton pump inhibitor was more effective in treating GERD than the proton pump inhibitor alone. "Further studies with longer follow-ups are required to confirm these findings."[11]

Proton Pump Inhibitors May or May Not Be Associated with Osteoporosis-Related Fractures

In a retrospective study published in the journal *CMAJ*, researchers from Canada wanted to determine the relationship between the use of proton pump inhibitors and the risk of osteoporosis-related fractures. Why is this important? Proton pump inhibitors are a frequently used treatment for GERD, and they may well be recommended for longer periods of time. Using data from the Population Health Research Data Repository, which contains comprehensive healthcare utilization data for nearly all of the residents of Manitoba, Canada, the researchers identified patients who had a fracture of the hip, vertebra, or wrist between April 1996 and March 2004. Based on age, sex, ethnicity, and comorbidity, each of the cases was matched to three controls. Included in the calculations were the number of years people used proton pump inhibitors. The researchers located 15,792 cases of osteoporosis-related fractures and matched those people to 47,289 controls, who had no history of these types of fractures. The researchers found no significant association between the use of proton pump inhibitors and osteoporosis-related fractures for those who used the medication for one to six continuous years. On the other hand, after seven years of continuous use, there was a statistically significant association between the use of proton pump inhibitors and any osteoporosis-related fractures. And, after five years of continuous proton pump inhibitors, the rate of hip fractures rose. The researchers commented that "this is not surprising because bone mineralization and resorption take place over many years, and the effect of a drug that has a subtle effect on bone mineralization may require several years of exposure before it has a measurable effect on clinical outcomes."[12]

In a study published in *JAMA Pediatrics*, researchers from Sweden, the UK, New York City, and Denmark examined the relationship between the use of proton pump inhibitors and the risk of fractures in children. The researchers used data from July 1, 2006, to December 31, 2016, from Sweden's National Patient Register on children under the age of eighteen years who used proton pump inhibitors. They were matched to children who did not use proton pump inhibitors. The cohort consisted of a total of 115,933 pairs of children. The mean age of the children who used proton pump inhibitors was 12.6 years and 61.1 percent were female. During a mean of 2.2 years of follow-up, there were 5,354 fractures among those taking proton pump inhibitors and 4,568 cases among those not taking these medications. The researchers found that proton pump inhibitors were associated with an increased risk of upper- and lower-limb fractures and other fractures, but not head or spine fractures. Furthermore, those taking proton pump inhibitors had a statistically significant 11 percent relative increased risk of any fracture. Most of the fractures tended to occur in children who were six years and older and in those who used these medications for longer periods of time. The researchers concluded that in their large cohort study, PPI [proton pump inhibitor] use was associated with a small but statistically significant increased risk of any fracture. "Risk of fracture should be taken into account when weighing the benefits and risks of PPI treatment in children."[13]

In another study published in the journal *Osteoporosis International*, researchers from Norway, Denmark, and the UK used data from the Norwegian Prescription Database, the third survey of the Nord-Trøndelag Health Study, and the Fracture Registry of Nord-Trøndelag to search for a link between the use of proton pump inhibitors and fractures. Their cohort consisted of 15,017 women and 13,241 men between the ages of fifty and eighty-five years. During a mean follow-up of 5.2 years, 266 women and 134 men had a first hip fracture and 662 women and 127 men had their first forearm fracture. Six people had fractures in both their forearm and hip. The fracture rate per one thousand person-years in women was 49.2 percent for users of proton pump inhibitors compared to 64.1 percent among non-users. The respective rates for men were 18.6 and 19.8 percent. So, unlike the two previous studies, the researchers in this study observed no increased risk of fractures among users of proton pump inhibitors. The researchers commented that the subjects in their study used proton pump inhibitors for six months to seven years, "which may be too short to cause a negative effect on bone." And, they noted that the type of proton pump inhibitor or the use of another type of medication might play a role in bone loss. The researchers concluded that the exposure to the four proton pump inhibitors in their study—pantoprazole, esomeprazole, lansoprazole, and omeprazole—"was not associated with increased risk of hip or forearm fractures."[14]

Use of Proton Pump Inhibitors May or May Not Cause Vitamin B12 Deficiency

In a cross-sectional trial published in the journal *Alimentary Pharmacology and Therapeutics*, researchers based in the Netherlands examined the association between levels of vitamin

B12 in the blood and the long-term use of proton pump inhibitors in the elderly. The cohort consisted of 124 long-term users of proton pump inhibitors who were sixty-five years or older and their partners, who did not use proton pump inhibitors. One additional "couple" was a mother and son. The median duration of proton pump inhibitor usage was six years. The subjects had been invited to participate by general practitioners. The proton pump inhibitor user and his or her partner had their blood drawn together in the same laboratory. The vitamin B12 status was determined by serum levels of vitamin B12, serum levels of homocysteine, and mean corpuscular volume. The researchers found the prevalence of vitamin B12 deficiency to be similar in both groups. The researchers commented that their findings "suggest that there is no need to screen elderly long-term PPI users for vitamin B12 deficiency, not even after six years of therapy."[15]

Meanwhile, in a cross-sectional trial published in the *Journal of the American Medical Directors Association*, researchers from the Bronx (New York City) also evaluated the use of proton pump inhibitors and vitamin B12 deficiency. Their cohort consisted of 542 adults between the ages of sixty and 102 years; 63 percent were female. The subjects were residents of long-term care facilities in the Bronx or community patients in the researchers' ambulatory geriatric clinic. All of the subjects were cared for by geriatricians or fellows in geriatric medicine. Data collection included patient interviews, physical examinations, medical histories, and medical records. The researchers learned that the subjects in this study tended to have low levels of serum vitamin B12. Additionally, when proton pump inhibitors were used for up to 72 months, the subjects had lower levels of vitamin B12. This was true for the subjects who used and did not use vitamin B12 supplementation. The researchers concluded "that there is a risk of gradual decline in B12 status during prolonged PPI use in older adults." And, they advised medical providers to periodically monitor the vitamin B12 status of their older adults who are taking proton pump inhibitors.[16]

Some Supplements May Help the Symptoms of GERD

In a trial published in the journal *GMC Gastroenterology*, researchers from Egypt wanted to learn if melatonin would be useful for the symptoms of GERD, such as heartburn, epigastric pain, and a significant decrease in lower esophageal sphincter pressure. They placed thirty-six subjects in one of four groups; each of the groups had nine subjects. After administration of medical histories and examinations, for four and eight weeks, nine patients with GERD were treated with melatonin alone, nine patients with GERD were treated with omeprazole alone, and nine patients with GERD were treated with melatonin and omeprazole. Nine healthy subjects comprised the control group and had no treatment. The researchers determined that the healthy subjects had significantly higher levels of melatonin than the subjects with GERD. The researchers also learned that all three types of treatments resulted in improvements in GERD symptoms. Still, GERD treatment was incomplete when the subjects were treated with melatonin alone or omeprazole alone for only four weeks. When each of these treatments continued for eight weeks or when the treatments were combined for four weeks, the treatment was complete. Additionally, the researchers noted that omeprazole alone was better than melatonin alone. The researchers concluded that "melatonin could be used in the treatment of

GERD either alone or in combination with omeprazole. The combination therapy of both melatonin and omeprazole is preferable as melatonin accelerates the healing effect of omeprazole and therefore shortens the duration of treatment and minimizes its side effects."[17]

In a single, blind, randomized trial published in the *Journal of Pineal Research*, a researcher from Brazil compared the treatment of people with GERD with two different agents—omeprazole and a supplement containing melatonin, L-tryptophan, vitamins B6 and B12, folic acid, methionine, and betaine. The cohort consisted of 351 people with GERD; they ranged in age from eighteen to eighty-eight years, with a mean age of forty-four years. They were from nineteen different cities and towns in five Brazilian states. For forty days, 175 subjects took 20 mg omeprazole and 176 subjects took the combination supplement. The researchers learned that all of the subjects taking the supplement experienced a total regression of their symptoms; some relief was even obtained after seven days on the supplement. Meanwhile, after nine days of treatment on omeprazole, 115 subjects obtained relief. An additional four subjects reported partial relief, and the remainder continued to experience all of their symptoms. Two subjects withdrew from the trial because of a persistent omeprazole-related headache. The differences between the two groups were statistically significant. The researchers commented that their findings "are highly significant because the patients who used the supplementation reported fewer side effects than patients who used omeprazole."[18]

REFERENCES AND FURTHER READING

Choi, Ji Min, Jong In Yang, Seung Joo Kang et al. "Association Between Anxiety and Depression and Gastroesophageal Reflux Disease: Results from a Large Cross-Sectional Study." *Journal of Neurogastroenterology and Motility* 24, no. 4 (2018): 593–602.

den Elzen, W. P. J., Y. Groeneveld, W. de Ruijter et al. "Long-Term Use of Proton Pump Inhibitors and Vitamin B12 Status in Elderly Individuals." *Alimentary Pharmacology and Therapeutics* 27, no. 6 (March 2008): 491–497.

Dharmarajan, T. S., M. K. Kanagala, P. Murakonda et al. "Do Acid-Lowering Agents Affect Vitamin B1 Status in Older Adults?" *Journal of the American Medical Directors Association* 9, no. 3 (March 2008): 162–167.

El-Serag, Hashem B., Stephen Sweet, Christopher C. Winchester, and John Dent. "Update on the Epidemiology of Gastro-Oesophageal Reflux Disease: A Systematic Review." *Gut* 63, no. 6 (2014): 871–880.

Friedenberg, Frank K., Jitha Rai, Vishwas Vanar et al. "Prevalence and Risk Factors for Gastroesophageal Reflux Disease in an Impoverished Minority Population." *Obesity Research & Clinical Practice* 4 (2010): e261–e269.

Fujiwara, Y., A. Machida, Y. Watanabe et al. "Association Between Dinner-to-Bed Time and Gastro-Esophageal Reflux Disease." *American Journal of Gastroenterology* 100 (2005): 2633–2636.

Gong, Yan, Qiang Zeng, Yi Yan et al. "Association Between Lifestyle and Gastroesophageal Reflux Disease Questionnaire Scores: A Cross-Sectional Study of 37,442 Chinese Adults." *Gastroenterology Research and Practice* 2019 (2019): 5753813.

Hoff, M., E. Skovlund, S. Skurtveit et al. "Proton Pump Inhibitors and Fracture Risk. The HUNT Study, Norway." *Osteoporosis International* 31 (2020): 109–118.

Kandil, T. S., A. A. Mousa, A. A. El-Gendy, and A. M. Abbas. "The Potential Therapeutic Effects of Melatonin in Gastro-Esophageal Reflux Disease." *BMC Gastroenterology* 10, no. 1 (2010): 7.

Li, Shujie, Shengying Shi, Feng Chen, and Jingming Lin. "The Effects of Baclofen for the Treatment of Gastroesophageal Reflux Disease: A Meta-Analysis of Randomized Controlled Trials." *Gastroenterology Research and Practice* 2014 (2014): 307805.

Mone, I., B. Kraja, A. Bregu et al. "Adherence to a Predominantly Mediterranean Diet Decreases the Risk of Gastroesophageal Reflux Disease: A Cross-Sectional Study in a South Eastern European Population." *Diseases of the Esophagus* 29 (2016): 794–800.

Murao, Tetsuya, Kouici Sakurai, Syuuichi et al. "Lifestyle Change Influences on GERD in Japan: A Study of Participants in a Health Examination Program." *Digestive Diseases and Sciences* 56 (2011): 2857–2864.

Pereira, Ricardo de Souza. "Regression of Gastroesophageal Reflux Disease Symptoms Using Dietary Supplementation with Melatonin, Vitamins and Aminoacids: Comparison with Omeprazole." *Journal of Pineal Research* 41, no. 3 (October 2006): 195–200.

Targownik, Laura E., Lisa M. Lix, Colleen J. Metge et al. "Use of Proton Pump Inhibitors and Risk of Osteoporosis-Related Fractures." *CMAJ* 179, no. 4 (August 12, 2008): 319–326.

Trinh, Dieu-Thuong Thi, An Hoa Tran, Minh-Man Pham Bui, and Nguyen Lam Vuong. "Thread-Embedding Acupuncture May Improve Symptom Resolution in Patients with Gastroesophageal Reflux Disease: A Randomized Controlled Trial." *Integrative Medicine Research* 12 (2021): 100971.

Wang, Yun-Han, Viktor Wintzell, Jonas F. Ludvigsson et al. "Association Between Proton Pump Inhibitor Use and Risk of Fracture in Children." *JAMA Pediatrics* 174, no. 6 (2020): 543–551.

Zhang, Chao-xian, Yong-mei Qin, and Bao-rui Guo. "Clinical Study on the Treatment of Gastroesophageal Reflux by Acupuncture." *Chinese Journal of Integrative Medicine* 16, no. 4 (August 2010): 298–303.

GASTROPARESIS

INTRODUCTION

Also known as delayed gastric emptying, gastroparesis is a disorder that slows or stops the movement of food from the stomach into the small intestine, even though there is no blockage in the stomach or intestine. The strong muscle contractions that normally propel food through the digestive tract fail to work properly. The stomach muscle contractions are weaker and slower than they should be. Food sits too long in the stomach.

Healthcare providers often classify gastroparesis into subtypes. So, gastroparesis that is a side effect of diabetes may be called diabetes-related gastroparesis. Gastroparesis that takes place after surgery may be called post-surgical gastroparesis. Gastroparesis that happens for no obvious reason is called idiopathic gastroparesis. Most cases of gastroparesis are considered to be idiopathic. In 1957, Paul Kassander, MD, a New Hampshire physician, first described diabetic gastroparesis in people with type 1 diabetes at a meeting of the American College of Physicians. A year later, in 1958, the *Annals of Internal Medicine* printed Dr. Kassander's detailed report.[1]

Diabetes is the most common single cause of gastroparesis. About one-third of the cases of gastroparesis are believed to be related to diabetes. Gastroparesis may occur when high levels of sugar damage nerves and the blood vessels that carry oxygen to tissues. When food sits too long in the stomach, blood sugar levels may drop too low. When the food is finally released, blood sugar levels may spike. But gastroparesis may also begin after surgery or when the vagus nerve (the nerve that controls the stomach muscles) has been damaged, as it may be with diabetes. A damaged vagus nerve is unable to send normal signals to the stomach muscles. Common surgical procedures that have caused post-surgical gastroparesis include the Nissen fundoplication, gastrectomy, gastric bypass surgery, pancreatectomy, vagotomy, and cholecystectomy. Gastroparesis-like symptoms may also be a response to the use of certain medications, such as opioid pain relievers, some antidepressants (amitriptyline, nortriptyline, and venlafaxine), some anticholinergics or medicines that block certain nerve signals, some medicines used to treat an overactive bladder, pramlintide (used to treat high levels of blood sugar), an infection usually from a virus, such as the Norwalk virus or rotavirus, an autoimmune disease, connective tissue disease such as scleroderma, nervous system diseases such as multiple sclerosis and

Parkinson's disease, endocrine disorders such as hypothyroidism, and treatments for high blood pressure and allergies.

SYMPTOMS, RISKS, AND COMPLICATIONS

People with gastroparesis may feel full minutes after starting to eat, and they feel full longer after ending a meal. It is not uncommon for them to be nauseous or vomit, even whole pieces of food. As a result, they may eat too little to maintain their health and a normal weight. In fact, they often lose weight. Other signs and symptoms include indigestion, abdominal bloating, abdominal pain, acid reflux, changes in blood sugar levels, loss of appetite, constipation, and malnutrition. Some people with gastroparesis do not have any noticeable symptoms.

A number of different complications have been associated with gastroparesis. These include severe dehydration, malnutrition, unpredictable blood sugar changes, decreased quality of life, and undigested food that hardens in the stomach, which is called a bezoar. The fermentation of undigested food may lead to bacterial overgrowth. And bezoars may cause an obstruction, nausea, severe vomiting, and reflux symptoms. Untreated gastroparesis may also worsen diabetes by altering blood sugar levels.

PREVALENCE

Although there appear to be few authoritative studies on the overall prevalence of gastroparesis in the United States, one impressive study conducted by researchers from Cleveland, Ohio, and Pittsburgh, Pennsylvania, appeared in the *Journal of Clinical Gastroenterology* in 2020. In this study, researchers surveyed a total of 43,827,910 medical records from 1999 to 2014. The survey was conducted using Explorys, a cloud-based platform, originally designed by the Cleveland Clinic Foundation, and was later acquired by IBM Watson. At the time of this study, Explorys had access to over 340 hospitals in the United States, comprising twenty-two different healthcare systems. The researchers determined that 69,950 patients had a diagnosis of gastroparesis, a prevalence rate of 0.16 percent. The highest rate of gastroparesis was seen in whites; that was followed by African Americans. Females accounted for 66.1 percent of the identified patients. People with type 1 diabetes had a higher prevalence of gastroparesis than people with type 2 diabetes. At the same time, the researchers found that medical records often failed to mention how gastroparesis was diagnosed. So, the actual prevalence of gastroparesis is unclear. "The rates of prevalence may be an overestimation as the diagnosis of GP [gastroparesis] has not been established with the recommended standard of care in many cases with this diagnosis."[2]

However, in an earlier study on the prevalence of gastroparesis published in the *Journal of Neurogastroenterology and Motility*, researchers from Rochester, Minnesota, and Spain commented that many people with "gastroparesis-like" symptoms have never actually had a gastric emptying test. Some of these people may well have undiagnosed gastroparesis. In order to determine an estimate of the percentage of people who have undiagnosed gastroparesis, the researchers developed a model to predict the rate of gastric emptying and then applied this model to community subjects. Ultimately, data from 450 subjects were analyzed. Of these, 330 were female; the cohort had a mean age of forty-six years. From these subjects, the researchers found that hidden gastroparesis may occur in 1.8 percent of community subjects. As a result, "the proportion of subjects with diagnosed gastroparesis may reflect only the tip of the iceberg in the community." In fact, "since the prevalence of diagnosed gastroparesis is low . . ., many subjects with gastroparesis may remain undiagnosed."[3]

On the other hand, the National Institute of Diabetes and Digestive and Kidney Diseases reports that for every 100,000 people, about ten men and forty women have gastroparesis. However, symptoms that are similar to those of gastroparesis occur in about one out of four adults in the United States.[4]

DIAGNOSIS AND TREATMENT OPTIONS

The diagnosis of gastroparesis usually begins with a description of the various symptoms. A blood test may be ordered to look for antibodies from a prior infection or autoantibodies that indicate an autoimmune disease. Then, imaging tests may be used to rule out an obstruction. These may include an upper endoscopy, a capsule endoscopy, an upper GI series, a CT scan, an MRI, and an abdominal ultrasound. Then, a gastric emptying scintigraphy (GES) may be used to measure gastric motility. A type of nuclear imaging test, medical providers add a small amount of radioactive material to a food or drink and then follow its progression through the digestive system. A gastric motility breath test (GEBT) tracks the progression of a meal through the digestive system by measuring gases in the breath. With this test, patients consume a special meal containing a carbon molecule (carbon-13) that produces a specific, measurable form of carbon dioxide (CO_2-13). After it reaches the intestine, this gas is measurable in the breath. Still, another test is the wireless motility capsule. With this test, patients swallow a pill-sized wireless electronic device. This device sends data to a receiver that the patient wears on his or her waist. After a few days, the wireless device will pass, and the receiver needs to be returned to the medical provider who ordered the test.

While there is currently no way to correct the damage caused by gastroparesis, there are medications that increase muscle contractions in the stomach and encourage the digestive system to empty. Prokinetic medications, which stimulate gastrointestinal motility, are the first line of treatment. Metoclopramide is the only FDA-approved medication to treat gastroparesis. While it stimulates muscle contractions in the stomach and helps relieve nausea, it has a black box warning because it has the potential to cause neurological problems including tremors and muscle twitching. As an alternative, your healthcare provider may recommend a motilin agonist, such as erythromycin or azithromycin. Though they are normally used as antibiotics, they may be prescribed for gastroparesis. Other potential treatment options include antiemetics for nausea and vomiting, proton pump inhibitors to treat acid reflux, pain relievers for stomach pain, and diabetes treatments to manage blood sugar.

Healthcare providers may also recommend dietary changes, such as eating a diet with less fiber and lower amounts of fat. In some severe cases, tube feeding or IV feeding may be advised. Some people may need IV fluids to rehydrate and correct electrolyte imbalances.

Surgery will only be advised as a last resort. During a pyloroplasty, a surgeon cuts into the pylorus muscle at the bottom of the stomach, which relaxes and expands the opening. One variety of this type of surgery is known as the G-POEM, which is an endoscopic procedure. Another type of gastroparesis surgery is the gastric bypass. During this procedure, known as a partial gastrectomy, part of the stomach is removed or closed off, and a new outlet is created from the stomach to the small intestine (gastrojejunostomy). Gastric bypass surgery may be especially helpful for people with type 2 diabetes who have obesity.

Some clinicians recommend that people with gastroparesis avoid taking opioids, tricyclic antidepressants, progesterone, anticholinergics, calcium channel blockers, amylin analogues, cyclosporine, clonidine, lithium, and antipsychotic medications, and they should not use nicotine or marijuana. It may be helpful to eat smaller meals four to six times per day and participate in some form of daily exercise.

RESEARCH FINDINGS

Metoclopramide and Erythromycin Are about Equally Effective for Gastroparesis in People with Diabetes

In a single-blind, crossover trial published in the journal *Diabetes Care*, researchers from Turkey compared the use of metoclopramide and erythromycin for treating thirteen patients with diabetes and severe gastroparesis. Of these thirteen, nine were treated with insulin and four were treated with oral hypoglycemic agents. No one had a history of gastric surgery. The patients began the trial by completing a questionnaire on their gastroparesis symptoms. For three weeks, the patients took either 10 mg of metoclopramide three times per day or 250 mg erythromycin three times per day—always thirty minutes before each meal. After a three-week washout period, they took the other medication for three weeks. Patients were seen weekly to review their clinical status and side effects. After each treatment was completed, the patients had gastric emptying tests. The researchers learned that the patients experienced significant improvement from both medications. Although no patient taking erythromycin reported any side effects, side effects from metoclopramide included weakness, sedation, leg cramps, palpitations, and drowsiness. The researchers noted that "both agents were found to have strong and similar gastrokinetic effects."[5]

Oral Metoclopramide Appears to Be Useful for Diabetic Gastroparesis

In a three-week, double-blind, randomized, placebo-controlled trial published in the journal *Diabetes Care*, researchers from several locations in the United States but based in New Haven, Connecticut, compared the use of oral metoclopramide and a placebo for treating diabetic gastroparesis. The initial cohort consisted of twenty-eight women and sixteen men, with a mean age of forty-one years. Thirty-seven patients had peripheral neuropathy, and thirteen had vascular complications. Five patients were receiving hemodialysis. Twenty patients took a total of 40 mg per day of metoclopramide and twenty-four took placebos. The patients in both groups had similar demographic characteristics. The researchers evaluated the following symptoms in the patients: intolerance of meals, fullness and bloating after meals, nausea, vomiting, anorexia, and early satiety. Two patients from each group did not complete the study. So, the final cohort was forty patients. The researchers determined that metoclopramide improved abdominal fullness and nausea. Levels of anorexia, meal intolerance, and early satiety improved in both groups. The researchers concluded that metoclopramide "appears to be a valuable adjunct in the therapy of gastric stasis due to diabetes mellitus."[6]

Risk of Parkinson Like Symptoms after Taking Metoclopramide Might Not Be as High as Some People Contend

In a study published in the *British Journal of Clinical Pharmacology*, researchers from Taiwan examined the actual risk of Parkinsonism in people who take metoclopramide. The researchers used data from the Longitudinal Health Insurance Database 2005, a subset of the Taiwan National Health Insurance Research Database. The researchers learned that from January 1, 2001, to December 31, 2011, there were 226,848 new users of metoclopramide. After excluding 7,917 users because of unknown prescription information, they had a total of 218,931 metoclopramide users and 218,931 age- and gender-matched non-user controls. Almost 60 percent of the groups were female, and the median age was forty-one years. During a one-year follow-up period, 122 users of metoclopramide and fifty-six non-users were diagnosed with Parkinsonism. Further, the researchers learned that people who took metoclopramide in higher doses or for longer periods of time had a higher risk of Parkinsonism than those who either took the standard dose of metoclopramide or took this medication for shorter periods of time. In this study, long-duration exposure accounted for the majority of high-exposure users.[7]

In a study published in the journal *Neurogastroenterology & Motility*, researchers from Sweden reexamined the belief that metoclopramide significantly increases the risk of Parkinsonian symptoms. According to these researchers, it has been estimated that people who use metoclopramide have an 1–10 percent increased risk for developing Parkinsonian symptoms. That is why the US Food and Drug Administration (FDA) issued a black box warning for this medication, restricting its use for no more than three months. The warning directly linked the development of Parkinsonian symptoms with the use of higher doses of this medication for longer periods of time, especially in elderly females. Meanwhile, the European Medicines Agency recommended that it only be used for up to five days. This warning led to a reduction in the use of metoclopramide and in a reduction in cases of medication-related Parkinsonian symptoms. But, one cannot help but ask, are the risks actually as high as the FDA contends? The researchers noted that data on the association between metoclopramide and Parkinsonian symptoms have been obtained from prescription databases, observational studies, and reports from specialized referral centers for involuntary movement in neurology. Yet, there are many studies indicating that the incidence is somewhat rare. For example, a report from the Swedish Adverse Drug Reactions Advisory Committee of eleven million people found only eleven cases over a five-year period of time. The researchers cited many more reports of exceedingly low rates of this disorder. And, they decided that the rate is in the range of 0.1 percent per 1000 patient years, far below previous estimates. Still, people taking metoclopramide should be aware of this potential side effect and should watch for early symptoms; they can then discontinue the medication and, hopefully, reverse the progression of Parkinsonian symptoms. This is especially true for those at highest risk, "elderly females, diabetics, patients with liver or kidney failure, and patients with concomitant antipsychotic drug therapy, which reduces the threshold for neurological complications."[8]

Erythromycin Seems to Be an Effective Treatment for Gastroparesis

In a trial published in the *New England Journal of Medicine*, researchers from Belgium studied ten patients with diabetes mellitus and gastroparesis (three men and seven women with a mean age of fifty-one years) and ten healthy subjects matched for age and sex. The researchers studied the emptying of liquids and solids on separate days after the administration of 200 mg of erythromycin or a placebo. After eating a meal, the patients with diabetes and gastroparesis received either erythromycin or a placebo infused over a fifteen-minute period of time. Measurements of gastric emptying were administered. The healthy subjects received neither a drug nor a placebo. All of the patients were subsequently treated for four weeks with erythromycin orally three times per day. On the morning of the last day of treatment, measurements were made of gastric emptying. The researchers determined that the intravenously administered erythromycin markedly improved the severely impaired gastric emptying of both liquids and solids in the ten patients. The drug was also effective when administered orally for four weeks. The researchers noted that after the intravenous administration of erythromycin, liquids and solids emptied at the same rate. In fact, their emptying rate was similar to the rate for liquids in the healthy subjects. The researchers concluded that "erythromycin markedly improves impaired gastric emptying in patients with severe diabetic gastroparesis."[9]

In a systematic review published in the *American Journal of Gastroenterology*, researchers from Chicago, Illinois, reviewed clinical trials on the ability of erythromycin to relieve the symptoms associated with gastroparesis. The researchers identified five clinical trials with sixty patients that met their criteria. Two studies evaluated patients with post-surgical or scleroderma-related gastroparesis. Three studies examined symptoms in patients with diabetic or idiopathic gastroparesis. Four of the five studies were open-label, and all of the studies were methodologically weak and highly subject to bias. The researchers assessed study design, dose of erythromycin and route of administration, duration of treatment, measures of gastric function, and symptom response. Improvement was reported in twenty-six patients (48 percent) and individual symptom scores were available for only twenty-three of the sixty patients. However, in these patients, total symptom scores were reduced by 25 percent or more in eleven of twenty-three (48 percent) of the subjects. The researchers commented that "one might look at a symptom response rate of forty-eight percent and be optimistic. This response rate, however, was obtained in a very small group of patients treated in unblinded fashion for short periods."[10]

But Azithromycin May Be a Better Choice Than Erythromycin

In a retrospective, case-control analysis published in the *Journal of Neurogastroenterology and Motility*, researchers from Gainesville, Florida, reviewed 120 patients who had a gastric emptying study for chronic abdominal pain or suspected gastroparesis. Once they were diagnosed with gastroparesis, the patients received either intravenous azithromycin or intravenous erythromycin. At baseline, both groups of patients had similar demographic characteristics. Thus, the mean age of the patients in the azithromycin group was forty-eight years, and the mean age of the patients in the erythromycin group was forty-seven years. The gastric emptying test results were similar for the two groups. The researchers learned that both azithromycin and erythromycin had similar positive effects on gastric emptying. But, azithromycin had fewer cardiac side effects and fewer overall drug-to-drug interactions. In addition, patients taking erythromycin often reported nausea, vomiting, and diarrhea. According to the researchers, these side effects are less likely to occur with azithromycin. The researchers added that they had found azithromycin useful in patients who have not been helped by metoclopramide or erythromycin. The researchers concluded that there is a need for "a larger randomized control study with a placebo arm to further evaluate the efficacy and safety" of azithromycin in the treatment of gastroparesis.[11]

It Is Probably Efficacious for Critically Ill Patients to Take Prokinetic Agents Such as Metoclopramide and Erythromycin

In a systematic review and meta-analysis published in the journal *Critical Care*, researchers based in Canada noted that prokinetic agents are frequently prescribed for critically ill patients who have delayed gastric emptying. Apparently, this is a common problem in critically ill people. The researchers wanted to determine the efficacy and safety of these medications for such ill patients, who are receiving enteral nutrition. The researchers located thirteen randomized controlled trials with 1,341 patients that met their criteria. The patients were all seriously ill with medical, surgical, and neurosurgical conditions. In these studies, the intervention groups received a prokinetic agent and the control groups received no intervention or a placebo. Eight trials used intravenous metoclopramide at different frequencies. Seven trials used erythromycin at a range of doses and administration schedules. Two studies were considered to be of high risk for bias; five studies were thought to be of low risk for bias. The researchers learned that the prokinetic agents were effective in improving feeding intolerance in critically ill patients.[12]

Prucalopride Seems to Be Useful for Gastroparesis

In a double-blind, randomized, placebo-controlled, crossover trial published in the *American Journal of Gastroenterology*, researchers from Belgium evaluated the ability of prucalopride to improve the symptoms of gastroparesis. The cohort consisted of thirty-four people with gastroparesis; there were twenty-six women. Twenty-eight cases were idiopathic, and the remaining subjects had diabetes. For four weeks, the subjects took either 2 mg per day of prucalopride or a placebo. Then, after a two-week washout period, they took the alternative option for four weeks. The subjects kept symptom and stool consistency diaries and completed questionnaires. And, gastric emptying tests were administered. Seven subjects dropped out of the trial; so, twenty-seven subjects completed the entire trial. One serious adverse event occurred; one of the subjects on prucalopride developed intestinal volvulus. Other side effects included diarrhea, headache, abdominal cramps, and cystitis. The researchers determined that solid but not liquid half-emptying times with prucalopride were significantly shorter than during placebo treatment. Daily diaries confirmed significant improvement for abdominal pain, postprandial fullness, bloating, early satiety, nausea, and overall symptom severity. The researchers concluded that "prucalopride showed symptomatic benefit of the drug in gastroparesis and in the subgroup of patients with idiopathic gastroparesis."[13]

People with Diabetic Gastroparesis May Benefit from Eating a Small Particle Size Diet

In a twenty-week, randomized, double-blinded, parallel group, controlled trial published in the *American Journal of Gastroenterology*, researchers from Sweden offered two different types of diet to fifty-six people with insulin-treated diabetes mellitus and the delayed gastric emptying seen in gastroparesis. The subjects in the intervention group ate a small particle diet that consisted of foods that were smaller than 2 mm in diameter, such as milkshakes, berry and fruit compote, mashed potatoes, smooth soups, and mashed turnips, or foods that could easily be processed into smaller sizes. The diet excluded foods with husks or peels, foods with membranes, stringy foods, seeds and grains, and compact, poorly digestible foods, such as pasta, rice, meat, raw vegetable salad, and cheese slices. The other group was told to follow the standard diet recommended for people with diabetes—fruit, vegetables, pasta and whole grain bread, meat, cheese, and nuts. Both groups were advised to eat only 25–30 percent of their calories from fat and limit the amount of fiber. Due to a worsening of their symptoms, five subjects in the intervention group left the study, and one subject in the second group died of a heart attack. So, fifty subjects completed the entire study. Among the assessments conducted were measurements of gastric emptying rate, severity of gastrointestinal symptoms, levels of anxiety and depression, and quality of life. All of the subjects on the intervention diet who completed the trial experienced a significant improvement in almost all of their gastrointestinal symptoms, such as nausea/vomiting, postprandial fullness, early satiety and bloating, and regurgitation/heartburn. The only exception was abdominal pain. They also had decreases in levels of anxiety. But the small particle diet did not improve their metabolic control. The researchers wondered if a longer trial might have yielded different metabolic control results. And the small particle diet had no effect on depression or quality of life. None of the subjects on the usual diet had any improvement in their gastrointestinal symptoms or in their levels of anxiety. The researchers concluded that information on the small particle diet should be shared with gastroparesis patients with diabetes. At the same time, there is a need for more research on the topic.[14]

Some Foods May Provoke Gastroparesis Symptoms and Other Foods May Alleviate Symptoms

In a study published in the journal *Digestive Diseases and Sciences*, researchers from Philadelphia, Pennsylvania, wanted to identify and characterize foods that provoked or alleviated symptoms of gastroparesis. The cohort consisted of forty-five patients, forty-one females and four males, with idiopathic or diabetic gastroparesis. They had a mean age of forty-one years. These subjects experienced symptoms such as the inability to finish a meal, feelings of fullness, upper abdominal discomfort, nausea, and loss of appetite. The subjects completed a demographic questionnaire, a patient assessment of upper gastrointestinal symptoms, and a food tolerance and aversion survey, which asked about their experiences eating certain foods. The researchers learned that the provoking foods had a higher fat content; they tended to be acidic, spicy, and roughage-based, while alleviating foods usually had a higher carbohydrate content and were often bland, sweet, salty, and starchy. Specifically, certain foods were found to exacerbate the symptoms of gastroparesis; these foods were orange juice, fried chicken breast, boiled cabbage, oranges, pork sausage, cheese pizza, sweet, raw peppers, boiled onions, canned tomato juice, romaine lettuce, brewed coffee, salsa, boiled broccoli, pork bacon, and deli-style roast beef. On the other hand, symptoms moderately improved with other foods. These included saltine crackers, jello, and graham crackers. Other foods, such as ginger ale, gluten-free foods, tea, sweet potatoes, pretzels, white fish, clear soup, salmon, potatoes, white rice, popsicles, and applesauce, did not provoke symptoms. Still, it is important to note that the differences between the two types of foods were not statistically different. The researchers concluded that their findings "provide . . . evidence for specific food items for a gastroparesis diet based on experience from patients with gastroparesis."[15]

In a trial published in the journal *Neurogastroenterology & Motility*, researchers from Philadelphia, Pennsylvania, investigated the effect of fat intake and solid and liquid meal consistency on the symptoms of gastroparesis. The cohort consisted of twelve patients, two males and ten females, with diabetic (n = 3) or idiopathic (n = 9) gastroparesis, who had an average age of 44.4 years and an average BMI of 29.6. They ate one of four different meals on four separate days—high-fat solid meal, high-fat liquid meal, low-fat liquid meal, and low-fat solid meal. With each meal, eight gastrointestinal symptoms were rated from zero (none) to four (very severe), every fifteen minutes, beginning before the meal and ending four hours after the meal. These symptoms were nausea, stomach fullness, bloating, stomach or belly visibly larger, upper and lower abdominal pain, heartburn, and chest discomfort. The researchers administered questionnaires on a number of different areas, including upper gastrointestinal symptoms, food frequency, and exercise habits. And they measured the body composition of the subjects. The researchers learned that the subjects had the worst symptoms after the high-fat solid meal. It was then that they had the most nausea, heartburn, stomach fullness, bloating, and their stomachs were visibly larger. And there were no significant differences in total symptom scores between the low-fat solid meal, the high-fat liquid meal, and the low-fat liquid meal. Still, the low-fat liquid meal appeared to have the least effect on the total symptom score. Interestingly, the symptom most affected by fat content and solid consistency was nausea. The researchers concluded that their findings "provide support for dietary recommendations that low-fat and more liquids may reduce symptoms in gastroparesis."[16]

There May Be an Association between Vitamin B12 Deficiency and Gastroparesis in People with Type 2 Diabetes

In a trial published in the journal *Diabetology & Metabolic Syndrome*, researchers from Egypt examined the association between vitamin B12 deficiency and gastroparesis in people with type 2 diabetes. The cohort consisted of 100 people who have had type 2 diabetes for more than ten years and fifty healthy controls, who were matched for age and sex. The people with type 2 diabetes were placed in one of two groups—those with gastroparesis (n

= 55) and those without this disorder (n = 45). All of the subjects had a medical history and clinical examination. The researchers determined that there were notable differences between the subjects with and without type 2 diabetes. For example, the subjects with type 2 diabetes had significantly higher BMI, waist circumference, and systolic and diastolic blood pressure than those without type 2 diabetes. Levels of vitamin B12 were significantly lower in subjects with type 2 diabetes than in the healthy controls. And the frequency of vitamin B12 deficiency was 54.5 percent in subjects with gastroparesis and 11.1 percent in those without gastroparesis. In fact, vitamin B12 proved to be an independent predictor for gastroparesis in subjects with type 2 diabetes.[17]

People with Idiopathic Gastroparesis May Have Multiple Dietary Deficiencies

In a trial published in the *American Journal of Gastroenterology*, researchers from Philadelphia, Pennsylvania, evaluated the intake of dietary protein, carbohydrate, fat, fiber, vitamins, and minerals in twenty-four subjects with symptomatic idiopathic gastroparesis (nineteen females with a mean age of forty-seven years) and twenty-four controls. For seven days, all of the subjects completed detailed records of their diets. The records were then given to the registered dietitian for an extensive evaluation. The researchers learned that the subjects with gastroparesis ate significantly less than the controls; they ate fewer carbohydrates, fats, and proteins than the controls. Furthermore, their dietary intake of various vitamins and minerals was below the recommended dietary allowance (RDA) for age and sex. Vitamins with intakes of less than 100 percent of the RDA were B, C, folate, niacin, riboflavin, and thiamine. Minerals with intakes of less than 100 percent of the RDA were calcium, copper, magnesium, iron, phosphorus, and zinc. Compared to controls, the intake of the mineral potassium was also significantly reduced among the subjects with gastroparesis. The researchers concluded that people with idiopathic gastroparesis consume "significantly fewer calories than their predicted requirements." Moreover, they consume "diets that are deficient in a number of essential vitamins and minerals." As a result, the researchers recommended more screening for gastroparesis among people with "functional" complaints.[18]

In a comprehensive trial published in the journal *Gastroenterology*, researchers from many locations but based in Philadelphia, Pennsylvania, discussed the nutritional deficiencies in patients with gastroparesis. The cohort consisted of 305 patients with diabetic or idiopathic gastroparesis enrolled in the National Institute of Diabetes and Digestive and Kidney Diseases Gastroparesis Registry. The patients completed dietary questionnaires at seven centers. The researchers learned that the average daily caloric intake of the subjects was 1,168, which was 58 percent of their daily energy expenditures. Overall, they were averaging only 1.4 meals per day. They tended to have smaller portions of food during the day. The daily intake was low in fat, low in fiber, and consisted of small food portions. More than five days per week, 10 percent of the group had nutrient drinks. Only five subjects followed a suggested gastroparetic diet. Deficiencies in the intake of vitamins and minerals from food ranged from 30 to 86 percent. While 38 percent of the subjects took multivitamins, the intake of other vitamins and supplements was much lower. Vitamin and mineral deficits were particularly notable for vitamins C, D, K, folate, and the minerals calcium, iron, magnesium, and potassium. Interestingly, subjects with diabetes had a higher daily caloric intake than those with idiopathic gastroparesis, and subjects with diabetes were more likely to consume a diet that had lower levels of carbohydrates and higher amounts of protein, fat, and fiber than subjects with idiopathic gastroparesis. And, subjects with idiopathic gastroparesis were more likely to have a lower percentage of most micronutrients than subjects with diabetes. Despite all these problems, only one-third of the subjects had nutritional counseling. The researchers noted that "diet compliance might be improved by several encounters [with a nutritional counselor] rather than a single visit."[19]

Acupuncture May Be Useful for People with the Symptoms of Gastroparesis

In a randomized, single-blinded, pilot trial published in the *Journal of Alternative and Complementary Medicine*, researchers from China investigated the ability of electroacupuncture to help people with type 2 diabetes who have had the symptoms of gastroparesis for at least three months. The cohort, which consisted of sixteen male and three female subjects, ranged in age from forty-one to seventy-four years. During four thirty-minute sessions that took place over a two-week period of time, nine subjects received electroacupuncture and ten received sham electroacupuncture. The Gastroparesis Cardinal Symptoms Index was used to evaluate symptom severity at baseline, at the end of the treatment, and two weeks after the treatment ended. The researchers determined that the half-emptying times in the nine patients with diabetic gastroparesis were significantly shortened by the electroacupuncture. At the same time, the half-emptying time did not change in the sham group. The symptom severity of postprandial fullness/satiety and bloating also improved significantly in the electroacupuncture group, but not in the sham group. And, electroacupuncture did not appear to improve nausea and vomiting. The researchers concluded that electroacupuncture "may have a future as a therapeutic option in the treatment of gastroparesis."[20]

REFERENCES AND FURTHER READING

Ahmed, Sally S., Hala A. Abd El-Hafez, Mohammed Mohsen et al. "Is Vitamin B12 Deficiency a Risk Factor for Gastroparesis in Patients with Type 2 Diabetes?" *Diabetology & Metabolic Syndrome* 15 (2023): 33.

Al-Saffar, Ahmad, Hans Lennernäs, and Per M. Hellström. "Gastroparesis, Metoclopramide, and Tardive Dyskinesia: Risk Revisited." *Neurogastroenterology & Motility* 31, no. 11 (November 2019): e13617.

Carbone, Florencia, Karenn Van den Houte, Egbert Clevers et al. "Prucalopride in Gastroparesis: A Randomized Placebo-Controlled Crossover Study." *American Journal of Gastroenterology* 114, no. 8 (August 2019): 1265–1274.

Erbas, Tomris, Eerhan Varoglu, Belkis Erbas et al. "Comparison of Metoclopramide and Erythromycin in the Treatment of Diabetic Gastroparesis." *Diabetes Care* 16, no. 11 (November 1993): 1511–1514.

Homko, C. J., F. Duffy, F. K. Friedenberg et al. "Effect of Dietary Fat and Food Consistency on Gastroparesis Symptoms in Patients with Gastroparesis." *Neurogastroenterology & Motility* 27, no. 4 (April 2015): 501–508.

Janssens, J., T. L. Peeters, G Vantrappen et al. "Improvement of Gastric Emptying in Diabetic Gastroparesis by Erythromycin – Preliminary Studies." *New England Journal of Medicine* 322 (1990): 1028–1031.

Larson, Jean M., Anna Tavakkoli, Walter E. Drane et al. "Advantages of Azithromycin Over Erythromycin in Improving the Gastric Emptying Half-Time in Adult Patients with Gastroparesis." *Journal of Neurogastroenterology and Motility* 16, no. 4 (October 2010): 407–413.

Lewis, Kim, Zuhoor Alqahtani, Lauralyn McIntyre et al. "The Efficacy and Safety of Prokinetic Agents in Critically Ill Patients Receiving Enteral Nutrition: A Systematic Review and Meta-Analysis of Randomized Trials." *Critical Care* 20 (2016): 259.

Maganti, Kalyani, Kingsley Onyemere, and Michael P. Jones. "Oral Erythromycin and Symptomatic Relief of Gastroparesis: A Systematic Review." *American Journal of Gastroenterology* 98, no. 2 (2003): 259–263.

McCallum, Richard W., Dominick A. Ricci, Hebert Rakatansky et al. "A Multicenter Placebo-Controlled Clinical Trial of Oral Metoclopramide in Diabetic Gastroparesis." *Diabetes Care* 6, no. 5 (September–October 1983): 463–467.

Ogorek, Carrie P., Laura Davidson, Robert S. Fisher, and Benjamin Krevsky. "Idiopathic Gastroparesis Is Associated with a Multiplicity of Severe Dietary Deficiencies." *American Journal of Gastroenterology* 86, no. 4 (1991): 423–428.

Olausson, Eva A., Stine Störsrud, Håkan Grundin et al. "A Small Particle Diet Reduces Upper Gastrointestinal Symptoms in Patients with Diabetic Gastroparesis: A Randomized Controlled Diet." *American Journal of Gastroenterology* 109 (2014): 375–385.

Parkman, Henry P., Katherine P. Yates, William L. Hasler et al. "Dietary Intake and Nutritional Deficiencies in Patients with Diabetic or Idiopathic Gastroparesis." *Gastroenterology* 141 (2011): 486–498.

Rey, Enrique, Rok Seon Choung, Cathy D. Schleck et al. "Prevalence of Hidden Gastroparesis in the Community: The Gastroparesis 'Iceberg.'" *Journal of Neurogastroenterology and Motility* 18, no. 1 (January 2012): 34–42.

Syed, Aslam R., Michael M. Wolfe, and Jorge Calles-Escandon. "Epidemiology and Diagnosis of Gastroparesis in the United States: A Population-Based Study." *Journal of Clinical Gastroenterology* 54, no. 1 (January 2020): 50–53.

Tsai, Shin-Chia, Shiow-Yunn Sheu, Li-Nien Chien et al. "High Exposure Compared with Standard Exposure to Metoclopramide Associated with a Higher Risk of Parkinsonism: A Nationwide Population-Based Cohort Study." *British Journal of Clinical Pharmacology* 84 (2018): 2000–2009.

Wang, Chung-Pang, Chia-Hung Kao, Wei-Kung Chen et al. "A Single-Blinded, Randomized Pilot Study Evaluating Effects of Electroacupuncture in Diabetic Patients with Symptoms Suggestive of Gastroparesis." *Journal of Alternative and Complementary Medicine* 14, no. 7 (2008): 833–839.

Wytiaz, Victoria, Carol Homka, Frank Duffy et al. "Food Provoking and. Alleviating Symptoms in Gastroparesis: Patient Experiences." *Digestive Diseases and Sciences* 60 (2015): 1052–1058.

HEMORRHOIDS AND FISSURES

INTRODUCTION

Also known as piles, hemorrhoids (pronounced hem-uh-roids) are irritated or swollen veins or blood vessels in and around the anus and lower rectum. They are very similar to varicose veins, and people who have varicose veins tend to have an increased risk of hemorrhoids. When hemorrhoids form inside the anus, they are termed internal hemorrhoids; when they form under the skin around the anus, they are called external hemorrhoids.

Fissures are tears or cracks in the anus. They are caused when the anal mucosa is stretched beyond its normal capacity, as may happen when trying to pass hard stools. Once the fissure occurs, it is repeatedly reinjured each time stool, especially hard stool, tries to pass. The exposed internal sphincter muscle beneath the tear experiences repeated spasms. The spasms pull the edges of the fissure apart, making it difficult for the wound to heal. Over time, the fissure may become chronic. In addition, the anus is surrounded by two circular muscles, the anal sphincters that help control bowel movements. If these muscles are too tight, they may add tension to the anal lining, making it easier to tear, and reducing blood flow to the area.

Though many people believe that hemorrhoids are a modern problem, that is not true. In fact, they were described in the four-thousand-year-old Babylonian Code of Hammurabi. And, they are alluded to in the *Edwin Smith Papyrus* (1700 BC), *Ebers Papyrus* (1500 BC), and the *Chester Beatty Papyrus* (1200 BC). But, it was not until 460 BC that Hippocrates coined the term "hemorrhoid"—a combination of the Greek *haema*, which means blood, and *rhoos*, which means flowing.[1]

Meanwhile, ancient people probably also had anal fissures. Still, they were not detailed in the medical literature until 1934, when they were described by the British surgeon John Percy Lockhart-Mummery.[2]

SYMPTOMS, RISKS, AND COMPLICATIONS

While the symptoms of hemorrhoids may vary from person to person, the most frequent symptoms include bright blood on the stool, toilet paper, and/or in the toilet bowl; pain and irritation around the anus; swelling or a hard lump around the anus; and itching.

Internal hemorrhoids are usually painless, but some people with internal hemorrhoids experience pain.

Symptoms of an anal fissure include sharp pain, burning, and itching during and after a bowel movement, a visible tear in the area, and bright red bleeding during or after a bowel movement. Some people find that their pain radiates to their buttocks, upper thighs, and lower back. While many people with hemorrhoids never experience any pain, just about everyone with anal fissures have pain. However, hemorrhoid pain tends to be constant, while anal fissure pain occurs in episodes.

There are a number of factors that place people at increased risk for hemorrhoids. These include frequent straining during bowel movements, a family history of hemorrhoids, aging, and chronic constipation or diarrhea. Other risk factors include sitting too long on the toilet, heavy lifting, an inactive lifestyle, failure to exercise regularly, anal intercourse, and obesity.

It is not uncommon for women to develop hemorrhoids during pregnancy and childbirth. The pressure of carrying the fetus places extra stress on the blood vessels in the pelvic area. If hemorrhoids do not form during pregnancy, they may well occur during delivery.

An article in *JAMA* noted that "in general, anything that puts pressure on the veins in the lower body can lead to hemorrhoids, including straining during a bowel movement, sitting on the toilet for long periods, constipation or diarrhea, being overweight, pregnancy, and age, which causes tissues to become weaker."[3]

There are several risk factors for anal fissures. These include constipation and straining to pass hard stool, eating a low-fiber diet, diarrhea, recent weight loss surgery, vaginal childbirth, minor trauma to the anal area, inflammatory conditions of the anal area, prior surgery, sexually transmitted infections, inflammatory bowel disease, anal cancer, tuberculosis, skin rash, and any medical problem or condition that affects bowel movement or the anus.

Hemorrhoids rarely trigger complications. Still, if they result in excessive bleeding, they have the potential to cause anemia, a condition in which there are insufficient numbers of red blood cells to carry oxygen to the body's cells, which may leave an individual feeling weak and tired. If a hemorrhoid prolapses and loses blood supply, it may become exceedingly painful and require surgical removal. This is known as a strangulated hemorrhoid. In addition, blood may pool in an external hemorrhoid and form a clot or thrombus. This may cause a hard, discolored lump near the anus, inflammation, swelling, and severe pain. The hemorrhoid may need to be drained by a primary care provider or specialist, such as a colorectal surgeon.

Complications associated with anal fissures include pain and discomfort, difficulty with bowel movements, potential for recurrence, clotting, uncontrolled bowel movements, flatulence, and reduced quality of life. Anal fissures that do not heal for an extended period of time may cause fecal impaction, anal stenosis (narrowing), and an anal fistula (abnormal passageway from inside the anus to the skin outside).

PREVALENCE

Hemorrhoids occur very often in both men and women. By the age of fifty, about half of all people have had hemorrhoids. An article in the journal *Clinics in Colon and Rectal Surgery* noted that hemorrhoid disease is the fourth leading outpatient gastrointestinal diagnosis; it accounts for about 3.3 million annual ambulatory care visits in the United States. Every year, about ten million Americans self-report that they have hemorrhoids. Both men and women have the highest occurrence rates between the ages of forty-five and sixty-five years. Hemorrhoids appear more often in Caucasians and in people with higher socioeconomic status.[4] They are thought to be more common in developed countries than developing countries. In addition to differences in diet, this may be a function of the posture assumed during bowel movements. In societies that have adopted Western practices, people sit on toilets; in developing societies, they tend to squat. People spend more time sitting on toilets than squatting.[5]

It has been estimated that 235,000 new cases of anal fissures are reported every year in the United States, and about 40 percent are chronic. But, these are only the reported cases. Large numbers of people probably self-treat their anal fissures (and hemorrhoids!) without ever seeking medical advice.[6]

DIAGNOSIS AND TREATMENT OPTIONS

Hemorrhoids are most frequently diagnosed by a digital rectal examination, in which a healthcare provider inserts a gloved, lubricated finger into the rectum. But, a medical provider may use an anoscope, or a hollow, lighted tube, or a proctoscope, a lighted tube, placed in the anus to diagnose them. If a more serious condition is suspected, a medical provider may conduct a sigmoidoscopy to view the lower third of the colon with a flexible lighted tube or complete a colonoscopy to view the entire colon with a flexible lighted tube.

Hemorrhoid treatments focus on reducing symptoms. Usually, medical providers recommend sitting in plain, warm water or a sitz bath several times a day. Or, they may suggest applying witch hazel pads or ice packs to reduce the swelling. Other initial treatments may include hemorrhoidal creams and/or suppositories, especially those containing hydrocortisone or lidocaine. Medical providers may also recommend adding more fruits and vegetables as well as whole grains to the diet, and they often suggest using stool softeners and a fiber supplement, such as psyllium or methylcellulose. When these measures fail to bring relief, a procedure may be advised. Internal hemorrhoids may be removed with a procedure known as rubber band ligation. A rubber band is placed around the base of the hemorrhoid; without circulation, the hemorrhoid shrinks and falls off. Unfortunately, this tends to be an uncomfortable procedure and frequently causes bleeding for a few days. With sclerotherapy, a chemical solution is injected into the blood vessel, and the hemorrhoid shrinks. Though there is little or no pain, it may not be as effective as the rubber band ligation. Sometimes, a special device is used to beam infrared light, burning the hemorrhoid. The hemorrhoid hardens and shrivels. This is known as electrical coagulation or infrared photo coagulation. Finally, it is sometimes necessary to conduct a more traditional surgical procedure to remove the hemorrhoids or groups of hemorrhoids. This is known as a hemorrhoidectomy. It is the most effective way to treat severe or recurring hemorrhoids. When a stapling device is used to remove the hemorrhoid(s), the procedure is termed a hemorrhoidopexy. Expect some postoperative pain, which may be treated with warm soaks and acetaminophen.

Though most anal fissures heal within a few weeks and respond well to drinking extra water, eating more fruits and vegetables, avoiding spicy foods, taking sitz baths, taking stool softeners and/or fiber supplements, and applying petroleum jelly and pain-relieving cream, such as one that contains lidocaine. If they last longer than six or eight weeks, they are considered chronic and require medical treatment. Medical treatment tends to focus on relaxing the anal sphincter muscles around the anal canal, allowing blood to return to the tissues and foster healing. Medical providers often begin by prescribing a nitroglycerin ointment, which makes blood vessels expand. Still, it may cause headaches in some people. Calcium channel blockers, which also dilate blood vessels, may be prescribed. A medical provider may inject Botox directly into the anal sphincter. During the three months that the injection lasts, the fissure has the opportunity to heal. If these treatments are not useful, surgery may be advised. During this procedure, which is known as an internal sphincterotomy, a surgeon cuts into the anal sphincter muscle to permanently release the tension. Complications associated with the surgery include the risk for infection, bleeding, persistent flatulence, fecal incontinence, and uncontrolled bowel movements.

RESEARCH FINDINGS

Fiber Supplements May Help Bleeding Internal Hemorrhoids

In a trial published in the journal *Hepato-Gastroenterology*, researchers from Spain wanted to learn if fiber supplements would help people dealing with internal bleeding hemorrhoids. The initial cohort consisted of fifty patients with internal bleeding hemorrhoids: twenty-nine males and twenty-one females, with a mean age of 48.3 years. They were randomly placed in one of two groups. For forty days, the twenty-three patients in the treatment group took a commercially available fiber supplement; the twenty-seven patients in the control group took a placebo. The researchers found that during the first fifteen-day period, the mean number of rectal bleeding episodes decreased from 5.2 to 4.8 in the treatment group and from 6.7 to 6.4 in the control group. During the second fifteen-day period, the mean number of bleeding episodes in the study group decreased to 3.1 and to 5.5 in the control group. During the last ten days of the study, there were 1.1 mean bleeding episodes in the treatment group and 5.5 in the control group. The researchers commented that "the addition of fiber to the diet significantly improved bleeding from internal hemorrhoids."[7]

In a systematic review and meta-analysis published in the *American Journal of Gastroenterology*, researchers from Spain, Canada, and Rockford, Illinois examined the impact of fiber for the treatment of symptomatic hemorrhoids. They located seven trials with 378 patients that met their criteria; all of the studies compared fiber supplements to placebos. Six were parallel studies and one was a crossover. Most of the patients had bleeding as their main hemorrhoid complaint. The researchers determined that the risk of not improving/persisting symptoms decreased by 47 percent in the people taking fiber. Studies with follow-ups, usually at six weeks and three months, demonstrated consistently good results. And, fiber also seemed to be useful for bleeding hemorrhoids. Fiber appeared to be most useful for people with less advanced hemorrhoids. Still, the researchers rated the quality of the evidence as moderate, and publication bias and funding were issues of concern. Nevertheless, the researchers concluded that "fiber is an effective treatment for symptomatic hemorrhoids (overall symptoms improvement and bleeding)." And, they underscored the need for additional larger trials on the usefulness of fiber for treating symptomatic hemorrhoids.[8]

But Fiber May Not Be as Useful as Some Suspect

In a double-blind trial published in the *British Journal of Surgery*, researchers from the UK tested the ability of a "bulk forming evacuant" (sterculia) to help people dealing with hemorrhoids. The initial cohort consisted of forty people with hemorrhoids. For three months, they were randomly assigned to take sterculia or a placebo. The subjects in both groups were similar in sex, age, symptoms, and degree of hemorrhoid prolapse. During the trial, symptomatic reviews were conducted monthly; during these reviews, the patients assessed each of their symptoms. Thirty-eight patients completed the trial; there were twenty in the fiber supplement group and eighteen in the control group. The researchers learned that 70 percent of the patients on the fiber supplement and 61 percent of those on the placebo noted improvements in bleeding. When asked about their overall opinion of treatment, twelve of those on the fiber and ten on the placebo indicated that they were better; this difference was not significant. About one-third of the patients had a shrinkage in their hemorrhoids, but, again, the difference between the two groups was not significant. The researchers concluded that "the lack of conclusive evidence of the value of bulk-formers is in keeping with out clinical experience. We find that once their symptoms have subsided only the minority of patients treated in a rectal clinic voluntarily continue to take bulk-formers indefinitely."[9]

People with Constipation, Strained Bowel Movements, and a Low-Fiber Diet Have an Increased Risk of Hemorrhoids

In a cross-sectional study published in the online journal *PLoS ONE*, researchers from several locations in the United States but based in Chapel Hill, North Carolina, examined the association between hemorrhoids and other factors such as constipation, strained bowel movements, a low-fiber diet, a sedentary lifestyle, and the use of aspirin or NSAIDs, alcohol, and cigarettes. The cohort consisted of 2,813 subjects who had a colonoscopy; of these, 1,074 were found to have hemorrhoids. The subjects were recruited from eleven centers in the United States and Puerto Rico. The researchers learned that the subjects with hemorrhoids were more likely to be older, nonwhite, less educated, and constipated. They were more likely to strain during bowel movements. On the other hand, frequent bowel movements, even as often as fifteen or more per week, did not increase the risk. And, people with higher intakes of dietary fiber had a lower risk for hemorrhoids. There did not appear to be an association between hemorrhoids and sedentary behavior, overweight or obesity, alcohol, smoking, and aspirin and NSAID use. The researchers concluded that their findings found only three conditions to be associated with hemorrhoids—constipation, straining with bowel movements, and a low-fiber diet.[10]

People with Hemorrhoids Are Less Likely to Think Their Bowel Habits Are Normal and Are More Likely to Have a Host of Problematic Symptoms

In a trial published in the *American Journal of Gastroenterology*, researchers from Sweden compared the functional bowel symptoms and anorectal complaints of people with hemorrhoids to those without hemorrhoids. One hundred consecutive patients who were about to have a hemorrhoidectomy completed a pre-surgery questionnaire on bowel and anorectal functional symptoms. Though they ranged in age from thirty-three to eighty-four years, they had a mean age of fifty-five years. There were fifty-one males and forty-nine females. In addition to this first group of patients, there were also two hundred age- and gender-matched control subjects and one hundred gender-matched consecutive patients undergoing an orthopedic procedure. The subjects in these two control groups also completed the same bowel questionnaire. While the researchers learned that bowel frequency was similar in all three groups, only 37 percent of the first group believed that their bowel frequency was normal, compared to 55 percent in the second group and 67 percent in the third group. Up to 37 percent of the first group reported bleeding, compared to eighteen and 26 percent in the second and third groups. Thirty-four percent of the first group had abdominal pain associated with bowel movements, but only three and 5 percent of the other groups had this symptom. And, those in the first group were more likely to have excessive straining, a feeling of incomplete bowel movements, repeated bathroom visits, soiling, itching, a reduced feeling of well-being, and a disturbed social life because of their bowel symptoms. As a result of their findings, the researchers theorized that up to half of the people with hemorrhoids probably have a coexisting functional bowel disease, such as irritable bowel syndrome. And, they concluded that "this knowledge might be important while selecting therapy for patients with hemorrhoids."[11]

People with Hemorrhoids May Be at Increased Risk for Hashimoto's Thyroiditis

In a study published in the journal *Frontiers in Endocrinology*, researchers based in Taiwan evaluated the association between hemorrhoids and Hashimoto's thyroiditis. Using Taiwan's Longitudinal Health Insurance Database, they compared the incident risk of hemorrhoids to the incident risk of Hashimoto's thyroiditis, the most common reason for hypothyroidism or low levels of thyroid hormone. The study cohort and comparison cohort consisted of 6,486 patients with hemorrhoids, and 25,944 without hemorrhoids. The mean follow-up time was about three years. Fifty-seven percent of the participants were men, and 39 percent were over fifty years old. The researchers learned that the incidence rate of Hashimoto's was higher in those who had hemorrhoids. While it was 5.37 per 1,000 person-years in those with hemorrhoids, it was 2.46 per 1,000 person-years in those without hemorrhoids. So, in this study, people with hemorrhoids appear to have about twice the risk of developing Hashimoto's thyroiditis. It should be noted that all of the patients with hemorrhoids had comorbidities such as constipation, cardiovascular disease, diabetes, and depression. The researchers concluded that "patients with hemorrhoids could be at increased risk of HT [Hashimoto's thyroiditis] compared with patients with other comorbidities of HT, such as cardiovascular disease."[12]

Rubber Band Ligation Seems to Be a Good Option for Treating Internal Hemorrhoids

In a retrospective study published in the *Indian Journal of Surgery*, a researcher from Yemen described treating almost nine hundred patients with second- and third-degree hemorrhoids with rubber band ligation. Eighty-five percent of the patients were male; they had a mean age of forty-five years. After their procedures, the patients were asked to return to the outpatient clinic for follow-up at two weeks, one month, and six months. They were then contacted by telephone every six months for two years. Slightly more than three-quarters of the patients (76 percent) were cured. Twenty percent had a recurrence of their symptoms. Only 4 percent had complications such as pain, rectal bleeding, and vasovagal symptoms (sudden drop in heart rate and blood pressure). The researchers concluded that rubber band ligation "is a simple, safe, and effective method for treating symptomatic second- and third-degree hemorrhoids and an outpatient procedure that contributes significant improvement in quality of life."[13]

Sitz Baths May Help Pregnant Women with Hemorrhoids Better Than Anorectal Cream

In a prospective, comparative trial published in the journal *Women and Birth*, researchers from Saudi Arabia compared the effectiveness of sitz baths and anorectal cream to treat hemorrhoids among pregnant Saudi Arabian women. The cohort consisted of 495 pregnant females with hemorrhoids. They ranged in age from sixteen to forty-four years. Two-thirds of the patients reported constipation. One group of 284 patients was told to take salty sitz baths, using 20 g of commercial salt, three times per day; the second group of 211 patients used an anorectal cream twice daily. The women in both groups used lubricant suppositories before moving their bowels and took Metamucil bulk-fiber. All of the patients in the sitz bath group achieved complete healing, while 179 (84.8 percent) of the patients in the anorectal cream group were completely healed. The researchers concluded that "a modified conservative treatment protocol for hemorrhoids during pregnancy, in which sitz bath is an essential modality, showed very promising outcomes compared to anorectal cream."[14]

A Sphincterotomy Appears to Be a Better Treatment Than Topical Nitroglycerin for Anal Fissures

In a randomized controlled trial published in the journal *Diseases of the Colon & Rectum*, researchers from Canada compared the long-term outcomes of patients who were treated with topical nitroglycerin to patients treated with a sphincterotomy for their chronic anal fissures. The initial cohort consisted of eighty-two patients with anal fissures. The patients using topical nitroglycerin applied the medication to the anal canal three times each day. All of the surgeries were performed by an experienced colorectal surgeon. The patients in both groups took psyllium seed and a stool softener. Of the original cohort, fifty-one patients were available for follow-up an average of 79.4 months after their treatment or surgery. There were twenty-seven patients in the nitroglycerin group and twenty-four in the surgery group. While the patients in both groups were demographically similar, there were significantly more females in the nitroglycerin group. The researchers learned that eleven of the twenty-seven subjects in the nitroglycerin group had persistent anal fissure symptoms within the previous year; none of those in the surgery group had symptoms. More than one-third of the subjects in the nitroglycerin group used medications for their anal fissures since the trial ended and 60 percent ultimately needed surgery. More than 90 percent of those having the surgery indicated that they would select the surgical procedure again, compared with 63 percent of the nitroglycerin patients. All of the patients in the surgery group were either "very" or "moderately" satisfied with their treatment, compared with 56 percent in the nitroglycerin group. The researchers concluded that "it seems that lateral internal sphincterotomy is a more durable treatment for chronic anal fissure compared with topical nitroglycerin therapy." And, there were no differences in fecal incontinence scores between the two groups.[15]

ProctoFiz, an Ointment Containing Hemp and Herbs, Appears Useful for Anal Fissures

In a single-arm, questionnaire-based, prospective trial published in the journal *Medical Cannabis and Cannabinoids*, researchers from Israel evaluated the use of ProctoFiz, an ointment containing hemp and herbs to treat anal fissures. The initial cohort consisted of ninety-two patients, 58.7 percent were female with a median age of 39 years. The patients were diagnosed over a period of eighteen months by a single senior colorectal surgeon at an ambulatory colorectal specialty clinic. All of the patients had anal fissures, and 96.8 percent had constipation and difficulty moving their bowels. For one month, the patients applied the ointment to the anal area three or four times per day. They also took a laxative and dietary supplemental fiber. During the month, there were two telephone assessments and one in-person assessment. The final analyses included eighty-nine patients. Eighty patients reported significant improvement after one week, and seventy-nine reported continued improvement after one month. After one week of treatment, the visual analogue score decreased by 6.6 points—from 8.9 to 2.3, with continuous improvement to a mean of 0.64 after one month. The researchers commented that "surgical intervention, although proven to be the most effective method of treatment, should be offered to patients only after pharmacological treatment has failed."[16]

Surgery Is Better for Treating Anal Fissures Than Zinc Oxide or Lidocaine

In a prospective, randomized trial published in the *International Surgery Journal*, researchers from India compared three different treatments for anal fissures—zinc oxide pomade, lidocaine pomade, and lateral internal sphincterotomy (surgery). The cohort consisted of ninety patients who were diagnosed with an anal fissure between January 2020 and January 2021. They were placed in one of three groups; each group had thirty patients. The patients in the first group took sitz baths and applied 15 percent zinc oxide pomade twice each day for six weeks; the patients in the second group took sitz baths and applied 5 percent lidocaine pomade twice each day for six weeks; and the patients in the third group had the surgery. There were no gender and age differences between the groups. The most notable symptom was pain. All of the patients were told to eat fiber-rich foods, and, if necessary, to take stool softeners. Assessments were conducted of healing rates, pain relief, recurrences, change in symptoms, and complications. Recovery was considered the absence of symptoms and anal fissures. The researchers learned that the patients treated with sitz baths and zinc oxide had a recovery rate of 23.33 percent; the patients treated with sitz baths and lidocaine had a recovery rate of 26.66 percent. At the same time, those treated with surgery had a recovery rate of 99 to 100 percent. "So lateral internal sphincterotomy is superior than zinc oxide and lidocaine pomade application in treatment of anal fissure."[17]

Topical Calcium Channel Blockers May Be Better Than Oral Channel Blockers for Anal Fissures

In a systematic review and meta-analysis of randomized controlled trials published in the *International Journal of Surgery*, researchers from Ireland compared the use of topical and oral calcium channel blockers for treating chronic anal fissures. The researchers located four trials with 279 patients (141 using topical and 138 using oral) that met their criteria. The researchers learned that 38.4 percent of those in the oral group and 21.3 percent in the topical group failed to heal. Side effects were also more common in the oral group; 39.1 percent in the oral group had side effects next to 15.6 percent in the topical group. The three trials that compared the recurrence rates found that it was 5.5 percent in the oral group and 5.4 percent in the topical group. The researchers concluded that "topical CCB [calcium channel blocker] is associated with improved healing and a superior side effect profile, but similar recurrence rates compared to oral CCB."[18]

Botulinum Injections (Botox) May Help People with Chronic Anal Fissures

In a prospective case series trial published in the *Journal of Family Medicine and Primary Care*, researchers from Iran evaluated the usefulness of injections of botulinum toxin for chronic anal fissures. The cohort consisted of 106 patients who suffered from chronic anal fissures or anal fissures they have had for more than six weeks; there were twenty-six males and ninety females, with a mean age of 38.56 years. All of the patients received a total of 30 units of botulinum toxin, and they were advised to eat a high-fiber diet and take laxatives. For two months, the patients were physically examined weekly and checked for bleeding, pain, hematoma, thrombosis, infection, incontinence, and healing of the fissure. At the end of the study, ninety patients (84.9 percent) were healed, with an average healing time of 4.68 weeks. The only complication in fourteen patients was "mild incontinence." Patients who were not fully healed at the end of two months were offered further injections or surgery. The researchers concluded that botulinum toxin "is a safe and effective modality for the treatment of chronic anal fissure, with a low complication rate."[19]

Sitz Baths May Not Provide Sufficient Relief for Anal Fissures

In a randomized, controlled trial published in the *ANZ Journal of Surgery*, researchers from India compared treating acute anal fissures with and without sitz baths. The initial cohort consisted of fifty-eight patients with acute anal fissures. All the patients had their anal fissures for two months or less. For four weeks, they were told either to take sitz baths in the morning and at night or to not take any sitz baths; everyone was told to take psyllium husk supplements. Each week, the patients were asked to assess their pain scores and the degree of healing. Twenty-seven patients in the sitz bath group and twenty-five in the control group completed the trial. Although the pain score was less in the sitz bath group, it failed to reach statistical significance. There were no differences between the groups in fissure healing. However, patients in the sitz bath group reported more satisfaction. The researchers concluded that "patients with acute anal fissures while receiving sitz baths, experienced approximately the same levels of pain when compared to those not receiving them; however, they reported a higher satisfaction score when compared with those not receiving sitz baths."[20]

There Does Not Appear to Be Sufficient Scientific Data to Support the Usefulness of Sitz Baths for Anorectal Disorders

In a literature review published in the journal *Diseases of the Colon & Rectum*, researchers from Los Angeles, California wanted to determine if there was scientific evidence to prove the usefulness of sitz baths for anorectal disorders. The researchers located thirty-six published articles that met their criteria. Twenty-seven were in English, five in German, two in Japanese, one in Korean, and one in Hebrew. Twenty-eight were in medical journals and eight in nursing journals. While some of the studies found clear benefits to sitz baths, such as more rapid healing and better pain relief, there were also reports of risks and complications, such as outbreaks of infection and burns from sitz baths that were too hot. The researchers concluded that there is an inadequate amount of scientific data to support the widespread use of sitz baths. More randomized, controlled studies are needed "to investigate whether this time-consuming recommendation is beneficial to patients suffering from anorectal conditions." At the same time, "patients should be given specific instructions on how to correctly perform sitz baths, including the temperature of the water and the device used."[21]

REFERENCES AND FURTHER READING

Aram, Fahmi Omer. "Rubber Band Ligation for Hemorrhoids: An Office Experience." *Indian Journal of Surgery* 78, no. 4 (August 2016): 271–274.

Beaty, Jennifer Sam and M. Shashidharan. "Anal Fissure." *Clinics in Colon and Rectal Surgery* 29 (2016): 30–37.

Brown, Carl J., Daniel Dubreuil, Laura Santoro et al. "Lateral Internal Sphincterotomy Is Superior to Topical Nitroglycerin for Healing Chronic Anal Fissure and Does Not Compromise Long-Term Fecal Continence: Six-Year Follow-Up of a Multicenter, Randomized, Controlled Trial." *Disease of the Colon & Rectum* 50 (2007): 442–448.

Gupta, Pravin J. "Randomized, Controlled Study Comparing Sitz-Bath and Non-Sitz-Bath Treatments in Patients with Acute Anal Fissures." *ANZ Journal of Surgery* 76, no. 8 (August 2008): 718–721.

Hsu, Sheng-Pang, Hsin-Hung Chen, Tzu-Yuan Wang et al. "Association of Hemorrhoids with Hashimoto's Thyroiditis and Associated Comorbidities: A Nationwide Population-Based Cohort Study." *Frontiers in Endocrinology* 11 (October 2020): 577767.

Johannsson, Helgri Örn, Wilhelm Graf, and Lars Påhlman. "Bowel Habits in Hemorrhoid Patients and Normal Subjects." *American Journal of Gastroenterology* 100 (2005): 401–406.

Kaushal, Manish, Arvind Shukla, P. Kovarthanan, and Yogesh Heremat Shivaprasad. "Zinc Oxide, Lidocaine, and Lateral Internal Sphincterotomy for Fissure-in-Ano: A Comparative Study." *International Surgery Journal* 9, no. 6 (June 2022): 1146–1150.

Madalinski, M. "Identifying the Best Therapy for Chronic Anal Fissure." *World Journal of Gastrointestinal Pharmacology and Therapeutics* 2, no. 2 (April 2011): 9–16.

Perez-Miranda, Manuel, Ana Gomez-Cedenilla, Teresa León-Colombo et al. "Effect of Fiber Supplements on Internal Bleeding Hemorrhoids." *Hepata-Gastroenterology* 43, no. 12 (1996): 1504–1507.

Peery, Ane F. Robert S. Sandler, Joseph A. Galanko et al. "RiskFactors for Hemorrhoids Screening Colonoscopy." *PLoS One* 10, no. 9 (2015): e0139100.

Ram, Edward, Yaniv Zager, Raanan Meyer et al. "Management of Chronic Anal Fissure with a Novel Topical Hemp-Herbal-Based Ointment: A Pilot Study." *Medical Cannabis and Cannabinoids* 6 (2023): 15–20.

Sahebally, Shaheel M., Khalid Ahmed, Raminta Cerneveciute et al. "Oral Versus Topical Channel Blockers for Chronic Anal Fissures – A Systematic Review and Meta-Analysis of Randomized Controlled Trials." *International Journal of Surgery* 44 (2017): 87–93.

Sandler, Robert S. and Anne F. Peery. "Rethinking What We Know About Hemorrhoids." *Clinical Gastroenterology and Hepatology* 17 (2019): 8–15.

Setareh Soltany, Hamid Reza Hemmati, Jafar Alavy Toussy et al. "Therapeutic Properties of Botulinum Toxin on Chronic Anal Fissure Treatment and the Patient Factors Role." *Journal of Family Medicine and Primary Care* 9 (2020): 1562–1566.

Shirah, Bader Hamza, Hamza Assad Shirah, Abdelelah Hussein Fallata et al. "Hemorrhoids During Pregnancy: Sitz Baths vs. Ano-Rectal Cream: A Comparative Prospective Study of Two Conservative Treatment Protocols." *Women and Birth* 31 (2018): e272–e277.

Sugarman, D. T. "Hemorrhoids." *JAMA* 312, no. 24 (December 24/31, 2014): 2698.

Sun, Zhifei and John Migaly. "Review of Hemorrhoid Disease: Presentation and Management." *Clinics in Colon and Rectal Surgery* 29 (2016): 22–29.

Tejirian, Talar and Maher A. Abbas. "Sitz Bath: Where Is the Evidence? Scientific Basis of a Common Practice." *Diseases of the Colon and Rectum* 48 (2005): 2336–2340.

HEPATITIS A, HEPATITIS B, AND HEPATITIS C

INTRODUCTION

Though many people are probably unaware, there are different types of hepatitis disease. The three most common and well known are hepatitis A, hepatitis B, and hepatitis C. Hepatitis A, hepatitis B, and hepatitis C vary in how they are spread, how they are treated, and how they may impact the long-term health and well-being of the body. Still, they all trigger inflammation of the liver and may affect the functioning of the liver. The word hepatitis actually means inflammation of the liver.

Hepatitis A is the most contagious of the three and the most likely to cause obvious symptoms, but it is the least likely to cause any serious problems. Hepatitis B and C are far more serious diseases that are increasingly spreading rapidly in many countries. Though less common in developed countries, they still affect millions of people and take a personal and financial toll on individuals, family members, workplace environments, and society at large. As a result, people, especially those at higher risk, should be vaccinated for hepatitis A and hepatitis B and do everything possible to prevent the transmission of all three types.

Hepatitis A

Hepatitis A is a highly contagious liver infection caused by the hepatitis A virus that lives in the blood and the stool of people who are infected. The virus spreads easily, and it is incredibly resistant. It may literally live unseen on a surface for months. Still, the virus does not spread through casual contact or by sneezing or coughing.

People are most likely to contract a hepatitis A infection from contaminated food or water or through close contact with an infected person or object. Cases of hepatitis A are often mild and generally don't require any special treatment. Most people recover from mild cases and have no permanent liver damage. In these instances, there is a good chance that the affected people have no idea they actually had a hepatitis A infection.

Preventing hepatitis A is relatively easy. There is a two-dose vaccine that is administered after a child has turned one year old. People with liver disease or who are considered at higher risk for hepatitis A who never received the vaccine may obtain it at a later date, even as an adult. The shots should be given six to eighteen months apart. Both shots are necessary for full protection. Practicing good hygiene, with frequent washing of hands with soap and water, is also a useful way to prevent this virus.

Diseases that sounded like hepatitis A were reported in both individuals and groups in China as early as five thousand years ago. Hippocrates described an illness he termed benign jaundice that seemed like hepatitis A. But, more specific symptoms of hepatitis A appeared in the seventeenth century associated with military campaigns. The first outbreak in the United States was in 1812 in Norfolk, Virginia, and it was quite common among the Union troops during the Civil War.[1]

Hepatitis B

Hepatitis B is a serious liver infection caused by the HBV. For most people, it is acute and lasts no more than six months. However, for others, it becomes chronic and lasts far longer, even for the rest of their lives. Sometimes, many years after recovering from an acute infection of hepatitis B, something causes the immune system of the body to weaken, and the virus reactivates. This reactivation may be brief or long-lasting. But, since it tends to occur in people who are immune-suppressed, it may be severe and cause liver failure.

People with hepatitis B are contagious for as long as the virus is active in their bodies. With acute hepatitis B, this may be as long as six months. For chronic hepatitis B, this may be years, decades, or a lifetime.

People with chronic hepatitis B have an increased risk of developing liver failure, liver cancer, or cirrhosis, which permanently scars the liver. Most adults with hepatitis B recover fully, even when they have severe symptoms. Children are more likely to develop long-lasting symptoms, a condition known as chronic infection. About 90 percent of infected infants become chronically infected, while two to 6 percent of adults develop chronic infection. So, it is crucial that infants receive their first vaccine as soon as possible after birth, and that anyone who may have a higher risk for this disease be vaccinated.

Hepatitis B is transmitted when blood, semen, or another body fluid from a person infected with the virus enters the body of someone who is not infected. This may occur through sexual contact, shared needles, syringes, or other drug equipment, or from mother to baby at birth. Hepatitis B is not easily transmitted through saliva. So, it is unlikely to be transmitted from sharing food or utensils or from someone coughing or sneezing.

A hepatitis B vaccine is very useful in preventing hepatitis B, but once a person is ill with hepatitis B there is no cure. Depending on the vaccine, it is usually given as three injections over six months or four doses over twelve months. This vaccine is strongly recommended for newborns, children and adolescents who were not vaccinated as newborns, people with liver disease and/or kidney disease, people who have sex with people who may have hepatitis B, men who have sex with men, people who are incarcerated or live in higher-risk group settings, travelers to high-risk areas, people who inject illegal drugs, people who work in certain higher-risk environments, and healthcare workers. There is also a combined hepatitis A and hepatitis B vaccine. The combined vaccine is usually given as three shots over a six-month period.

An article in the journal *Biomolecules* noted that the hepatitis B virus has existed for between two and three thousand years. Today, worldwide, the chronic form of this disease affects about 300 million people.[2]

Hepatitis C

Hepatitis C (HCV) is a viral infection that causes liver swelling or inflammation. It spreads through contact with blood that contains the virus. There are two main types of hepatitis C—acute and chronic. Both types of infection begin with acute hepatitis C, which may start from two weeks to six months after exposure to the virus. In about 15–25 percent of cases, the body clears acute hepatitis C, and the virus does not progress to a chronic phase. This is called spontaneous viral clearance. When hepatitis C continues for an extended period of time, it is termed chronic hepatitis C. Once it is in the chronic phase, hepatitis C is usually damaging the liver. This occurs in about 75–85 percent of cases. The risk of cirrhosis after chronic hepatitis C infection is 20 percent within twenty years and 30 percent within thirty years. Cirrhosis-related mortality from hepatitis C ranges from 2–5 percent per year. And, in people with hepatitis C cirrhosis, liver cancer occurs in about 3–10 percent per year. Chronic hepatitis C infection is the leading cause of liver transplants in the United States.

Around the world, there are seven or eight types of hepatitis C, called genotypes, and sixty-seven subtypes. The most common hepatitis C genotype in the United States, Europe, and Latin America is type 1.

Hepatitis C was first recognized in 1975 when Steve Feinstone, MD, determined that transfusion-associated hepatitis was not associated with the hepatitis A virus or the hepatitis B virus. He defined the disease as non-A, non-B hepatitis. It was later termed hepatitis C.[3]

SYMPTOMS, RISKS, AND COMPLICATIONS

Hepatitis A

Many people with hepatitis A never have any symptoms. Yet, when symptoms appear they may include unusual tiredness and weakness, nausea, vomiting, diarrhea, abdominal pain and discomfort (especially on the right side), off-white or gray stool, loss of appetite, low-grade fever, dark urine, joint pain, yellowing of the skin (jaundice), and intense itching. It is important to realize that people with hepatitis A are contagious for up to two weeks even if they do not have symptoms, and they remain contagious for up to two weeks after the symptoms appear.

Certain lifestyle actions increase the risk of hepatitis A infection. These include traveling to Mexico, Central America, and South America where the virus is common, eating at a restaurant where there has been a hepatitis A outbreak, and being in close contact, including sexual contact, with someone who has had hepatitis A. Other risks include eating food handled by people with the virus who do not thoroughly wash their hands after using the restroom, failing to adequately wash one's own hands after using the restroom or changing a baby's diaper, drinking contaminated water or ice, and eating some raw or undercooked fish, including raw shellfish from polluted waters. People who have HIV and people who use recreational drugs have a higher risk, as do men who have sex with other men. People receiving dialysis and those on medications that suppress the immune system after an organ transplant have higher risks. Even those who have an abnormal but unexplained liver enzyme test should be aware of their higher risk.

Unlike hepatitis B and hepatitis C, people who have hepatitis A tend not to have complications, and hepatitis A is normally not an ongoing or chronic infection. However, in rare instances, hepatitis A has caused an acute and sudden loss of liver function, particularly in older people and those with chronic liver disease. Acute liver failure requires hospitalization, and in even rarer instances, a person may need a liver transplant.

Hepatitis B

Not everyone with hepatitis B has symptoms. With or without symptoms, people with hepatitis B are contagious. Still, there are a number of symptoms associated with hepatitis B; they range from mild to severe. These include abdominal pain, dark urine, fever, joint pain, loss of appetite, nausea and vomiting, weakness and fatigue, and yellowing of the skin and whites of the eyes (jaundice). These symptoms tend to appear about one to four months after infection, although they may well appear sooner. Some people, especially children, may have no symptoms.

A number of factors increase the risk of exposure to hepatitis B. These include unprotected sex with someone who is infected, unprotected sex with multiple sex partners, having the hepatitis C virus, sharing needles and syringes, being housed in a group setting, incarceration or past incarceration, and accidental needle sticks, which is of particular concern for healthcare workers, and childbirth, when an infected mother may pass the virus to an infant. Each year, thousands of infants are born to mothers infected with hepatitis B. Up to 25 percent of people infected at birth die prematurely of hepatitis B-related causes. That is why pregnant women should always be tested for the hepatitis B infection, and infants should be immunized shortly after birth. People who live with someone who has hepatitis B have a higher risk, as do men who have sex with other men. In the United States, about 2 percent of people with HIV are also infected with hepatitis B. Although it is considered highly unlikely in the United States, transmission is possible from a blood transfusion or during surgery.

People who are infected with hepatitis B may develop a number of complications. These include the previously noted scarring of the liver (cirrhosis), liver cancer, liver failure, as well as kidney disease, inflammation of blood vessels, or reactivation of the hepatitis B virus in people on immunosuppressive medications, such as high-dose corticosteroids and chemotherapy. People with HIV are at increased risk for complications and death from hepatitis B infection. That is why all people with HIV should be tested for hepatitis B and, if negative, should receive the hepatitis B vaccination.

Hepatitis C

In its acute phase, hepatitis C rarely has any symptoms. Many people are totally unaware that they have an infection. If there are symptoms, they tend to be jaundice, fatigue, nausea, fever, and muscle aches. Even chronic hepatitis C may have no symptoms for many years. Symptoms may appear only after the virus has actually damaged the liver.

Then, the symptoms may include easy bleeding and bruising, fatigue, loss of appetite and weight loss, yellowing of the skin (jaundice), dark-colored urine, a fluid backup in the stomach area termed ascites, leg swelling, and confusion, drowsiness, and slurred speech or hepatic encephalopathy, and spiderlike veins on the skin, known as spider angiomas.

Although it is generally recommended that all adults be screened for hepatitis C, certain people have an increased risk. These include anyone who has injected, snorted, or inhaled an illegal drug, anyone who has atypical results from a liver screening, babies born to a mother with hepatitis C, pregnant women, healthcare workers who may have been in contact with blood or sustained a needlestick, people who have had tattoos or body piercings performed with unsterilized equipment, people who share a razor or toothbrush with someone who may have bled while using it, people with hemophilia who were treated with clotting factors before 1987, people on long-term hemodialysis, people who donated blood or organ transplants before 1992, sexual partners of anyone diagnosed with hepatitis C, people with HIV, men who have sex with other men, and anyone who has been incarcerated.

There are a few potential complications associated with hepatitis C. These include scarring of the liver, called cirrhosis, which makes it harder for the liver to function, liver cancer, and liver failure, where the liver may stop functioning entirely.

PREVALENCE

Hepatitis A

Worldwide, especially in parts of the world where sanitation is poor and food and water are often contaminated, hepatitis A is incredibly common. In the United States, where sanitation is far better and vaccination tends to be encouraged, the rates of hepatitis A have declined markedly. Currently, they are as low as 1.2 cases per 100,000 population. The greatest reductions have been seen in children and in states with higher rates of vaccination. Because the prevalence is much higher in Mexico, states that border Mexico also have higher rates of hepatitis A.

Hepatitis B

In the United States, it is estimated that between 880,000 and 1.89 million people have chronic hepatitis B infection.[4] About 20,000 new cases occur each year. New hepatitis B infections are highest among people between the ages of thirty and fifty-nine years. Unfortunately, many people in this group, even those at higher risk, have not been vaccinated. About 70 percent of the new cases of hepatitis B are seen in people born outside the United States, especially those born in Asia, the Pacific Islands, and Africa.

Hepatitis B is the most common liver infection in the world. As many as one-third of the world's population (about two billion people) have been infected. About 250 million people worldwide are living with the infection. Large numbers of these people are unaware that they are infected. Many have probably never heard of hepatitis B.

Hepatitis C

Although statistics vary, several years ago, it was estimated that, worldwide, about 60 to 170 million people are living with hepatitis C. Even if those figures are too high, they still represent a staggering number of people. In an average year, about 20,000 people die of hepatitis C-related liver disease. In the United States, about 1 percent of the population is infected. That represents nearly four million people. People between the ages of twenty and thirty-nine have the highest risk. In the United States, injection drug use is the most common mode of acquisition. Worldwide, transmission often occurs in medical settings with unsterilized equipment. Groups with the highest risk include American Indians, Alaskan Natives, and non-Hispanic white populations.

DIAGNOSIS AND TREATMENT OPTIONS

Hepatitis A

Medical providers diagnose hepatitis A based on the symptoms and a blood test. The blood test will look for antibodies to the hepatitis A virus called immunoglobulin M (IgM) antibodies. A positive test means the patient has hepatitis A. If the blood test finds antibodies to the hepatitis A virus that are immunoglobulin G (IgG) antibodies, then the patient is immune to hepatitis A, either from a past hepatitis A infection or a hepatitis A vaccination.

Typically, treatment for hepatitis A infection begins with rest, drinking lots of fluids, and eating an especially healthful diet, with lots of fruits and vegetables. Because certain medications, such as acetaminophen (Tylenol), may further harm an inflamed liver, check with a healthcare provider before using any medications. Until fully healed, no alcohol should be consumed.

Hepatitis B

Hepatitis B is diagnosed with two blood tests, the hepatitis B surface antigen and the IgM hepatitis B core antibody, which are able to detect the virus long before any symptoms may appear. It has been estimated that almost 70 percent of those who are infected are unaware of their infection. In some cases, additional tests will be ordered. These include a liver ultrasound, in which an ultrasound called a transient elastography may locate the amount of liver damage, and a liver biopsy, in which a medical provider uses a thin needle to remove a small amount of liver tissue.

Treatment for acute hepatitis B is similar to that for hepatitis A. Medical providers recommend lots of rest, healthier nutrition, and plenty of fluids, which enable the body to fight the infection. In severe cases, hospitalization may be required.

While there is no cure for chronic hepatitis B, which is defined as having the hepatitis B surface antigen present for six or more months, there are several antiviral treatments that may reduce the risk of developing more serious illness and liver cancer. These treatments reduce the amount of virus in the body and lower the chance of developing cirrhosis, liver failure, or hepatocellular carcinoma. The US FDA has approved three nucleoside analogues and two interferon alpha drugs for the treatment of chronic hepatitis B in adults. People with chronic hepatitis B infection will probably need to remain on treatment for life. Livers that have been damaged beyond any hope of repair may require a liver transplant. During this surgery, a surgeon replaces the liver with a healthier one. Most of these are obtained from people who have died, but sometimes they may be obtained from a live donor who donates a portion of their liver. As might be expected, there are always shortages of available livers for transplantation.

It is important to underscore the fact that people who may have been exposed to hepatitis B should contact their healthcare provider without delay. In certain cases, such as an unvaccinated person sustaining a needlestick injury from someone with active hepatitis B, an injection of the hepatitis B immunoglobulin within twenty-four hours of exposure may help prevent the development of hepatitis B. It should be administered at the same time as an injection of the hepatitis B vaccine.

Hepatitis C

Hepatitis C is diagnosed with two tests—the antibody test and the PCR or polymerase chain reaction test. The antibody test determines if the body has been exposed to the hepatitis C virus. A positive result means that exposure occurred, and that the body has produced antibodies against the virus. But, this exposure may have occurred in the more distant past, and the body may no longer be infectious. The only way to tell if a person is currently infectious is the second test, the PCR, which determines if the virus is reproducing in the body and the person is still infectious.

Most people with acute and chronic hepatitis C virus are now treated with newer antiviral medications, with the aim to treat the virus during the acute phase rather than waiting six months to determine if the patient has a chronic infection. In many cases, these medications are able to cure the infection. They may well stop the acute infection from developing into a chronic infection.

RESEARCH FINDINGS

Hepatitis A

Rates of Hepatitis A Are Elevated among the Homeless

In a study published in the journal *Public Health Reports*, researchers from Atlanta, Georgia, Cambridge, Massachusetts, and San Francisco, California, used serologic and questionnaire data to examine the prevalence and risk factors for the presence of hepatitis A antibodies among the homeless and marginally housed in San Francisco. Of the 1,138 adults surveyed, the researchers learned that 52 percent had antibodies to hepatitis A, indicating that at some point they were exposed to the virus. That was 58 percent higher than might be expected from the expected prevalence of the general population. The longer the years of homelessness, the higher the prevalence. Those who were homeless for one year or less had a rate of 46 percent, while those homeless for five years or more had a rate of 61 percent. But, other variables were also associated with positive hepatitis A antibodies. These included drug use, being born in another country, race (Hispanics had the highest rate, followed by whites and Black individuals), and increasing age. Other factors did not appear to impact the presence of hepatitis A antibodies. These included gender, sex-related behaviors, and non-injection drug-related behaviors such as smoking or snorting. Although many homeless people have drug or sex-related medical problems, the researchers determined that homelessness appeared to be an independent risk factor for hepatitis A. And, they concluded that "studies on the cost-effectiveness and impact of various strategies, such as vaccinating homeless people based on age or duration of homelessness, could be used to guide these considerations."[5]

Despite Widespread Recommendations Very Few People Appear to Actually Receive Hepatitis A Vaccinations

In a retrospective study published in the *American Journal of Gastroenterology*, researchers from Rockford, Illinois wanted to learn about how many patients actually receive hepatitis A vaccinations. Why is this important? According to the researchers, from 2017 to 2020, the rate of hepatitis A infections in the United States increased by nearly 300 percent. At the same time, more than thirty states reported nearly 19,000 hepatitis A-related hospitalizations. "Therefore, recognizing patients who are most at risk of HAV-related complications is crucial." The researchers commented that the Centers for Disease Control and Prevention recommend certain people should be vaccinated. These include people with a history of intravenous drug use, unstable housing, incarceration, international travel, hepatitis B/C infections, chronic liver disease, and diagnosis of cirrhosis, as well as men who have sex with other men. That is why the researchers retrospectively studied 19,363 patients from northern Illinois and southern Wisconsin, areas that included both urban and rural populations. All of the patients with positive hepatitis serologies were excluded. Data were obtained for age, gender, race, median household income, insurance, accessibility to PCP, and indication for hepatitis A vaccination. The researchers determined that only 15n percent of the people surveyed had received a hepatitis A vaccination, "despite appropriate indication." The highest percentages of those receiving the vaccine were white, non-Hispanic, and native English speakers. But, Asians had the highest rates of vaccination; Hispanics were the least likely. People under the age of thirty-five were much more likely to be vaccinated than older people. And, people with private insurance and Medicaid had higher rates of vaccination than those on Medicare. There were no statistically significant differences in gender. The researchers concluded that an "astoundingly low percentage of patients" actually received the hepatitis A vaccination. It is important that the hepatitis A vaccine be offered to all patients who meet the guidelines, "irrespective of race, gender, age, or insurance status."[6]

In the Midst of a Hepatitis A Outbreak, an Emergency Department Effectively Vaccinated Hundreds of Community Residents

In a retrospective review published in the *Western Journal of Emergency Medicine*, physicians from Camden, New Jersey, and Philadelphia, Pennsylvania, described their response to an outbreak of hepatitis A. In August 2019, the Philadelphia Department of Public Health declared that an outbreak of hepatitis A had caused a public health emergency in Philadelphia. At that time, 154 cases of hepatitis A were identified; in prior years, the number had been fewer than ten. As a result, in conjunction with the Philadelphia Department of Public Health, which paid for the vaccines, the Department of Emergency

Medicine at Temple University Hospital offered a free vaccination program for community members. It was held from July 16 to October 8, 2019. During the period studied, there were a total of 10,033 Emergency Department visits, with 5,009 of them prior to the implementation of the vaccination program and 5,024 after the program began. Six hundred and sixty-nine hepatitis A vaccines were administered. Before the vaccination program began, seventy-three patients were diagnosed with hepatitis A, of whom sixty-seven were hospitalized. After the program began, thirty-nine patients were diagnosed with hepatitis A, and thirty-one were admitted. The researchers concluded that "a partnership between the ED [emergency department] and the local public health department resulted in the vaccination of 669 patients in six weeks in the midst of an outbreak of a vaccine preventable illness, with the corresponding drop in ED visits and hospital admission for acute hepatitis."[7]

Certain Symptoms Are Most Often Seen in Children with Hepatitis A

In a trial published in the journal *Cureus*, researchers from India wanted to determine which symptoms were most often seen in children with hepatitis A. The cohort consisted of one hundred children between the ages of one and eighteen years who presented with hepatitis A at a tertiary care center in western India. Almost half of the patients were between the ages of one and five years. Forty percent were between the ages of six and ten years. Fifty-one percent were male, and 49 percent were female. Seventy-eight percent lived in rural areas, and 22 percent were from urban areas. Sixty-five percent primarily used tap water, and 35 percent had well water. Only serologically confirmed cases were enrolled in the trial. The researchers learned that the children presented with symptoms including fever, nausea, dark-colored urine, anorexia, vomiting, jaundice, liver enlargement, and abdominal pain. In almost all of the patients, the illness lasted more than five days; in only three patients, it lasted for less than five days. The highest number of cases were seen from June to September, which is the monsoon season in India, and the socioeconomic status of most of the families was lower or upper lower. The researchers commented that their study "adds to the literature regarding the clinical profile of symptomatic patients."[8]

The Hospitalization Costs Associated with an Outbreak of Hepatitis A Are Considerable

In a study published in the journal *Emerging Infectious Diseases*, researchers from Atlanta, Georgia, used the Healthcare Cost and Utilization Project data to estimate the average cost associated with a hepatitis A-related hospitalization in 2017. Although the researchers acknowledged that the hepatitis A vaccine has dramatically lowered the rates of hospitalization, there were still 3,366 cases reported in the United States in 2017. And, state health departments reported more than 31,000 associated cases from July 1, 2016, to February 7, 2020. Of these, 18,900 had reportedly been hospitalized. The researchers determined that the average cost per hepatitis A-related hospitalization was $16,232. But, the average costs ranged from $12,921 to $19,680. The researchers noted that their findings emphasized "the importance of improving hepatitis A vaccination coverage among at risk adults."[9]

Hepatitis B

Hepatitis B Vaccine Seems to Remain Effective for Long Periods of Time

In a systematic review and meta-analysis published in the journal *Vaccines*, researchers from Italy studied the long-term effectiveness of the hepatitis B vaccination in healthcare students in "highly" developed countries. While the researchers noted that the vast majority of these students were probably vaccinated as babies and young children, they wanted to learn if the students continued to be protected against this virus. Why is this important? Because in the course of their studies and work, these students are likely to be exposed to blood and other bodily fluids. The researchers identified forty-six studies with 52,749 participants that met their criteria. The studies were published in English or Italian from January 1, 2000, to November 30, 2021. Thirty-nine articles were published after 2010. Twenty-two were performed in Italy, four in Japan, three in the United States and Saudi Arabia, two in Germany, and one each in Australia, Cyprus, Greece, Hong Kong, Israel, Malaysia, the Netherlands, South Korea, Spain, Switzerland, Turkey, and the United Arab Emirates. Twenty-six studies included overall healthcare students, eighteen included medical students and trainees, and two studies focused on nursing students. Sample sizes ranged from one hundred to 10,294. The mean age ranged from nineteen to 29.9 years; the female gender ratio ranged from 33.7 percent to 79.4 percent. The prevalence of the completed primary cycle of hepatitis B vaccination ranged from 40.3 percent to 100 percent, and the time since primary cycle completion ranged from 0.08 to 21.4 years. The researchers determined that three out of every four students had protection against hepatitis B infection. Among those who did not initially show protection, the protection rate rose to over 90 percent after receiving a "challenge" dose. Only very small numbers of students failed to acquire protection from the vaccine. The researchers suggested that this number may be as low as 0.1 percent. The researchers commented that healthcare providers should focus their attention on vaccination of groups of people with increased risks, such as those working in healthcare settings, living in prisons and homeless shelters, people who inject drugs, and migrants from endemic areas. And, they concluded that "healthcare students vaccinated with the complete HBV primary cycle maintain an effective humoral immunity against this pathogen for over two decades."[10]

Alcohol Users Have Higher Rates of Hepatitis B

In a systematic review and meta-analysis published in the journal *Alcohol and Alcoholism*, researchers from Brazil investigated the prevalence of hepatitis B among users of alcohol. They identified eighteen studies with 12,204 users of alcohol that met their criteria. The majority of the subjects were men, and eleven of the studies were deemed to have a low risk of bias. The heterogeneity among the studies was "substantial." More than half of the studies described the cut-off value of the amount of alcohol consumption per day and that ranged from 12 or more grams per day to more than 80 grams per day. In most of the studies, the prevalence of hepatitis B among alcohol users was not the primary goal, but it was possible to obtain that information. Nine studies noted the minimum duration of alcohol consumption, and that ranged from two weeks to over ten years. However, only three studies evaluated the mean duration of alcohol consumption, and it ranged from nineteen to twenty-seven years. Fourteen of the studies included data from hospitals.

One was a community-based cohort, and the other three were from addiction or mental health units. Sample sizes ranged from 58 to 2,720, with a mean of 678 and a median of 317. Only six studies mentioned the mean age of the alcohol users, and in those studies, it was 44.6 years. In the eleven studies that mentioned gender, the vast majority were males. Six studies were from Europe, three from the American continent, eight from Asia, and one from Africa. The estimated worldwide prevalence of hepatitis B was 20 percent. The researchers noted that the high rate may be partially explained by the fact that more than half of the studies included patients with chronic liver disease or cirrhosis. Among users of alcohol, the lowest prevalence of hepatitis B was 10 percent. However, it tended to be higher than in the general population. The researchers suggested that alcohol use might make more people vulnerable to at-risk actions such as unsafe sex and drug use. The researchers concluded that the prevalence of hepatitis B infection in alcohol users was high. And, because alcohol and hepatitis B are known to be associated with liver disease, "adult alcohol users should be carefully monitored with serological screening."[11]

Cognitive Behavioral Therapy Does Not Appear to Improve the Quality of Life in People with Hepatitis B, but Did Improve Emotional Well-Being

In a trial published in *Modern Care Journal*, researchers from Iran examined the use of cognitive behavioral therapy to improve the quality of life in people with hepatitis B infection. The cohort consisted of sixty patients with hepatitis B who were recruited from a private infectious disease clinic. Thirty patients were placed in the intervention group and thirty in the control group. The two groups were similar. Patients in the intervention group received eight forty-five-minute sessions of cognitive behavioral therapy; the patients in the control group received no cognitive behavioral therapy. All of the patients completed a thirty-six-item survey before and after the intervention. The researchers determined that the interventions had no significant effect on the quality of life of the patients. However, they did improve the emotional well-being of the patients with hepatitis B. According to the researchers, this insignificant effect of cognitive behavioral therapy may be attributable "to the high prevalence of severe mental problems such a depression and anxiety due to the intake of medications such as interferon, tenofovir, and lamivudine." Such psychiatric problems are known to impair quality of life issues.[12]

There Does Not Appear to Be an Association between Hepatitis B Infections and Postpartum Depression in Chinese Women

In a retrospective cohort study published in the journal *Frontiers in Public Health*, researchers from China evaluated the association between hepatitis B infection and postpartum depression in Chinese women. The cohort consisted of 3,808 Chinese women who gave birth in a hospital in southern China. The hepatitis B positive group had 278 women, and the control group had 3,530 women. Six weeks after delivery, 453 women (11.9 percent) were considered to have postpartum depression. The researchers learned that women with hepatitis B were more likely to have postpartum depression, but they did not have a significantly higher rate than the control women. The researchers concluded that hepatitis B infection did not increase the risk of postpartum depression in women with no psychiatric or family history. "The absence of an association may be explained by the diversity of sociological, behavioral, and psychological factors that affect the mental health of puerperal women."[13]

Overall, Interferon Therapy Appears Useful for People with Chronic Hepatitis B

In a cross-sectional trial published in the journal *Scientific Reports*, researchers from China examined the overall usefulness of treating patients with chronic hepatitis B infection with interferon therapy. The researchers commented that while interferon has proven to be the most effective treatment for achieving a clinical cure for hepatitis B, treatment outcomes remain uncertain, there are multiple side effects, and the therapy is expensive. These problems have the potential to affect a patient's quality of life. The researchers evaluated one hundred chronic hepatitis B patients receiving interferon, one hundred patients receiving nucleoside/nucleotide analogues, and eighty-seven receiving non-antiviral treatment. Various scales were used to measure the overall usefulness of the different medications. These included the Hepatitis B Quality of Life Instrument and the Connor Davidson Resilience Scale. The researchers found that a number of factors affected the quality of life of the patients. Among these were level of education, profession, health insurance, hair loss, antiviral treatment, absenteeism, presenteeism, overall work impairment, activity impairment, resilience, tenacity, strength, and optimism. When compared to the other two treatments, chronic hepatitis B patients treated with interferon scored higher for quality of life (and other factors such as psychological well-being, anticipation, stigma, vulnerability, transmission, and viral response) than the patients on the other medications. As a result, the researchers concluded that "the impact of interferon therapy on the daily lives and work of CHB patients does not appear to be a major cause for concern."[14]

Patients with Chronic Hepatitis B Experience Varied Psychological Reactions

In a qualitative trial published in the *Journal of Caring Sciences*, researchers from Iran wanted to learn more about the varied emotions experienced by people ill with chronic hepatitis B. The cohort consisted of ten men and eight women with chronic hepatitis B; they ranged in age from twenty-three to fifty years, with a mean age of thirty-five years. Most of these patients were diagnosed after a blood donation or routine pregnancy test. Data were collected during unstructured in-depth interviews in medical centers in three cities of Iran. All of the interviews were recorded, typed, and analyzed. The researchers learned that the primary problem was "psychological instability," which included the three sub-themes of grief reaction, emotional challenges, and inferiority complex. Grief reaction included responses such as stupor, denial, anger, and aggression; emotional challenges included worry and apprehension, contradiction with beliefs, fear of deprivation, fear of stigma, waiting for death, and prognosis ambiguity; and inferiority complex included social withdrawal, a sense of humiliation and embarrassment, and a sense of guilt and blame. The researchers commented that the patients in this study were clearly not prepared for the consequences of their screenings and suffered profound emotional distress, somewhat similar to people who are dying. The researchers concluded that there is a need for medical providers to better inform their patients about the hepatitis B infection. "Ongoing education of the patients, the medical staff and the population at risk with the use of appropriate informing strategies and standard education and consultation programs before and after screening test by the medical centers and the mass media are recommended."[15]

Adding Traditional Chinese Medicine to the Treatment of Hepatitis B with Related Cirrhosis May Reduce the Development of Hepatocellular Cancer in Patients

In a systematic review and meta-analysis published in the journal *Heliyon*, researchers from China and Malaysia wanted to learn if traditional Chinese medicine could play a role in reducing the incidence of hepatocellular cancer in people with chronic hepatitis B and related cirrhosis. The researchers identified ten randomized controlled trials with a total of 2,702 patients—1362 experimental and 1,340 controls—that met their criteria; the studies were all published between 2013 and 2023. The heterogeneity between the studies was low, and all of the patients were diagnosed with chronic hepatitis B liver fibrosis. The patients in the experimental groups were treated with both Western and traditional Chinese medicine; the patients in the control groups were treated only with Western medicine. The researchers learned that compared to the control groups, the incidence of hepatocellular cancer in patients treated with both types of medicine was reduced by 39 percent. In subgroup analysis, the researchers noted that after one year, three years, and five years, the patients in the combined group had significantly less hepatocellular cancer. The researchers concluded that the combination therapy "showed the promising potential of reducing the incidence of HCC [hepatocellular carcinoma] in patients with hepatitis B cirrhosis, by improving liver function and enhancing the viral response." Still, the researchers added "the observed effects should be interpreted with caution and the limitations must be considered."[16]

There Seems to Be an Association between Low Levels of Serum Vitamin D and High Viral Loads in Patients with Chronic Hepatitis B

In a systematic review and meta-analysis published in the journal *BMC Gastroenterology*, researchers from China compared the vitamin D serum levels of people with chronic hepatitis B and healthy controls. They identified seven studies with 814 chronic hepatitis B patients and 696 healthy controls that met their criteria. The included studies, which were all observational in design and in English, were published between 2012 and 2017. Five studies were conducted in Asia, one in the Middle East, and one in Europe. One study included only pregnant women, and another study only included men. The researchers determined that vitamin D levels were lower in people with chronic hepatitis B than in the controls, and people with lower levels of vitamin D had higher levels of the hepatitis B virus. The researchers underscored the need for more research on this association, especially since they were only able to locate a relatively small number of studies. "Considering the limitations of the present study, further well-designed comprehensive researchers are needed to address the remaining issues."[17]

Vitamin E May Be an Useful Addition to the Treatment of Chronic Hepatitis B

In a pilot trial published in the journal *Antiviral Research*, researchers from Italy analyzed the usefulness of vitamin E as a treatment for chronic hepatitis B. The initial cohort consisted of thirty-two patients. They were randomly placed on 300 mg vitamin E twice daily (n = 15) or no vitamin E supplementation (n = 17). At baseline, the two groups were similar. The patients were seen monthly for the first three months and then quarterly for an additional twelve months. By the end of the trial, the patients in the intervention group experienced notable improvements. In fact, a "complete response" was observed in seven of the patients taking vitamin E and in none of the controls. The researchers concluded that their findings "indicate that, at the dosage tested, vitamin E is potential interest in the treatment of chronic hepatitis B." Further, "considering the good tolerability and low price, it might represent an alternative or additional treatment to other therapies."[18]

Hepatitis C

People with Hepatitis C May Benefit from Dietary Interventions

In a randomized, controlled trial published in the *Nutrition Journal*, researchers from Romania wanted to learn if people with chronic hepatitis C would benefit from changes in their diet and levels of physical activity. The initial cohort consisted of 120 patients with chronic hepatitis C who were over the age of thirty-five—with an average age of fifty-four—and had a BMI over 25. So, they were all overweight or dealing with obesity. At baseline, the subjects were similar in both groups, and all of the subjects were sedentary, not involved in any form of exercise. For one year, they were placed on either a low-calorie or low-fat diet. The researchers performed a variety of tests such as anthropometric measurements, fasting glucose profiles, serum lipids, liver profiles, and blood counts. Ten of the subjects did not complete the trial. Most of the non-completers were in the low-fat diet group. The researchers learned that after six and twelve months, the people in both groups had significant decreases in caloric consumption. At six months, weight loss was greater in the low-calorie group. However, at one year, weight loss was similar in both groups. Both diets were associated with reductions in the prevalence and severity of steatosis (fat in the liver). The researchers found that the subjects with chronic hepatitis C benefited from both diets. They improved a number of important medical concerns including insulin resistance and liver fibrosis. In addition, the subjects tended to become more physically active during the first half of the trial, although that decreased during the second half, especially in the low-fat group. The researchers concluded that the subjects who were overweight or were dealing with obesity "had significant improvements in body weight, lipid and hepatic profiles."[19]

There Seems to Be an Association between Levels of Serum Vitamin D and the Hepatitis C Virus

In a systematic review and meta-analysis published in the *World Journal of Gastroenterology*, researchers from Brazil and Spain examined the association between levels of serum vitamin D and the levels of the hepatitis C virus in the body. The researchers located eight observational studies and three interventional studies that met their criteria. The eight studies addressed vitamin D levels before and after antiviral therapy, while the three studies involved the intake of vitamin D supplementation. These studies included 1,575 subjects; 1,117 of these subjects were infected with hepatitis C. Most of the studies included people only infected with hepatitis C who ranged in age from thirty-eight to fifty-six years. Four studies had subjects infected with hepatitis C and HIV. Most of the studies were conducted in Europe, and only one was from North America. The researchers determined that the subjects with higher levels of vitamin D had levels of hepatitis C that were no longer detectable in the blood (sustained virological response or SVR). While the researchers underscored the need for more research on this topic, they concluded that "vitamin D supplementation improves SVR in HCV infected individuals."[20]

In Some Instances, Acupuncture May Increase the Risk of Hepatitis C Transmission

In a systematic review and meta-analysis published in the *Korean Journal of Gastroenterology*, researchers based in Korea reviewed the possibility that hepatitis C may be transmitted during acupuncture treatments. They located twenty-eight studies with 194,826 participants and 178,583 controls that met their criteria. There were 16,243 users of acupuncture. Fourteen of the studies were cross-sectional case-control, but twelve were cross-sectional, and two were cross-sectional cohort in design. Sixteen studies included Asian populations, and twelve included non-Asian individuals. Thirteen studies analyzed hospital samples, and nine were from the general population. Except for three studies that obtained data from medical records, the majority of the studies collected data from questionnaires. The researchers learned that those who used acupuncture had a significantly higher rate of hepatitis C transmission than the controls. The researchers concluded that their findings indicated that "acupuncture potentially increases the HCV transmission rate." Further, "unsafe medical procedures and social practices, including acupuncture, should be performed with caution."[21] (It should be parenthetically noted that when disposable, single-use needles are used and other routine safety precautions are practiced, the probability of such transmission is considered remote.)

On the Other Hand, Veterans with Hepatitis C Seem Pleased with Their Acupuncture Treatments

In a pilot trial published in the *European Journal of Integrative Medicine*, researchers from Portland, Oregon, noted that veterans are increasingly requesting and using complementary and alternative medicine. The researchers compared the usefulness of acupuncture treatments for sixteen veterans with hepatitis C who were receiving antiviral therapy, and thirty veterans with hepatitis C who were not receiving antiviral therapy. Forty-one of the veterans were male, and the mean age of the veterans was fifty-eight years. For eight weeks, the veterans attended two weekly acupuncture sessions. Quantitative data were collected at seven time points. The researchers found that the veterans who were receiving antiviral therapy were less likely to see improvement, and they had less improvement as the treatment progressed. On the other hand, a trend toward improvement was seen in the veterans not receiving antiviral therapy. The researchers commented that the antiviral therapy may result in "considerable physical, mental, and social burdens." So, they were not surprised that the veterans in this group did not experience improvements. Still, the researchers noted that all of the veterans "reported having a positive experience with acupuncture and would recommend it to others."[22]

Anxiety and Depression Seem to Be Relatively Common in People with Hepatitis C

In a trial published in the journal *General Hospital Psychiatry*, researchers from Ireland examined a group of ninety patients awaiting interferon treatment for hepatitis C. They wanted to estimate the prevalence of anxiety and depression. Among the ninety subjects were twenty-three women, and forty-two subjects in the cohort had contracted hepatitis C through injecting drugs. The median age for the men was thirty-seven, and the women had a median age of forty-four years. Forty percent of the subjects were HIV positive. Twenty-four percent had an anxiety disorder; 86 percent of these were previously undiagnosed, and 28 percent had a depressive disorder, and 72 percent were previously undiagnosed. The prevalence of depressive disorder was higher in women than men, although the difference was of borderline statistical significance. The prevalence of anxiety disorders was similar in men and women. The prevalence of coexisting anxiety and depressive disorders was significantly higher in women than men. The researchers commented that people with hepatitis C, like people with other significant medical illnesses, have high rates of psychological problems and a reduced quality of life. The researchers concluded that their findings underscored "the significant prevalence of underdiagnosed mood disorder in persons with hepatitis C, with significant levels of psychiatric disorder across all patient subgroups." As a result, patients with hepatitis C should be considered at risk for a psychiatric disorder, and their medical management should include psychiatric evaluation and, if necessary, treatment.[23]

In a trial published in the *Brazilian Journal of Psychiatry*, researchers from Spain and Brazil studied the incidence of depression in a group of patients with hepatitis C who were being treated with antiviral therapy. The initial cohort consisted of fifty-four subjects with hepatitis C; at baseline, they were considered to be without a mood disorder. Forty-six subjects received antiviral therapy for twelve weeks, and eight received this therapy for twenty-four weeks. All were evaluated through a depression module of the Patient Health Questionnaire at three time points—baseline, four weeks, and end of treatment. The researchers learned that the cumulative incidence of major depression and any depressive disorder during the antiviral treatment was 12.9 percent and 46.3 percent, respectively. The researchers concluded that their findings emphasize the need to screen patients receiving antiviral therapy for depressive disorders and to identify any potential risk factors.[24]

Patients with Hepatitis C Improve Their Health-Related Quality of Life If They Participate in Exercise

In a cross-sectional, observational trial published in the journal *BMJ Open Gastroenterology*, researchers from the UK wanted to learn more about the association between physical activity and exercise, cardiovascular disease risk, and health-related quality of life in people with hepatitis C. The researchers noted that it has been shown that people with hepatitis C have increased risks of cardiovascular disease and a reduced health-related quality of life. The researchers recruited eighty-six patients; 74 percent were men and 94 percent were white. The average age was fifty-two years. Forty-two percent reported that they were currently active, and 44 percent were inactive. The gender, ethnicity, and socioeconomic status between the two groups were similar. Although the overall health-related quality of life tended to be low, patients who were active had a better health-related quality of life than those who were not. While the metabolic and cardiovascular characteristics between the two groups were similar, the patients categorized as active scored significantly higher on the psychological and social interaction subscales than those who were inactive. The researchers observed that their findings suggest that physical activity and exercise should be promoted as a potential therapeutic tool to improve health-related quality of life in patients with hepatitis C, "even if participation may not result in improved cardiometabolic and biochemical parameters." And, they concluded that "addressing specific motivators/barriers to exercise for patients will be key to designing effective PA/exercise interventions in this patient population to ensure maximum uptake and adherence."[25]

REFERENCES AND FURTHER READING

Andreone, Pietro, Sirio Fiorino, Carmela Cursaro et al. "Vitamin E as Treatment for Chronic Hepatitis B: Results of a Randomized Controlled Pilot Trial." *Antiviral Research* 49 (2001): 75–81.

Baloch, L., G. Patel, R. Collins-Cronkright et al. "Who Really Receives Hepatitis A Vaccinations?" *American Journal of Gastroenterology* 116 (October 2021): S548.

Bukh, Jens. "The History of Hepatitis C Virus (HCV): Basic Research Reveals Unique Features in Phylogeny, Evolution and the Viral Life Cycle with New Perspectives for Epidemic Control." *Journal of Hepatology* 65, no. 1 Supplement (October 2016): S2–S21.

Egmond, Elfi, Zoe Marino, Ricard Navines et al. "Incidence of Depression in Patients with Hepatitis C Treated with Direct-Acting Antivirals." *Brazilian Journal of Psychiatry* 42, no. 1 (January–February 2020): 72–76.

Feinstone, Stephen M. "History of the Discovery of Hepatitis A Virus." *Cold Spring Harbor Perspectives in Medicine* 9, no. 5 (May 2019): a031740.

Golden, Jeannette, Anne Marie O'Dwyer, and Ronan M. Conroy. "Depression and Anxiety in Patients with Hepatitis C: Prevalence, Detection Rates and Risk Factors." *General Hospital Psychiatry* 27 (2005): 431–438.

Golden, Sara E., Diane Miller, Lissi Hansen et al. "The Experience of Veterans with Hepatitis C and Acupuncture: A Mixed Methods Pilot Study." *European Journal of Integrative Medicine* 10 (February 2017): 8–18.

Hallsworth, Kate, Shion Gosrani, Sarah Hogg et al. "Association of Exercise Participation Levels with Cardiometabolic Health and Quality of Life in Individuals with Hepatitis C." *BMJ Open Gastroenterology* 8 (2021): e000591.

Hennessey, Karen A., David R. Bangsberg, Cindi Weinbaum, and Judith A. Hahn. "Hepatitis A Seroprevalence and Risk Factors Among Homeless Adults in San Francisco: Should Homelessness Be Included in the Risk-Based Strategy for Vaccination?" *Public Health Reports* 124, no. 6 (November–December 2009): 813–817.

Hofmeister, Megan G., Shaoman Yin, Maria V. Aslam et al. "Hepatitis A Hospitalization Costs, United States, 2017." *Emerging Infectious Diseases* 26, no. 5 (May 2020): 1040–1041.

Hu, Ye-Chao, Wei-Wei Wang, Wei-Yun Jiang et al. "Low Vitamin D Levels Are Associated with High Viral Loads in Patients with Chronic Hepatitis B: A Systematic Review and Meta-Analysis." *BMC Gastroenterology* 19 (2019): 84.

Huang, Wei, Xiaoli Wu, Zhenzhen Yao et al. "Investigating the Relationship Between Hepatitis B Virus Infection and Postpartum Depression in Chinese Women: A Retrospective Cohort Study." *Frontiers in Public Health* 11 (2023): 1214151.

Hyunb, Myung Han, Ji Hoon Kim, Jeong Won Jang et al. "Risk of Hepatitis C Virus Transmission Through Acupuncture: A Systematic Review and Meta-Analysis." *Korean Journal of Gastroenterology* 82, no. 3 (September 2023): 127–136.

Kaigh, Caroline, Andrea Blome, Kraftin E. Schreyer, and Megan Healey. "Emergency Department-Based Hepatitis A Vaccination Program in Response to an Outbreak." *Western Journal of Emergency Medicine* 21, no. 4 (July 2020): 906–908.

Magri, Mariana Cavalheiro, Arielle Karen da Silva Nunes, Bianca Peixoto Dantas et al. "Meta-Analysis of the Prevalence of HBV Infection Among Alcohol Users Worldwide." *Alcohol and Alcoholism* 55, no. 2 (2020): 136–143.

Murlidharan, S., A. L. Sangle, M. Engade, and A. B. Kale. "The Clinical Profile of Children with Hepatitis A Infection: An Observational Hospital-Based Study." *Cureus* 14, no. 8 (August 2022): e28290.

Ogunnaike, M., S. das, S. S. Raut et al. "Chronic Hepatitis B Infection: New Approaches Towards Cure." *Biomolecules* 13, no. 8 (August 2023): 1208.

Rahmani, A.., A. Montecucco, B. K. Vitturi et al. "Long-Term Effectiveness of Hepatitis B Vaccination in the Protection of Healthcare Students in Highly Developed Countries: A Systematic Review and Metal-Analysis." *Vaccines* 10 (2022): 1841.

Riyahi, Nasrin, Masood Ziaee, and Reza Dastjerdi. "The Effects of Cognitive Behavioral Therapy on Quality of Life among Patients with Hepatitis B." *Modern Care Journal* 15, no. 3 (July 2018): e82748.

Rusu, Emilia, Mariana Jinga, Georgiana Enache et al. "Effects of Lifestyle Changes Including Specific Dietary Intervention and Physical Activity in the Management of Patients with Chronic Hepatitis C – A Randomized Trial." *Nutrition Journal* 12 (2013): 119.

Tu, An, Xiaoning Zhu, Paniz Zarghami Dastjerdi et al. "Evaluate the Clinical Efficacy of Traditional Chinese Medicine as the Neoadjuvant Treatment in Reducing the Incidence of Hepatocellular Carcinoma in Patients with Hepatitis B-Related Cirrhosis: A Systematic Review and Meta-Analysis." *Heliyon* 10, no. 3 (February 15, 2024): e24437.

Valizadeh, L., V. Zamanzadeh, R. Negarandeh et al. "Psychological Reactions Among Patients with Chronic Hepatitis B: A Qualitative Study." *Journal of Caring Sciences* 5, no. 1 (2016): 57–66.

Villar, Livia Melo, Jose Antonio Del Campo, Isodora Ranchal et al. "Association Between Vitamin D and Hepatitis C Virus Infection: A Meta-Analysis." *World journal of Gastroenterology* 19, no. 35 (September 21, 2013): 5917–5924.

Zhang, Mengdi, Meijuan Wan, Wen Wang et al. "Effect of Interferon Therapy on Quality of Life in Patients with Chronic Hepatitis B." *Scientific Reports* 14 (2024): 2461.

INGUINAL HERNIA

INTRODUCTION

Caused by a weakening of the muscles in the lower abdomen that allows intra-abdominal contents to pass through the resulting opening, an inguinal hernia is a bulge in the groin region of the body, the area between the lower section of the abdomen and the thigh. Inguinal hernias, which are also known as groin hernias, occur in the inguinal canal, which is a passageway that runs down either side of the pelvis into the sex organs. Most often, inguinal hernias contain fat or a section of the small intestine.

In the abdomen, three layers protect the intestines. The first is a thin layer known as the peritoneum; the second is made up of the abdominal muscles, and the third is the skin. An inguinal hernia forms when the intestines and peritoneum push through the muscles and appear as a bulge in the skin.

Though they form on the right side more often than the left, inguinal hernias may occur on both sides of the body and at any age. In fact, infants may be born with an inguinal hernia; about five out of every one hundred infants are born with one.

There are two main types of inguinal hernias. The most common type, known as indirect inguinal hernias, occurs in men and women. It is associated with a defect in the lower abdominal wall that is present at birth. In men, the hernia starts in the abdomen and descends through an opening to the groin area and reaches the scrotum, the sac that contains the testicles. If this opening does not close at birth, a hernia develops. In women, this type of hernia occurs when a weakening of the abdominal muscles causes a reproductive organ or section of the small intestine to slide into the groin area. On the other hand, direct inguinal hernias, which normally only occur in men, are caused by a weakening of the abdominal muscles.

The word "hernia" originates from the Latin word for "prolapse," and the earliest evidence of an inguinal hernia was recorded in approximately 1552 BC in ancient Egypt. The term "groin hernia" was first used by Henri Fruchaud, a French surgeon and anatomist, in the 1950s.[1]

SYMPTOMS, RISKS, AND COMPLICATIONS

The main symptom of an inguinal hernia is a bulge in the groin area. In men, it may extend into the scrotum and cause an enlarged scrotum. Small inguinal hernias may slide back and forth through an opening in the abdomen and not cause any symptoms. Larger inguinal hernias may sometimes be massaged back into the abdomen. Inguinal hernias that are unable to be moved back into the abdomen are called incarcerated hernias. When people strain, inguinal hernias increase in size, and they decrease in size when someone is lying down. These hernias may cause sudden pain and/or a feeling of weakness, pressure, burning, a dragging sensation, or aching in the groin area, which may worsen when bending over, coughing, or lifting. At the same time, many inguinal hernias, even larger ones, may have no noticeable pain. Signs and symptoms of an inguinal hernia in infants include crying, coughing, or straining during a bowel movement, as well as irritability and decreased appetite. In an older child, an inguinal hernia may be more obvious when the child coughs, strains during a bowel movement, and stands for longer periods of time.

While genetics clearly play a role in the development of inguinal hernias, other factors also place people at increased risk. For example, inguinal hernias are far more common in men than women, and they are more often seen in infants born before their due date. People who are white have an increased risk, as do older people, pregnant women, and people who have previously had a hernia. Inguinal hernias are more likely to occur in people who increase pressure on the walls of abdominal muscles by excessive coughing, who stand for long periods of time, have a connective tissue disorder, have a lower body mass index, work in hard manual labor, participate in frequent strenuous exercise, lift heavy weights, and strain to pass bowel movements. They are also more common in males who have had a prostatectomy.

Although they may appear to be benign, inguinal hernias should never be ignored. They tend to grow larger, and the intestine may become trapped inside the bulge and lose its blood supply. This is known as a strangulated inguinal hernia; such a hernia may lead to inflammation and infection of the tissue, and, eventually, gangrene and death. A strangulated inguinal hernia requires emergency attention; it must be evaluated by a medical provider and/or surgeon. Symptoms of such hernia include severe intense pain, a hernia bulge that is turning red, purple, or dark, fever, rapid heart rate, an inability to move the bowels or pass gas, and nausea and vomiting.

PREVALENCE

In the United States, inguinal hernias are very common. It has been estimated that there are about 800,000 inguinal hernia surgeries performed each year. They account for about 75 percent of all abdominal wall hernias. The incidence is most common in children from birth to age five and in seniors after the age of seventy years. Two-thirds of these hernias are indirect. Males account for about 90 percent of all inguinal hernias. Over a lifetime, an inguinal hernia will affect nearly 25 percent of men and less than 2 percent of women.[2] Indirect inguinal hernias affect up to 4.5 percent of children, including 2 percent of babies assigned male at birth and 1 percent of babies assigned female at birth. Premature babies are up to 30 percent more likely to develop one.

DIAGNOSIS AND TREATMENT OPTIONS

Inguinal hernias are usually diagnosed during the physical examination that follows a medical history. Often, a medical provider asks the patient to stand and cough. The medical provider will want to see and feel the hernia. In children, inguinal hernias are most obvious when they cry, cough, or stand. When the history suggests that there is an inguinal hernia, but the medical provider is unable to locate one, other tests, such as an ultrasound, CT imaging, or an MRI may be ordered.

In adults, small hernias that are not causing any problems are usually simply watched. Surgery is recommended for larger, symptomatic inguinal hernias in adults and all inguinal hernias in children. The goal of inguinal hernia surgery is to move the hernia contents back into the abdominal cavity and close the defect. This is called herniorrhaphy. There are two main types of surgery for inguinal hernias. In an open repair surgery, an incision is made into the groin area. The surgeon moves the hernia back inside the abdomen and closes the defect in the abdominal wall with stitches. Sometimes, a piece of mesh is used to strengthen the closure and reduce the risk of recurrence. This is called hernioplasty. In the second type of surgery, known as laparoscopic surgery, the surgeon makes a few tiny incisions and inserts a thin scope with a tiny camera into these incisions. Using the scope and camera, the surgeon repairs the hernia. Mesh is normally used in this procedure. Because there is minimal cutting, there is less pain and a faster recovery with this type of surgery. Though there are surgeons who specialize in hernia surgery, most general surgeons have repaired many inguinal hernias. Inguinal hernia surgery is normally an outpatient procedure. It may be performed under general, regional, or local anesthesia. Pediatricians tend to recommend treating all children with inguinal hernias, as they have a higher risk of complications. Expect some postoperative pain, which may be treated in many cases with over-the-counter pain relievers. Potential complications for adults and children include injury to nearby organs, blood vessels, or nerves; bleeding, infection, problems with wound healing, blood clots; and reactions to anesthesia. After inguinal hernia surgery, some people have a problem urinating, and about 10 percent have chronic pain in the groin area, which may be caused by nerve damage or a sensitivity to the mesh insert. Hernias tend to recur in up to 10 percent of adults; hernias tend not to recur in children.

RESEARCH FINDINGS

Family History Is a Key Determinant Factor in the Risk of Inguinal Hernias in Adult Males

In a case-control trial published in the journal *Surgery*, researchers from Hong Kong evaluated the risk factors for the development of primary inguinal hernias in adult males. The cohort consisted of 1,418 male patients who were recruited at the general surgical or hernia clinic of a university-affiliated teaching hospital in Hong Kong. There were 709 patients with an inguinal hernia and 709 without an inguinal hernia. Each patient was interviewed by a research assistant who used a standardized questionnaire. The researchers noted that the patients with an inguinal hernia had significantly lower body weights and a shorter body heights, but there were no significant differences between the two groups for body mass indices and educational achievement. The researchers learned that the most important determining factor for primary inguinal hernia was a family history of hernias. Other factors associated with primary inguinal hernias were chronic obstructive airway disease (COPD) and strenuous physical activity. Still, they concluded that the development of primary inguinal hernias "is probably a multifactorial process."[3]

Family History Seems to Play a Role in the Early Recurrence after Inguinal Hernia Repair

In an observational cohort study published in the journal *BMC Surgery*, researchers from Germany evaluated issues such as family history, age, and male gender that may play a role in an early recurrence of an inguinal hernia after a surgical repair. The cohort consisted of seventy-five patients who had at least two recurrent inguinal hernias; there were sixty-seven males and eight females. Data were collected by a single research assistant on gender, age, smoking, comorbidity, medication, and family history. Statistical analyses were carried out using the Statistical Package for the Social Sciences. The researchers determined that thirty-three of the seventy-five inguinal hernia patients had similarly affected relatives. The onset of the primary hernia was at the age of forty-one years for patients with a family history and at the age of forty-eight years for patients without a family history. So, hernia recurrence occurred about seven years earlier in patients with a family history. The researchers commented that their findings determined that family history is not only a factor in the occurrence of primary inguinal hernias but also in their recurrence. "Family history as a risk factor for early recurrence would support the hypothesis that collagen gene or genes associated to collagen metabolism play a role for hernia disease."[4]

But, There Are Also Other Risk Factors for Inguinal Hernias in US Adults

In a retrospective, case-control study published in the journal *Hernia*, researchers from California and New York investigated demographic, clinical, and behavioral risk factors for undergoing inguinal hernia repair surgery. The researchers used data on 302,532 members of a large, integrated healthcare delivery system with electronic health records. From 2007 to 2020, 7,314 (2.42 percent) of the people in this group had inguinal hernia surgery. The incidence was 6.31 percent in men and 0.53 percent in women. The majority of the patients who had this surgery were non-Hispanic white (85 percent), followed by Hispanic/Latinos (6.6 percent), East Asians (5 percent), and African American (2.7 percent). Older men, especially those between the ages of seventy and eighty years, and those who participated in more vigorous physical activity were more likely to have inguinal hernia surgery. People who drank alcohol and women who smoked also had higher rates of this surgery. In contrast, the rates of inguinal hernia surgery were lower in people who were overweight or had obesity. The researchers concluded that their findings may help identify people who are at higher risk for inguinal hernia repair surgery.[5]

In another study published in the *American Journal of Epidemiology*, researchers from Silver Spring and Bethesda, Maryland examined risk factors for incident inguinal hernias among adults in the United States. Their cohort consisted of 5,316 men and 8,136 women who participated in the first National Health and Nutrition Examination. Almost twenty years later, they were followed for a hospital or physician diagnosis of an inguinal hernia. The researchers learned that during this long period of time, 13.9 percent of the men and 2.1 percent of the women were diagnosed with an inguinal hernia. Older men were more likely to have inguinal hernias than younger men. Thus, the incidence was 7.3 percent among men between the ages of twenty-four and thirty-nine years and 22.8 percent among men aged sixty to seventy-four years. White men were almost twice as likely as Black men to have an inguinal hernia. Heavier men were less likely to have an inguinal hernia. Factors that were unrelated to the risk for inguinal hernia included recreational and non-recreational physical activity, constipation or bowel movement frequency, chronic cough, chronic obstructive pulmonary disease, alcohol intake, minimum adult weight, weight loss or weight gain, height, and education. Less information was provided on the risk in women. Still, the risk increased among women who were older, lived in rural areas, were taller, had a chronic cough, and had an umbilical hernia. The researchers concluded that in the US inguinal hernia "is a common condition among men that increases substantially with aging. The lower risk among overweight and obese men was an unexpected finding that bears further study."[6]

Smaller Inguinal Hernias Appear to Be an Independent Risk Factor for Developing Chronic Postoperative Inguinal Pain

In a study published in the journal *Annals of Surgery*, researchers from Switzerland and Germany investigated the association between the size of an inguinal hernia and the development of chronic postoperative inguinal pain (CPIP). They obtained a cohort of 57,999 male patients from the Herniamed Registry, a multicenter, internet-based hernia registry with 644 participating hospitals and surgeons in private practice in Germany, Austria, and Switzerland. Also recorded in this registry were the European Hernia Society classification of the size of the hernia, the postoperative complications that occurred up to thirty days after the surgery, and the findings of a one-year follow-up questionnaire, which asked about recurrences, pain at rest, pain on exertion, and chronic pain requiring treatment. The researchers determined that smaller inguinal hernias are a risk factor for developing chronic postoperative inguinal pain. This occurred irrespective of the patient's age, hernia repair technique, or other risk factors. Moreover, smaller inguinal hernias were correlated with significantly higher rates of pain at rest, pain on exertion, and chronic pain requiring treatment one year after the surgery. Compared with older patients, the patients who were younger than fifty-five years had higher rates of pain at rest, pain on exertion, and pain requiring treatment "with the same significant association of smaller inguinal hernias and higher risk of developing CPIP [chronic postoperative inguinal pain]." The researchers concluded that "smaller inguinal hernias have been identified as an independent patient-related risk factor for developing CPIP."[7]

After Laparoscopic Inguinal Hernia Surgery, Three Factors Seem to Contribute to the Length of Convalescence

In a single-center trial published in *Surgery*, researchers from Denmark wanted to learn what factors contribute to the length of convalescence after laparoscopic inguinal hernia surgery. The cohort consisted of 162 male patients; they ranged in age from twenty to eighty-five years. In total, ninety-two patients were employed, and seventy patients were not employed. Forty-three patients had a sedentary to light physical workload, and forty-nine patients had a moderate to strenuous workload. Ninety-nine patients had a sedentary to light level of leisure activity, and sixty-three patients had a moderate to strenuous level of leisure activity. Convalescence days, or days before returning to work and leisure activities, averaged five and three days, respectively. The researchers learned that planned sick leave, pain, and fatigue were the main reasons activities were not resumed earlier. "Postoperative, self-registered planned sick leave, and complaints of pain and fatigue were the dominant reasons for not resuming normal activities within the first three days after operation."[8]

Electroacupuncture May Reduce the Pain Experienced Following Inguinal Hernia Surgery

In a prospective, randomized, double-blinded, placebo-controlled trial published in the *Korean Journal of Pain*, researchers from Iran examined the use of acupuncture to reduce the pain experienced after inguinal hernia surgery. The cohort consisted of ninety male patients who were about to have inguinal hernia surgery. They were randomly divided into two equal groups. The patients in both groups had similar demographic characteristics; they ranged in age from twelve to fifty-five years, with a mean age of twenty-five years. The anesthesia techniques were the same for all of the patients. The patients in one group received electroacupuncture, and the patients in the other group served as a control group. The researchers determined that the patients in the electroacupuncture group had lower levels of pain, and they requested morphine, a narcotic pain medication, less often than the patients in the control group, and the difference was statistically significant. The patients in the electroacupuncture group also took statistically lower doses of morphine. And, probably because they took less morphine, the subjects in the electroacupuncture group had statistically less dizziness and nausea. The researchers concluded that "acupuncture in patients, after inguinal surgery, can reduce the need for analgesics, which also directly reduces the complications that may occur when analgesics are used in relieving pain postoperatively."[9]

Apparently, Whenever Possible, It Is Better to Postpone Hernia Surgery in Pregnant Women

In a cluster-wide, retrospective, descriptive study published in the journal *Surgical Practice*, researchers from Hong Kong examined factors associated with the presence of hernias in pregnant women. They collected data on forty-one pregnant women with hernias from January 2002 to January 2022; twenty-two of these hernias were inguinal hernias. The median age of hernia onset was thirty-one years. All of the women either developed hernias while pregnant, or they knew they had unrepaired hernias prior to pregnancy. No patient developed complications during pregnancy or delivery. Fourteen (63.6 percent) of the twenty-two women with inguinal hernias developed during pregnancy reported hernia disappearance after delivery. But, five of these women had a hernia recurrence: one at the fifth year, one at the seventh year post-delivery, and the remaining three during subsequent pregnancies. Eighteen women (43.9 percent) had hernia surgery after delivery; none had perioperative or postoperative complications, and there were no hernia recurrences, even among those women who had subsequent pregnancies. The researchers concluded that "hernia has few complications during pregnancy and delivery. Repair could be safely delayed until post-partum."[10]

Another study on hernias during pregnancy was published in the *Journal of the American College of Surgeons*. This study described twelve female patients with inguinal or umbilical hernias that were seen by a single surgeon at the Mount Sinai Medical Center in New York City. The women ranged in age from twenty-seven to forty-one years, with a mean age of thirty-five years. Fifty-eight percent of the women had inguinal hernias, and almost all of the hernias were on the right side. Ninety-two percent of the patients had a bulging mass and 67 percent had pain. None of the women needed a hernia repair while still pregnant, but they all had surgery after they delivered their babies. None had any complications. And, during a mean follow-up of seventeen months, no one had a recurrent hernia. Four of these women had subsequent uncomplicated pregnancies. The researchers commented that their findings support the belief that pregnant women with hernias should be monitored, and the surgical repair should take place after the baby has been delivered. They support the "watchful waiting" strategy during pregnancy, with a plan for postpartum herniorrhaphy."[11]

But Some Pregnancy Inguinal Hernias May Not Be Real Inguinal Hernias

In a study published in *Hernia*, researchers from Austria described a consecutive series of eighteen pregnant women who were referred to surgeons because of the "gradual onset of inguinal swelling and groin ache." All of the women, who had a median age of 28.5 years, were examined during and after their pregnancies by at least two surgeons. Four of the suspected hernias occurred toward the end of the first trimester, twelve occurred in the second trimester, and two in the last trimester. The women did not have any of the usual risk factors for the development of hernias, such as chronic obstructive pulmonary disease and smoking. Most of the women were referred by their gynecologists, and none had previously had surgery for an inguinal or femoral hernia. Though the surgeons found no inguinal hernias in any of the women, they did find large varicose veins in the area normally occupied by the hernias. Apparently, the inguinal hernia-like symptoms subsided in all of the women within weeks after delivery. The median follow-up time was eleven months. The researchers concluded that "the diagnosis of an inguinal hernia with a first symptomatic onset during pregnancy may be wrong in most cases."[12]

A Person's Work May Contribute to the Development of an Inguinal Hernia

In a systematic review and meta-analysis published in *Hernia*, researchers from the Netherlands investigated the relationship between the work that people do and their risk for developing a lateral inguinal hernia. The researchers located fourteen studies that met their criteria. Two studies were case reports, one had a cross-sectional design, five had a case-control design, one had a retrospective cohort design, and five had a prospective cohort design. Three of these studies with 621 workers were included in the meta-analysis. The researchers determined that there was an association between men who completed physically demanding work that included standing and walking for more than six hours each day or lifting cumulative loads of more than 4,000 kg per workday and an increased risk for the development of a lateral inguinal hernia. Thus, the researchers commented that there is a direct association between the development of a lateral inguinal hernia and "physically demanding work that is characterized by standing/walking and lifting."[13]

A Surgical Repair of an Inguinal Hernia with a Mesh Insert Appears Preferable to a Repair without a Mesh Insert

In a study published in the *British Journal of Surgery*, researchers from the Netherlands wanted to learn if the surgical repair of an inguinal hernia with a mesh insert would help lower recurrence rates. During a three-year period, 289 patients who were scheduled for inguinal hernia surgery at one of six hospitals were randomized to have a mesh insert (n = 146) or to have the repair without the insert (n = 143). (The mesh group had a small number of "conversions" to non-mesh, and the non-mesh group had a small number of "conversions" to mesh.) During a long-term follow-up of about ten years, one-third of the patients died. None of the deaths was associated with the hernia surgery. The researchers learned that while only one person in the mesh group had a recurrence, eighteen in the non-mesh group had a recurrence. At the same time, there was no significant correlation between recurrence and age, obesity, history of pulmonary disease, constipation, or prostate disease. The researchers noted that their findings "provided evidence that mesh repair of inguinal hernia is superior to non-mesh repair in the long term." And, they concluded that "non-mesh primary inguinal hernia repair should be completely abandoned in adults if recurrence rates are to be reduced."[14]

In a systematic review with a meta-analysis published in the *World Journal of Surgery*, researchers from Tunisia compared repairing a strangulated inguinal hernia with or without a mesh. The researchers located nine studies that met their criteria; there were two randomized controlled trials, three nonrandomized prospective studies, and four retrospective studies. From five studies with 413 patients, the researchers learned that there were twenty-six reported wound infections. There were seven in the mesh patients and nineteen in the non-mesh patients. So, the wound infection rate was lower in the mesh patients than in the non-mesh patients, but the difference was not statistically significant. From three studies with a total of 260 patients, the researchers determined that the patients with the mesh insert had lower rates of recurrence. There were two recurrences in the mesh patients and twenty-five in the non-mesh patients. As in the previous studies, the researchers determined that using a mesh insert during inguinal repair surgery improves the overall results. The researchers concluded that the "mesh repair technique is a good option for the treatment of strangulated inguinal hernias in adults, giving an acceptable wound infection rate and fewer recurrences than non-mesh repair."[15]

Though Inguinal Hernias Commonly Occur in the Elderly, Not All Elders Are Good Candidates for Hernia Repairs

In an article published in the *Journal of the American Medical Directors Association*, researchers from Chapel Hill, North Carolina, noted that some research studies on inguinal hernias in the elderly had advised "watchful waiting." After all, most inguinal hernias have a low risk of complications, and there is an increased risk of morbidity and mortality when operating on people sixty-five years of age or older. The researchers examined which elders were better candidates for inguinal hernia repairs. The researchers noted that chronological age alone is not necessarily a measure of a patient's fitness for surgery. Rather, physical and cognitive frailty is far more important. It is also crucial to factor in preexisting conditions such as cardiac, renal, pulmonary, hepatic, and neurological problems, as well as nutritional, socioeconomic, and affective status. And, general anesthesia has been known to trigger cognitive decline. So, if possible, it is better to use local anesthesia with the elderly. On the other hand, elderly patients who present with incarcerated, obstructed, or strangulated inguinal hernias are, in all likelihood, to require immediate surgery. So, in many cases, it is best to repair an inguinal hernia before it becomes an emergency. "It behooves the heath care provider, both medical and surgical, to weigh the risks of pursuing elective repair rather than await an impending emergency."[16]

REFERENCES AND FURTHER READING

Buch, Kerri E., Parissa Tabrizian, and Celia M. Divino. "Management of Hernias in Pregnancy." *Journal of the American College of Surgeons* 207, no. 4 (2008): 539–542.

Chiu, Hon Yu, Tsz Ting Law, Lily Ng, Kin Yuen Wong. "Hernia in Pregnancy – Does It Matter?" *Surgical Practice* 26, no. 4 (November 2022): 257–261.

Cowan, B., M. Kvale, J. Yin et al. "Risk Factors for Inguinal Hernia Repair Among US Adults." *Hernia* 27 (2023): 1507–1514.

Hentati, Hassen, Wajih Dougaz, and Chadli Dziri. "Mesh Repair Versus Non-Mesh Repair for Strangulated Inguinal Hernia: Systematic Review with Meta-Analysis." *World Journal of Surgery* 38 (2014): 2784–2790.

Hoffmann, Henry, Daniela Walther, Reinhard Bittner et al. "Small Inguinal Hernias Are Independent Risk Factors for Developing Chronic Postoperative Inguinal Pain(CPIP)." *Annals of Surgery* 271, no. 4 (April 2020): 756–764.

Hori, Tomohide and Daiki Yasukawa. "Fascinating History of Groin Hernias: Comprehensive Recognition of Anatomy, Classic Considerations for Herniorrhaphy, and Current Controversies in Hernioplasty." *World Journal of Methodology* 11, no. 4 (July 20, 2021): 160–186.

Jansen, P. L., U. Klinge, M. Jansen, and K. Junge. "Risk Factors for Early Recurrence After Inguinal Hernia Repair." *BMC Surgery* 9 (2009): 18.

Kuijer, P. P. F. M., D. Hondebrink, C. T. J. Hulshof, and H. F. Van der Molen. "Work-Relatedness of Inguinal Hernia: A Systematic Review Including Meta-Analysis and GRADE." *Hernia* 24 (2020): 943–950.

Lau, Hung, Christian Fang, Wai K. Yuen, and Nivritti G. Patil. "Risk Factors for Inguinal Hernia in Adult Males: A Case-Control Study." *Surgery* 141 (2007): 262–266.

Lechner, M., R. Fortelny, D. Öfner, and F. Mayer. "Suspected Inguinal Hernias in Pregnancy – Handle With Care!" *Hernia* 18 (2014): 375–379.

Perez, Arielle j. and Shannelle Campbell. "Inguinal Hernia Repair in Older Persons." *Journal of the American Directors Association* 23 (2022): 563–567.

Ruhl, Constance E. and James E. Everhart. "Risk Factors for Inguinal Hernia Among Adults in the US Population." *American Journal of Epidemiology* 165 (2007): 1154–1161.

Taghavi, Rahim, Kamyar Tavakoli Tabasi, Nasser Mogharabian et al. "The Effect of Acupuncture on Relieving Pain After Inguinal Surgery." *Korean Journal of Pain* 26 (2013): 46–50.

Tolver, M. A., P. Strandfelt, G. Forsberg et al. "Determinants of a Short Convalescence After Laparoscopic Transabdominal Preperitoneal Inguinal Hernia Repair." *Surgery* 151, no. 4 (2012): 556–563.

van Veen, R. N., A. R. Wijsmuller, W. W. Vrijland et al. "Long-Term Follow-Up of a Randomized Clinical Trial of a Non-Mesh *versus* Mesh Repair of Primary Inguinal Hernia." *British Journal of Surgery* 94 (2007): 506–510.

INTESTINAL OBSTRUCTION

INTRODUCTION

Also known as a bowel obstruction, an intestinal obstruction is a partial or complete blockage that keeps food or liquid from passing through the small or large intestine (colon). When this occurs, feces, digestive juices, and gas may be stuck behind the blockage, damaging the tissue.

There are two main types of intestinal obstructions. The first is a small bowel obstruction, which accounts for about 80 percent of obstructions. These happen in the small intestine, the organ that connects the stomach to the large intestine. The second occurs in the large intestine, the organ that connects to the small intestine and ends with the rectum and anus. There are also partial obstructions, in which food, digestive juices, and gas are still able to pass, and complete obstructions, in which food, digestive juices, and gas are completely blocked. There is even a phenomenon known as a pseudo-obstruction in which people experience the symptoms of an obstruction when they do not actually have one. Researchers believe that pseudo-obstructions are caused by nerve signaling problems.

There are several different causes of intestinal obstructions. These include adhesions—which are fibrous bands of tissue that may form after abdominal or pelvic surgery, hernias, or portions of the intestine that protrude into another part of the body; colon cancer and twisting of the colon; impacted feces; ingestion of a foreign object that is unable to be broken down; or strictures from an inflamed intestine caused by certain conditions such as Crohn's disease or diverticulitis. In the United States, abdominal adhesions are the leading reason for small bowel obstructions, hernias are the second most common cause, and colon cancer is the main cause of large bowel obstructions. In children younger than three years, intussusception is the main cause of bowel obstructions. With this condition, one segment of the intestine collapses inside another segment. The collapsed segments may block the bowel and blood flow. And, some infants are born with a congenital condition called malrotation. With this medical problem, the intestines do not form properly, and they may twist (volvulus), causing a blockage.

Historical records indicate that cases of intestinal obstruction were documented in ancient texts like the Ebers Papyrus (1550 BC) and by Hippocrates, who indicated that the condition was recognized and described in early medical history.

SYMPTOMS, RISKS, AND COMPLICATIONS

There are a number of signs and symptoms associated with an intestinal obstruction. These include crampy abdominal pain that initially comes in waves but eventually becomes constant, a loss of appetite, an overall feeling of illness, severe constipation (a sign of complete blockage) or diarrhea (a sign of partial blockage), rapid heartbeat, dark-colored urine, nausea and vomiting, dehydration, fever, an inability to have a bowel movement or pass gas, and the swelling of the abdomen. The pain from a small bowel obstruction is more likely to come in short intermittent waves, and it is likely to feel concentrated in one place. The cramping from a large bowel obstruction tends to be more continuous, and it is more likely to feel spread out. Infants and children may have the same signs and symptoms, but they may also have blood in the stool, green or yellow vomit, and a swollen, firm abdomen.

A number of factors increase the risk of an intestinal obstruction. These include abdominal or pelvic surgery, which may cause adhesions, a common intestinal obstruction, Crohn's disease, which may cause the walls of the intestine to thicken, thus narrowing the areas for feces to pass, and abdominal cancer.

Left untreated, an intestinal obstruction has the potential to cause serious, life-threatening complications. These include the cutting off of the blood supply to part of the intestine, which will cause the intestinal wall to die, tear, leak, and trigger an infection or peritonitis. Peritonitis is a life-threatening condition that requires immediate attention and often surgery. When an infection spreads throughout the body, it is called sepsis. Strangulation with tissue death is another life-threatening complication. With strangulation, an intestinal obstruction prevents parts of the intestine from obtaining a sufficient amount of blood. Eventually, the tissue dies and gangrene forms. Without intensive care, a person may die.

PREVALENCE

Small bowel obstructions are a frequent reason that people seek medical care in an emergency department, and they are considered a common surgical emergency. In fact, it has been estimated that there are about 300,000 such surgeries in the United States every year. Uncommon in the general population, large bowel obstructions are most often seen in people with colon cancer. About 40 percent of people with colon cancer are diagnosed because of the symptoms of an obstruction. Bowel obstructions are more often seen in older people.

DIAGNOSIS AND TREATMENT

Diagnosis of a bowel obstruction begins with a medical history and physical examination to check for a swollen abdomen. A stethoscope may be used to listen for bowel sounds. Blood tests will be ordered, including a complete blood count to look for an infection and an electrolyte analysis to indicate severe dehydration. A breath test may be ordered to determine how fast digesting food is moving through the intestine. Imaging tests will enable the medical provider to view the obstruction. These may include X-rays of the abdomen, which will outline blockages and areas of the intestine that may have already died. Detailed horizontal images may be provided by a CT scan, and a barium enema X-ray, which fills the large intestine with a liquid before X-ray images are taken, may also be useful. Since both the CT scan and barium enema X-ray use radiation, women who are or may be pregnant and children may be advised to have MRI, which uses a large magnet rather than radiation to take images of the body.

Most people with bowel obstructions require prompt treatment in the hospital. Normally, complete obstructions require emergency surgery. During surgery, the surgeon removes adhesions or tumors that are causing the blockage. In rare instances, they remove diseased segments of tissues. On occasion, a stent or tube mesh is placed in the intestine to keep it open and resolve the obstruction without additional surgery. A stent may also be used as a temporary solution until the patient is sufficiently healthy for additional surgery.

With partial bowel obstructions, medical providers have more time to stabilize the condition, and surgery may sometimes be avoided, at least temporarily. Patients tend to be treated for dehydration with intravenous (IV) fluids, and a nasogastric tube may be used to suction out fluids and air backed up from the blockage. Medications are used to treat and prevent nausea and vomiting and to treat pain. Sometimes, in order to let the bowel rest, patients are told to stop eating and drinking; they may be allowed to drink a liquid that contains nutrients people normally obtain from food.

Without treatment, the blocked parts of the intestine may die, leading to serious problems. However, with prompt medical care, an intestinal obstruction may often be successfully treated.

RESEARCH FINDINGS

Patients Who Have Surgeries for Small Bowel Obstructions Caused by Adhesions Have a Risk of Recurrence

In a study published in the journal *Annals of Surgery*, researchers from Norway wanted to understand the patterns of recurrence that may take place after one or more episodes of small bowel obstruction due to adhesions. That is why they analyzed more than forty years of hospital records of 500 patients who had operations for small bowel obstructions caused by adhesions; there were 240 men and 260 women with a median age of fifty-six and fifty-five years, respectively. The patients were followed until death, loss to follow-up, or the end of the study. The median follow-up was ten years, and the maximum follow-up was forty-one years. Twenty-eight percent of the patients were followed for twenty years or longer. The total number of admissions for small bowel adhesion obstructions was 686. A questionnaire on recurrences and abdominal complaints was sent to all living patients. The researchers learned that the cumulative recurrence rate for patients operated on for one small bowel adhesion obstruction was 18 percent after ten years and 29 percent after thirty years. The cumulative recurrence rate reached 81 percent for patients with four or more such admissions. Most recurrent episodes took place within five years of the previous one, but the risk was still present ten to twenty years after an episode. And, this risk was, according to the researchers, "considerable."[1]

A Low-Fiber Diet Appears to Help People Manage Inoperable Malignant Bowel Obstructions

In a mixed methods single-arm feasibility trial published in the *Journal of Human Nutrition and Dietetics*, researchers from the UK wanted to determine if a low-fiber diet consisting primarily of clear fluids, thin liquids, and pureed and soft foods would be helpful for patients with inoperable malignant bowel obstructions. Would this diet enable them to better manage their symptoms, was it easy to follow, and would it improve quality of life and reduce hospital admissions? Eligible patients included those with at least one symptom, such as pain, bloating, early satiety, nausea, and vomiting, and who were able to tolerate an oral diet. The cohort consisted of twenty-four female and six male patients between the ages of eighteen and eighty-five years; they had a mean age of sixty years. Nineteen of the cohort had colorectal cancer, and eleven had gynecological cancer. Information on symptoms and quality of life were collected on the first and last day of this twenty-eight day trial. Twenty-six patients completed the trial, and twenty-five found the diet very easy or easy to understand. And the results were notable. For example, while 96 percent of the patients had pain on day one of the trial, 63 percent had pain on day twenty-eight. The number of people reporting severe or very severe symptoms decreased between baseline and the end of the study, and the mean number of hospital admissions and corresponding bed days were all reduced during the trial. All but two of the patients who responded to the quality of life question had either an improvement in their quality of life or no change from baseline to day twenty-eight. The researchers concluded that their study demonstrated "that a modified-consistency low-fibre diet is easily followed, reduces symptoms of MBO [malignant bowel obstruction], may have an impact on admissions to hospital and improve QOL [quality of life]."[2]

Early Small Bowel Obstructions Seem to Be a Rare Complication of a Benign Hysterectomy

In a retrospective, nested, cohort study published in the *American Journal of Obstetrics & Gynecology*, researchers from Cleveland, Ohio evaluated the incidence of and risk factors for early small bowel obstructions following a hysterectomy for benign indications. Data were obtained from the American College of Surgeons National Surgical Quality Improvement Program, which included data on patient demographics and clinical and surgical factors. From this information, the researchers learned that of 47,937 hysterectomies, there were 286 patients with small bowel obstructions, a rate of 5.9 per one thousand hysterectomies. Of these, 125 patients developed small bowel obstructions during their initial hospital stay and sixty-six had a repeat surgery. The median number of days from the time of surgery to the development of a small bowel obstruction was five. When the researchers compared the patients with and without small bowel obstructions, they found that the patients with obstructions were older, forty-nine versus forty-six years, and they were more likely to smoke. In addition, the patients with small bowel obstructions were more likely to have a history of prior abdominal surgery and to have medical comorbidities, such as hypertension and dyspnea (difficulty with breathing). Operative time was thirty minutes longer in the small bowel obstruction group, and the patients with small bowel obstructions had higher rates of contaminated or infected wounds. Uterine weight was greater in the small bowel obstruction group, and patients with small bowel obstructions were almost twice as likely to have surgery by a gynecologic oncologist and less likely by an obstetrician-gynecologist. Patients with small bowel obstructions were far more likely to have abdominal hysterectomy than laparoscopic or vaginal hysterectomy. Despite all these facts, small bowel obstructions remain a relatively rare occurrence in patients undergoing a hysterectomy for benign indications. "Although route of hysterectomy was not found to be a significant risk factor for early SBO [small bowel obstruction], variables that are typically more often associated with abdominal hysterectomy compared to minimally invasive hysterectomy, higher wound class, larger uteri, and perioperative transfusion were strongly correlated with subsequent development of early obstruction."[3]

Patients Have an Increased Risk of Early Postoperative Small Bowel Obstructions after Colorectal Surgery

In a trial published in the *Euroasian Journal of Hepato-Gastroenterology*, researchers from India examined the incidence of early postoperative small bowel obstruction following colorectal surgery. The cohort consisted of one hundred patients who had colorectal surgery at a tertiary center in India; they had a mean age of 50.39 years. Seventy-six percent were male and 24 percent were female. Sixty percent lived in urban areas and 40 percent lived in rural locales. Of the one hundred patients, open and laparoscopic methods were used in 25 and 75 percent of the cases, respectively. Seventy-five percent of the patients had elective surgery and 25 percent had emergency surgery. In 74 percent of the cases, surgery lasted less than one hour; in 26 percent of the cases, surgery was longer than one hour. In 93 percent of the cases, there was less than 300 mL of blood loss. Most of the cases were stapler stitched. Following surgery, 11 percent of the patients developed early postoperative small bowel obstruction. The average time of obstruction onset was 4.30 days. The researchers found several factors associated with early postoperative small bowel obstructions. These included age, BMI, anemia, history of previous bowel habits, smoking status, neoadjuvant chemoradiotherapy (chemoradiotherapy before surgery), bowel preparation, operative procedure, surgery duration, and type of anastomosis (surgical connection between two structures). However, they also determined that certain factors played the strongest role in the development of these obstructions. They were as follows: history of previous bowel habits, history of previous abdominal surgeries, perioperative bowel preparation, and blood transfusions. Overall, according to these researchers, their findings suggested that early postoperative small bowel obstruction is a significant complication of colorectal surgery. And, they "highlight the importance of conducting a thorough assessment and management of individuals who have a history of irregular bowel movements, history of prior operations, or perioperative bowel preparation."[4]

Colorectal Patients with an Intestinal Obstruction Have a Lower Survival Rate

In a study published in the journal *Epidemiology and Health*, researchers from Malaysia examined the association between colorectal cancer and intestinal obstructions. Data on 4,501 patients with colorectal cancer were obtained from the national colorectal registry;

3,908, 86.8 percent did not have intestinal obstructions, and 593 or 13.2 percent did. Most of the colorectal cancer patients with intestinal obstructions were in the sixty to sixty-nine years age group, followed by the seventy or more age group. Most of the patients with intestinal obstructions were male. Using this data, the researchers compared the survival rate of colorectal patients with intestinal obstructions to those without such obstructions. Intestinal obstructions were reported in more than 13 percent of the patients. After treatment, the three-year survival rate for patients with intestinal obstructions was 48.3 percent and 54.9 percent for patients without intestinal obstructions. The five-year survival rate for patients with intestinal obstructions was 37.3 percent and 45.6 percent for patients without intestinal obstructions. The researchers concluded that "colorectal cancer patients without intestinal obstruction showed a tendency to live longer than those with intestinal obstruction, and the difference between the two groups was significant."[5]

Delaying Emergency Surgery to Treat a Small Bowel Obstruction Results in Higher Rates of Medical Problems and Mortality

In a study published in the *British Journal of Surgery*, researchers based in the UK noted that small bowel obstructions are a common reason for an emergency laparotomy—the surgical incision into the abdomen. That is why the researchers wanted to determine if it is better to proceed quickly with the surgery or to delay the surgery for a day or longer. Using data from the National Emergency Laparotomy Audit, the researchers examined a cohort of 9,991 patients who had an emergency laparotomy for small bowel obstructions during a two-year period of time. The primary outcome measure was the thirty-day mortality, with death data obtained from the Office for National Statistics. Patients were grouped according to the time between admission and surgery—less than twenty-four hours, twenty-four to seventy-two hours, and more than seventy-two hours. The majority of the laparotomies (6,879 or 68.9 percent) were performed twenty-four or more hours after admission. The researchers determined that the overall thirty-day mortality rate was 7.2 percent (722 patients). Despite patients treated within twenty-four hours being in the highest risk group, their unadjusted thirty-day mortality rate was only slightly higher than that in patients treated in twenty-four to seventy-two hours. But, the rate in the group of patients treated more than seventy-two hours after admission was "substantially higher." So, people who waited longer periods of time for their surgeries had higher rates of mortality. In fact, patients who had their operations more than seventy-two hours after hospital admission had a 39 percent higher mortality rate than those who had surgery less than twenty-four hours after admission. According to the researchers, "the timing of laparotomy is an independent predictor of all-cause thirty-day mortality."[6]

Bowel Obstructions May Be Caused by Phytobezoars

In a case report published in the *Iranian Journal of Public Health*, researchers from Iran described the case of a sixty-one-year-old man who presented to the emergency department of a hospital in Iran with a bowel obstruction. Apparently, a few days before, the man, who had no history of previous abdominal surgery, ate a large amount of pomegranate seeds. During a laparotomy, it was determined that the seeds had formed a phytobezoar, a hard, indigestible mass in the gastrointestinal tract that primarily consisted of plant materials. The phytobezoar, which caused a complete obstruction of the small intestine, was removed. After an unremarkable postoperative course, the man was discharged, and at his two-month follow-up visit was found to be doing well. The researchers commented that "patients with small bowel obstruction that have a history of recent consumption of vegetables or food with high fiber content and no past history of surgery, phytobezoar should be kept in mind with high index of suspicion."[7]

Another phytobezoar case was reported by researchers from Australia and published in the *Journal of Surgical Case Reports.* In this case, a man in his seventies presented with a one-day history of abdominal pain and vomiting. He was unable to move his bowels or pass gas. His medical history included complicated surgical procedures for adhesions and the recent consumption of an entire packet of peanuts, which was about to expire. A bowel obstruction was suspected, and for the next forty-eight hours, the man was admitted for a trial of conservative management. However, the obstruction failed to resolve, and the man had increasing levels of pain and began to develop peritonitis. At that point, the man had emergency surgery, and the peanut phytobezoar was located and removed. Although the postoperative recovery was slow, the man was eventually discharged on postoperative day eight. The researchers concluded that "intestinal obstruction due to bezoar is a rare but important phenomenon that may be difficult to identify on imaging. Rapid ingestion of large volumes of organic matter in patients presenting with SBO [small bowel obstruction] should raise suspicion."[8]

Still another report of a phytobezoar causing a bowel obstruction was published in the *Journal of International Medical Research.* In this case, researchers from Taiwan described an eighty-year-old man with diabetes mellitus who had been undergoing hemodialysis for five years. He presented with a one-day history of colicky pain, bilious vomiting, and abdominal distension. While his vital signs were stable, physical examination revealed a distended abdomen without surgical scars or hernias and hyperresonance upon percussion, decreased bowel sounds, and tenderness over the right lower quadrant without rebounding pain. The patient had gastroparesis that had altered his gastrointestinal motility for many years. Meanwhile, hoping to improve his constipation, the man ate several whole guavas, but his advanced age made them hard to chew. He was diagnosed with phytobezoar-induced mechanical small bowel obstruction. After a few days of medical management, the man's symptoms resolved, and he was discharged. According to the researchers, "dyspeptic symptoms are common in patients undergoing dialysis. . . . Therefore, early presentations of gastric phytobezoars may easily be overlooked, which may result in subsequent obstruction." The researchers concluded that "phytobezoar-induced SBO remains an uncommon etiology of SBO. It can occur in the absence of previous gastric surgery and can be overlooked without clinical suspicion."[9]

Physiotherapy May Reduce the Rate of Recurrent Bowel Obstructions

In a trial published in the *World Journal of Gastroenterology*, researchers from several locations in the United States but based in Phoenix, Arizona, wanted to learn if a certain type of physiotherapy, known as the Clear Passage Approach, would reduce the rate of recurrent small bowel obstructions. One hundred and three subjects, between the ages of nineteen and eighty-nine years, who had a history of recurrent adhesive small bowel obstructions were treated with the Clear Passage Approach, a type of manual physiotherapy that focuses on decreasing adhesive crosslinking in abdominopelvic viscera. Pre- and post-therapy data that measured obstructions and quality of life were compiled and then compared to 136 untreated control subjects. Subjects in the treatment group were significantly older. Despite histories of more prior hospitalizations, obstructions, surgeries, and years impacted by bowel issues, the 103 Clear Passage Approach treated subjects reported a significantly lower rate of repeat small bowel obstructions than the 136 untreated controls. Subjects treated with the therapy demonstrated significant improvements in diet, pain, gastrointestinal symptoms, quality of life, and pain severity. Only medication remained unchanged. The researchers commented that "manual physical therapy can provide adjunct therapy for known adhesions where there is no other available therapy proven to decrease recurrent SBO [small bowel obstructions] or to treat pain associated with adhesive disease." The Clear Passage Approach "appears to be a valuable conservative option for patients who previously were told that there was nothing that they could do to reduce their chances of recurrent SBO."[10]

REFERENCES AND FURTHER READING

Ahmad, Bilal, Mohd Fazl Ul Haq, Mubashir Ah Shah et al. "Early Postoperative Small Bowel Obstruction After Colorectal Surgery: Incidence and Exploratory Analysis of Potential Risk Factors." *Euroasian Journal of Hepato-Gastroenterology* 14, no. 1 (2024): 70–74.

Akrami, Majid and Mohammad Reza Sasani. "Dietary Habits Affect Quality of Life: Bowel Obstruction Caused by Phytobezoar." *Iranian Journal of Public Health* 45, no. 8 (August 2016): 1080–1082.

Allan, Lindsey, Naomi Hatchett, Simon S. Skene et al. "Management of Inoperable Malignant Bowel Obstruction Using 4-Step BOUNCED Diet." *Journal of Human Nutrition and Dietetics* 38 (2025): e13388.

Fevang, Bjørg-Tilde Svanes, Jonas Svanes, Stein Atle Lie et al. "Long-Term Prognosis After Operation for Adhesive Small Bowel Obstruction." *Annals of Surgery* 240, no. 2 (August 2004): 193–201.

Mohd Suan, Mohd Azri, Wei Leong Tan, Shahrul Aiman Soelar et al. "Intestinal Obstruction: Predictor of Poor Prognosis in Colorectal Carcinoma?" *Epidemiology and Health* 37 (March 2015): e2015017.

Peacock, O., M. G. Bassett, A. Kuryba et al. "Thirty-Day Mortality in Patients Undergoing Laparotomy for Small Bowel Obstruction." *British Journal of Surgery* 105 (2018): 1006–1013.

Rice, Amanda D., Kimberly Patterson, Evette D. Reed et al. "Decreasing Recurrent Bowel Obstructions, Improving Quality of Life with Physiotherapy: Controlled Study." *World Journal of Gastroenterology* 24, no. 19 (May 21, 2018): 2108–2119.

Sealey, Andrew J. and Ngee-Soon Lau. "Peanut Phytobezoar: An Unusual Cause for Small Bowel Obstruction." *Journal of Surgical Case Reports* 8 (2024): rjae564.

Sheyn, David, C. Emi Bretschneider, Sangeeta T. Mahajan et al. "Incidence and Risk Factors of Early Postoperative Small Bowel Obstruction in Patients Undergoing Hysterectomy for Benign Indications." *American Journal of Obstetrics & Gynecology* 220, no. 3 (March 2019): 251.e1–251.e9.

Wei, Kuang-Yu, Chih-Chien Sung, and Shih-Hua Lin. "Phytobezoar-Induced Small Bowel Obstruction in an Elderly Patient Undergoing Dialysis: A Case Report *Journal of International Medical Research* 48, no. 10 (October 2020): 0300060520962942.

IRRITABLE BOWEL SYNDROME (IBS)

INTRODUCTION

Irritable bowel syndrome (IBS) is a disorder in which there is abdominal pain, cramping, and changes in bowel movements. Symptoms of IBS, which is both a functional problem and a neurogastrointestinal disorder, range from mild to severe. While the symptoms of IBS may begin at any age, they most often first emerge in adolescence or early adulthood. They rarely begin after the age of fifty years.

There are four main types of IBS—IBS with diarrhea (IBS-D), IBS with constipation (IBS-C), IBS with both diarrhea and constipation, termed mixed (IBS-M), and IBS that does not fall into the previous three classes; it is IBS unclassified (IBS-U).

Researchers still do not know the exact causes of IBS. It may begin following a bacterial or parasitic infection of the intestines. This is known as postinfectious IBS. But, other triggers, such as stress, are known to cause this medical problem. The intestine is connected to the brain by nerves, and nerve signals go back and forth between the brain and the gastrointestinal tract. During stress, these connections become stronger and more sensitive. It is believed that IBS is related to the hypersensitivity of the nerves found in the wall of the gastrointestinal tract.

William Osler, the famous Canadian physician, described the nineteenth-century version of irritable bowel syndrome, which was then known as mucous colitis, as occurring primarily in psychiatrically disordered young women and accompanied by the passage of mucus. Osler's belief that there was a psychiatric basis for IBS continued for decades. By the 1970s, when IBS was termed spastic colon, it was still seen as having a "substantial psychiatric component." Since then, progress has been made. Current concepts should "embrace the interplay between abnormal, visceral, function, peripheral and central abnormalities of the perception and handling of painful stimuli and the impact of social and psychological factors, all of which contribute both to illness onset and to the persistence of symptoms."[1]

SYMPTOMS, RISKS, AND COMPLICATIONS

There are a whole host of symptoms of IBS, including abdominal pain, cramping, fullness, bloating, changes in bowel movements, gas, mucus in the stool, feeling of incomplete evacuation, diarrhea, constipation, or both. Specifically, there must be belly pain and discomfort averaging at least one day a week in the last three months. There must be at least two of the following: pain and discomfort related to defecation, a change in the frequency of defecation, or a change in stool consistency. The symptoms of IBS-D include frequent, loose, watery stools. It is not uncommon to have an urgent need to have bowel movements. The symptoms of IBS-C include a hard time passing stool and fewer bowel movements. Bowel movements may require straining, and only small amounts of stool may pass.

Many people experience the symptoms of IBS every day; for others, these symptoms tend to occur only during flare-ups. But, the symptoms generally reemerge periodically.

There appears to be a genetic component to IBS. Many people with the symptoms of IBS have additional family members with the same or similar symptoms. It is known that IBS does not damage the digestive tract or increase the risk of colon cancer. Large numbers of people tolerate their symptoms very well and complete their daily activities. But, others find that their symptoms prevent them from having a normal quality of life.

People with IBS have an increased risk for other medical problems. These include fibromyalgia, chronic fatigue syndrome, and chronic pelvic pain.

PREVALENCE

Whether it is mild, moderate, or severe, IBS is a very common disorder in the United States. In fact, IBS is the most common medical problem that gastroenterologists diagnose. It has been estimated that it affects up to 15 percent of the population. Only about 5–7 percent see a medical provider to receive a diagnosis.

IBS is twice as common in people assigned female at birth, and it is rarely seen in people who are not stressed, anxious, depressed, or dealing with past or present post-traumatic stress disorder. IBS is believed to be associated with childhood stress, including physical, sexual, and emotional abuse. IBS is more often seen in people who have had bowel surgery or an illness that slows digestion, such as diabetes.

DIAGNOSIS AND TREATMENT OPTIONS

There are no specific tests to diagnose IBS. Generally, IBS is diagnosed based on symptoms. Still, medical providers tend to order a few tests, primarily to rule out other gastrointestinal problems. These may include blood tests to check for anemia and celiac disease and stool samples to look for blood, infections, and parasites. Breath tests may be used to check for an intolerance for lactose, the sugar found in dairy products, and/or bacterial overgrowth in the small intestine. In an attempt to determine the cause of belly pain, a CT scan may be ordered. To rule out other problems, such as Crohn's disease and colon cancer, a medical provider may recommend a colonoscopy in which a flexible tube is inserted through the anus to examine the colon.

It is known that certain foods may trigger IBS. These include fatty foods, such as French fries, and caffeine-containing foods or beverages such as coffee and tea. One frequently advised suggestion is to keep a food intake and IBS symptom diary. That may enable the identification of foods and drinks that are problematic. For example, dairy products are a frequent culprit for people with IBS. And, larger meals may easily trigger IBS. So, many advise eating smaller, more frequent meals. Extra fiber may help with both IBS-C and IBS-D. Adding fiber-rich foods and a fiber supplement may be useful. Laxatives may be beneficial for tough cases of IBS-C. A low FODMAP diet that reduces the amount of hard-to-digest carbohydrates may relieve some symptoms. Medical providers may also recommend the removal of certain other foods from the diet, such as those that contain gluten or foods that foster the creation of gas in the intestine, such as beans, brussels sprouts, cabbage, and carbonated beverages. Since it is strongly believed to have a psychological component, exercise, meditation, and yoga may be effective, as well as an antidepressant medication. And, it is important to drink sufficient fluids and get enough sleep.

Medical providers may recommend certain medicines. To control intestinal muscle spasms, there are several anticholinergic medicines, such as dicyclomine (Bentyl), propantheline, belladonna, and hyoscyamine (Levsin). Some providers advise low-dose tricyclic antidepressants and/or probiotics and/or the antibiotic rifaximin (Xifaxan). Medications for IBS-D include loperamide (Imodium A-D), alosetron (Lotronex), and eluxadoline (Viberzi); medications for IBS-C include Phillips' Milk of Magnesia, Miralax, lubiprostone (Amitiza), bisacodyl, plecanatide (Trulance), and linaclotide (Linzess). Many providers suggest some form of psychotherapy, such as cognitive behavioral therapy.

Some medical providers may also advise experimenting with certain types of complementary and alternative medicine, such as acupuncture, massage therapy, biofeedback, meditation, hypnosis, and traditional Chinese medicine.

RESEARCH FINDINGS

Peppermint Oil Seems to Be Helpful for the Symptoms of IBS

In a prospective, multicenter, open-label, single-arm trial published in the journal *BioPsychoSocial Medicine*, researchers based in Japan noted that peppermint oil is widely used in Europe for IBS. However, in Japan, there has been no clinical evidence for the use of peppermint oil, and it has not been approved as a treatment. The cohort consisted of sixty-nine patients with IBS; there were thirty-seven males and thirty-two females who ranged in age from seventeen to sixty years. They were treated with an enteric-coated capsule containing 187 mg of peppermint oil. For four weeks, the drug was administered orally before meals, three times per day. Sixty-seven subjects completed the trial. By the end of the second week of the trial, the severity scores of the following seven symptoms were significantly lower—abdominal discomfort, abdominal distension, borborygmi (rumbling sounds), flatulence, incomplete defecation, defecation urgency, and straining. By the end of the trial, the severity scores of all of these seven symptoms as well as heartburn were significantly lower. Adverse events occurred in fourteen subjects; they were mild or moderate in severity. The researchers concluded that their "findings suggest that peppermint oil may be effective in the Japanese population and that it has an acceptable safety profile."[2]

In a systematic review and meta-analysis published in the *Journal of Clinical Gastroenterology*, researchers from Ontario, Canada, and La Jolla, California, studied the usefulness of peppermint oil for IBS. The researchers located nine studies with 726 subjects that met their criteria; in all of the studies, the treatment period continued for at least two weeks. Seven of these studies were double-blind, placebo-controlled parallel group trials in adult patients with active IBS. One study was a double-blind, placebo-controlled parallel group trial in pediatric patients with active IBS. And, the final study was a double-blind, placebo-controlled crossover trial that provided outcomes for the first crossover. These studies used various doses of peppermint oil. Most of the studies appeared to be of high methodological quality. The reported adverse events included heartburn, dry mouth, belching, peppermint taste, peppermint smell, rash, dizziness, headache, increased appetite, and a cold perianal sensation. The subjects who received an enteric-coated peppermint oil capsule were significantly more likely to experience an adverse event than those who took a placebo. The researchers determined that their study found "moderate quality evidence" that peppermint oil is a safe and effective treatment for IBS. The subjects had "significant global improvement" of IBS symptoms and improvement in abdominal pain. The researchers concluded that "peppermint oil is a safe and effective short-term therapy for active IBS."[3]

Acupuncture May Be Useful for IBS-D, Even If It Is Only Because of the Placebo Effect

In a multicenter, randomized pilot trial published in *JAMA Network Open*, researchers from China evaluated the use of acupuncture for IBS-D. The initial cohort consisted of ninety patients (fifty-four males and thirty-six females), with a mean age of 34.5 years. They were placed in one of three groups—one group used specific acupoints, a second group used nonspecific acupoints, and a third group used sham acupuncture. Each of the groups had thirty subjects. Over four consecutive weeks, the subjects in all three groups received three thirty-minute sessions per week. The treatments were administered by certified acupuncturists. Real needles were used in the acupuncture groups and blunt-tipped placebo needles were used in the sham group. Seventy-nine subjects completed the trial. Although the researchers determined that the subjects in the two acupuncture groups had "clinically meaningful improvement in IBS-D symptoms," there were no significant differences between responses of the subjects in the three groups. Considering that only one group of subjects actually received acupuncture to treat IBS-D, why was the response so positive? According to the researchers, "placebo effects are considered a part of the efficacy of acupuncture, and clinical trials in IBS are themselves associated with high placebo response rates." The researchers noted that there is a need for larger, sufficiently powered trials to assess the feasibility of acupuncture.[4]

Similarly, Chinese Herbal Medicine May Be Useful for IBS-C

In a randomized, double-blind, placebo-controlled trial published in the journal *Clinical Gastroenterology and Hepatology*, researchers from Australia studied the efficacy and safety of a standardized, specifically formulated Chinese herbal medication for IBS-C. The initial cohort consisted of 125 patients with IBS-C who were recruited from thirteen medical centers in New South Wales, Australia; they were divided into two demographically similar groups. For eight weeks, sixty-one subjects took a preparation containing seven Chinese herbs, and sixty-four took a placebo. The herbs were selected to address the symptoms of IBS-C, including constipation, abdominal pain, cramping, and bloating, and to reduce abdominal spasms and flatulence. The subjects were followed for a total of sixteen weeks. Fifty subjects in the herbal group and fifty-eight in the placebo group completed the trial. The researchers determined that there were clinical and statistical improvements in the subjects who took the herbal preparation. But, not all of the IBS-C symptoms were resolved. While the subjects saw improvements in the frequency of bowel movements and stool consistency, they still had abdominal pain and distention. The researchers concluded that "further CHM [Chinese herbal medicine] studies are warranted for IBS, including subgroups of IBS-D, mixed IBS, and also the related disorder of functional constipation."[5]

Probiotics Appear to Reduce Pain and the Symptoms Severity of IBS

In a randomized, double-blind, three-arm, placebo-controlled trial published in the journal *BioMed Research International*, researchers from Italy assessed the use of multispecies probiotics to treat IBS-C. The researchers enrolled a total of 157 male and female Caucasian subjects with IBS-C; they had a mean age of 37.4 years. The subjects were divided into three demographically similar groups. For sixty days, the subjects in two of the groups took different probiotic formulations; the subjects in the third group took a placebo. Seven of the subjects did not complete the trial. So, there were fifty subjects in each group. During the trial, the subjects were periodically evaluated, and they were seen again thirty days after the trial ended. The researchers found that the subjects taking probiotics had more improvement in their symptoms than those taking the placebos, and the improvement was maintained during the follow-up period. The researchers commented that "multispecies probiotics may have a variety of different beneficial effects particularly on IBS symptoms because each species acts in a particular way on the gastrointestinal tract, and two or more species eating together may have a synergistic effect." Still, there is a need for more clinical trials on the use of probiotics for the symptoms of IBS.[6]

Repeat Treatment with Rifaximin Seems to Be Safe and Effective for IBS-D

In a trial published in the journal *Gastroenterology*, researchers from several US cities, but based in Boston, Massachusetts, evaluated the safety and efficacy of a repeat treatment of IBS-D with the nonsystemic antibiotic rifaximin. The phase three trial included adults with IBS-D who relapsed after an effective treatment with rifaximin. For fourteen days, the 636 patients were randomly assigned to receive rifaximin 550 mg three times per day (n = 328) or a placebo three times per day (n = 308). The researchers determined that the percentage of responders was significantly higher in the rifaximin group than the placebo group, 38.1 percent versus 31.5 percent. Significant improvements were also seen in other problems, such as abdominal pain and bowel movement urgency. Although the trial results were clearly positive, the researchers nevertheless commented that "questions remain about the role of nonsystemic antibiotics in the long term, particularly when patients with IBS-D may require years of symptom management."[7]

Linaclotide Appears Useful for IBS-C

In a multicenter, open, observational, non-interventional trial published in the journal *BMJ Open*, researchers from Switzerland, the UK, Germany, and Austria evaluated the effectiveness and tolerability of linaclotide for IBS-C. The trial, which took place in thirty-one primary, secondary, and tertiary centers in Switzerland and Austria, included 138 patients eighteen years or older with moderate to severe IBS-C. The mean age of the patients was fifty years, and more than 75 percent were female. The trial in Austria consisted of a four-week treatment period, and the trial in Switzerland continued for sixteen weeks. The medication was given in doses of 290 mg. At baseline, more than 90 percent of the patients reported abdominal pain and bloating. They had a mean of 2.1 bowel movements per week. During the trial, a total of thirty-seven patients discontinued the medication, noting that it was ineffective or had adverse effects. The most common adverse effect was diarrhea. The patients in both countries had reductions in abdominal pain and bloating and increases in the number of bowel movements. The physicians treating these patients rated the effectiveness and tolerability of linaclotide as "good" or "excellent" for the majority of their patients. The researchers concluded that linaclotide is a safe and effective treatment of IBS-C. "Patients with IBS-C receiving linaclotide experienced effective treatment of moderate-to-severe symptoms in routine clinical practice."[8]

In a randomized, double-blind, placebo-controlled, phase three trial published in the *American Journal of Gastroenterology*, researchers from Ann Arbor, Michigan, Boston and Cambridge, Massachusetts, and Jersey City, New Jersey, examined the use of linaclotide for people with IBS-C. Their cohort consisted of 804 patients with a mean age of forty-four years; 90 percent were female and 78 percent were white. The twenty-six-week trial was conducted at 102 clinical centers in the United States. The patients, who were randomized to receive 290 mg of linaclotide or a placebo, were seen periodically throughout the trial. A total of 655 patients (81.5 percent) completed the first twelve weeks of the treatment period, and 599 (74.4 percent) completed the entire trial. Although the placebo group had more men, the two groups were well balanced with respect to demographic and bowel and abdominal symptoms. The researchers learned that, compared to the patients in the placebo group, the patients in the linaclotide group had statistically significant improvements in their IBS-C symptoms. By the end of their treatment, 45 percent of those in the linaclotide group were either "very" or "quite" satisfied with their treatment compared to 20 percent in the placebo group. And, 56 percent of those in the linaclotide group and 33 percent of those in the placebo group reported "adequate relief." As for their degree of relief of IBS-C symptoms, 72 percent of the linaclotide group said they were "somewhat, considerably, or completely" relieved compared to 45 percent of the placebo patients. A total of 263 (65.4 percent) of the linaclotide group and 228 (56.6 percent) of the placebo group had at least one adverse event. The most frequently reported adverse event was diarrhea. Still, only eighteen patients in the linaclotide group and one in the placebo group discontinued the trial because of diarrhea. The researchers concluded that "linaclotide has the potential to offer relief for the multiple symptoms from which patients with IBS-C suffer."[9]

Plecanatide Also Seems Useful for IBS-C

In a study published in the *International Journal of General Medicine*, researchers from several locations in the United States but based in Chicago, Illinois, pooled two identically designed randomized, double-blind, placebo-controlled, phase three clinical twelve-week trials on the efficacy and safety of plecanatide for IBS-C. The combined cohort consisted of 2,176 patients with IBS-C; 74 percent were female, and they had a mean age of 43.5 years. The patients were divided into three groups: 724 took 3 mg plecanatide, 723 took 6 mg plecanatide, and 729 took a placebo. The researchers learned that a significantly higher percentage of patients in the plecanatide groups responded to the treatment than those in the placebo group, and the medication was generally well tolerated. There were significant improvements in abdominal discomfort, abdominal fullness, abdominal pain, bloating, and cramping, and these occurred as early as the first week and were maintained throughout the study. The most commonly reported adverse event was diarrhea, which occurred in 4.3 percent of patients treated with 3 mg and 4 percent of those treated with 6 mg, compared with 1 percent of those treated with placebo. The researchers concluded that "plecanatide is safe and effective for the treatment of global and individual symptoms in adults with IBS-C."[10]

Low-Dose Imipramine May Help People with IBS

In a randomized, double-blind trial published in the *World Journal of Gastroenterology*, researchers from Lebanon evaluated the use of low-dose imipramine for the symptoms of IBS. The initial cohort consisted of 107 patients; it was divided into two demographically similar groups. For twelve weeks, they took either low-dose imipramine (n = 59) or a placebo (n = 48). In cases where the responses were unsatisfactory, doubling the dose was permitted once at week two. After the trial ended, there was a four-week follow-up period. At that point, there were thirty-one subjects in the imipramine group and twenty-five in the placebo group. More people in the imipramine group dropped out because of adverse events. The imipramine group reported an 80.6 percent relief of symptoms, while the placebo group reported a far lower 48 percent relief rate. For both groups, the highest rate of relief was achieved at week four, with 90.3 percent for imipramine and 68 percent for placebo. The researchers concluded that imipramine reduced the symptoms of IBS and improved the quality of life. "Gradual dose escalation, perhaps in small increments of 10 mg, and close monitoring are likely to result in a better therapeutic response."[11]

Alverine Citrate May or May Not Be Useful for IBS

In a six-month randomized, double-blind, placebo-controlled, pragmatic trial published in the *International Journal of Clinical Practice*, researchers from France examined the use of the combination of alverine citrate and simethicone for IBS. The initial cohort consisted of 436 patients, with a mean age of 54.4, 73.4 percent women, with moderate or severe IBS; eighty-seven general practitioners treated them with either the alverine citrate/

simethicone preparation or the medication(s) preferred by the general practitioner. When IBS episodes occurred, the patients in the combination group (n = 222) took one soft capsule that contained 60 mg alverine citrate and 300 mg simethicone three times per day before meals until the episode had resolved. The patients in the usual treatment group (n = 214) could use any treatment that did not contain alverine citrate or simethicone. These usual treatments tended to include at least one or more antispasmodics as well as laxatives, analgesics, and bulking agents. Sometimes psychotropic agents were prescribed. Forty patients did not complete the trial; twenty-three of these were in the combination group and seventeen in the usual treatment group. The researchers learned that the severity of IBS symptoms, especially abdominal pain and bloating, decreased significantly in both groups. However, the improvement was "more pronounced" in the combination alverine citrate/simethicone group. The researchers concluded that the alverine citrate/simethicone treatment "led to a greater improvement of QoL [quality of life], reduced the burden of the disease, and was more effective for IBS symptom relief than the usual treatments."[12]

On the other hand, in a three-center, twelve-week, double-blind, randomized, placebo-controlled trial published in the journal *Alimentary Pharmacology and Therapeutics*, researchers based in the UK had different results. The initial cohort consisted of 107 patients with IBS; 36 percent had only minor pain, 51 percent had moderately severe pain, and 13 percent had severe pain. Sixty-five percent described their pain as frequent, and 12 percent had very frequent pain. For twelve weeks, fifty-three patients took alverine citrate and fifty-four took a placebo. At baseline, both groups were demographically similar. All of the subjects were Caucasian, with a mean age of 39.6 years, and 80 percent were female. Eighty-seven patients completed the trial; there were forty-two in the alverine citrate group and forty-five in the placebo group. The researchers determined that 66 percent of the patients treated with alverine citrate improved, compared with 58 percent of the placebo group. This difference was not statistically significant. Further, there were also no significant differences between the groups with regard to other factors, such as the improvement in the severity and frequency of symptoms. Twenty-one patients in the alverine citrate group and twenty-six in the placebo group experienced adverse events; none was serious. By the end of the trial, the majority of the patients in both groups noted their symptoms had improved. "However, no statistically significant difference between the treatment groups was note in symptoms score reduction for any of the variables studied."[13]

When First-Line Therapies Fail to Bring Relief, Low-Dose Amitriptyline May Be Useful for IBS

In a randomized, double-blind, placebo-controlled, phase three trial published in the journal *Lancet*, researchers from the UK evaluated the usefulness of low-dose amitriptyline, a tricyclic antidepressant, for IBS when first-line therapies have failed to bring relief. (First-line therapies included lifestyle changes and medications such as antispasmodics, laxatives, and anti-diarrheals.) The six-month trial was conducted at fifty-five general practices in England; the initial cohort consisted of 463 subjects with IBS, with a mean age of 48.5 years. There were 315 females and 148 males. Over 80 percent had IBS-D or IBS-M. Two hundred and thirty-two were assigned to take low-dose amitriptyline, and 231 were assigned to take a placebo. In total, 338 (73 percent) completed the entire treatment—173

(75 percent) in the amitriptyline group and 165 (71 percent) in the placebo group. One hundred and five of the subjects discontinued their trial medication before six months—forty-six (20 percent) in the amitriptyline group and fifty-nine (26 percent) in the placebo group. The most frequent reason for stopping the trial was an adverse event, followed by a perceived lack of benefit. The researchers learned that low-dose amitriptyline was better than the placebo as a "second-line" treatment for IBS. Moreover, it was safe and well tolerated. And, they concluded that "general practitioners should offer low-dose amitriptyline to patients with IBS whose symptoms do not improve with first-line therapies."[14]

People with IBS May Improve If They Follow a Low FODMAP Diet

In a randomized, controlled, single-blind, crossover trial published in the journal *Gastroenterology*, researchers from Australia wanted to determine if a low FODMAP diet would improve the symptoms of IBS. (FODMAP foods are fermentable carbohydrates that do not absorb well in the small intestine. Examples are wheat, onions, garlic, legumes, and some fruits and vegetables.) The cohort consisted of thirty patients with IBS and eight healthy controls, who were matched for demographics and diet. The researchers began by collecting dietary data on the subjects for one week. The participants were then assigned to receive a low FODMAP diet or a typical Australian diet for 21 days. After a washout period, they were all assigned to the alternative diet. Daily symptoms were rated with a visual analogue scale. The researchers determined that the subjects with IBS who ate a lower FODMAP diet had improvements in their symptoms. In fact, their symptoms were reduced by more than one-half, and "all measured symptoms were reduced to a level that arguably is considered good symptoms control." Among the controls, symptoms were minimal and unaltered by either diet. The researchers concluded that "the low FODMAP diet has efficacy in the vast majority of patients with IBS and support its use as a first-line therapy."[15]

In a trial published in the *Journal of Human Nutrition and Dietetics*, researchers from London, England, assessed the responses of eighty-two patients with IBS who attended a follow-up dietetic outpatient visit for dietary management of their symptoms. Questionnaires were completed by forty-three patients who received counseling on a low FODMAP diet and thirty-nine patients who received the usual dietary advice. At baseline, there were no significant differences between the groups in age, gender, and the prevalence of symptoms. The patients rated symptom changes for bloating, abdominal pain and discomfort, flatulence, diarrhea, constipation, nausea, and levels of energy. While 74 percent of the patients in the low FODMAP group reported satisfaction with their symptom response, a much lower 54 percent of the standard dietary advice group were satisfied. A higher percentage of patients in the low FODMAP group reported improvement for each of their assessed symptoms. And, when all the symptoms were combined into a composite symptom score, there was a significant difference between the groups. The researchers noted that "low FODMAP dietary advice implemented by trained dietitians is more successful in improving composite symptoms and that patient satisfaction with symptoms is also greater." Further, "markedly fewer patients reported no change or worsening of symptoms in response to the low FODMAP diet compared to those receiving standard dietary advice."[16]

REFERENCES AND FURTHER READING

Abdul-Baki, Heitham, Ihab I. El Hajj, Lara ElZahabi et al. "A Randomized Controlled Trial of Imipramine in Patients with Irritable Bowel Syndrome." *World Journal of Gastroenterology* 15, no. 29 (2009): 3636–3642.

Bensoussan, Alan, John E. Kellow, Suzannah J. Bourchier et al. "Efficacy of a Chinese Herbal Medicine in Providing Adequate Relief of Constipation-Predominant Irritable Bowel Syndrome: A Randomized Controlled Trial." *Clinical Gastroenterology and Hepatology* 13 (2015): 1946–1954.

Brenner, Darren M., Spencer D. Dorn, Ronald P. Fogel et al. "Plecanatide Improves Symptoms of Irritable Bowel Syndrome with Constipation: Results of an Integrated Efficacy and Safety Analysis of Two Phase 3 Trials." *International Journal of General Medicine* 16 (2023): 3769–3777.

Chey, William D., Anthony J. Lembo, Bernard J. Lavins et al. "Linaclotide for Irritable Bowel Syndrome with Constipation: A 26-Week, Randomized, Double-Blind, Placebo-Controlled Trial to Evaluate Efficacy and Safety." *American Journal of Gastroenterology* 107 (2012): 1702–1712.

Ducrotte, P., J. C. Grimaud, M. Dapoigny et al. "On-Demand Treatment with Alverine Citrate/Simeticone Compared with Standard Treatments for Irritable Bowel Syndrome: Results of a Randomised, Pragmatic Study." *International Journal of Clinical Practice* 68, no. 2 (February 2014): 245–254.

Ford, Alexander C., Alexandra Wright-Hughes, Sarah L. Alderson et al. "Amitriptyline at Low-Dose and Titrated for Irritable Bowel Syndrome as Second-Line Treatment in Primary Care (ATLANTIS): A Randomised, Double-Blind, Placebo-Controlled, Phase 3 Trial." *Lancet* 402 (2023): 1773–1785.

Halmos, Emma P., Victoria A. Power, Susan J. Shepherd et al. "A Diet Low in FODMAPs Reduces Symptoms of Irritable Bowel Syndrome." *Gastroenterology* 146 (2014): 67–75.

Jones, Roger. "Irritable Bowel Syndrome: Management of Expectations and Disease." *British Journal of General Practice* 54, no. 504 (July 1, 2004): 490–491.

Khanna, Reena, John K. MacDonald, and Barrett G. Levesque. "Peppermint Oil for the Treatment of Irritable Bowel Syndrome: A Systematic Review and Meta-Analysis." *Journal of Clinical Gastroenterology* 48 (2014): 505–512.

Lembo, Anthony, Mark Pimentel, Satish S. Rao et al. "Repeat Treatment with Rifaximin Is Safe and Effective in Patients with Diarrhea-Predominant Irritable Bowel Syndrome." *Gastroenterology* 151 (2016): 1113–1121.

Matsueda, K., S. Fukudo, M. Ogishima et al. "Efficacy and Safety of Peppermint Oil for the Treatment in Japanese Patients with Irritable Bowel Syndrome: A Prospective, Open-Label, and Single-Arm Study." *BioPsychoSocial Medicine* 18 (2024): 3.

Mezzasalma, V., E. Manfrini, E. Ferri et al. "A Randomized, Double-Blind, Placebo-Controlled Trial: The Efficacy of Multispecies Probiotic Supplementation in Alleviating Symptoms of Irritable Bowel Syndrome Associated with Constipation." *BioMed Research International* 2016 (2016): 4740907.

Mitchell, S. A., A. S. Mee, G. D. Smith et al. "Alverine Citrate Fails to Relieve the Symptoms of Irritable Bowel Syndrome: Results of a Double-Blind, Randomized, Placebo-Controlled Trial." *Alimentary Pharmacology and Therapeutics* 16, no. 6 (June 2002): 1187–1195.

Pohl, Daniel, Michael Fried, Dominic Lawrence et al. "Multicentre, Non-Interventional Study of the Efficacy and Tolerability of Linaclotide in the Treatment of Irritable Bowel Syndrome with Constipation in Primary, Secondary and Tertiary Centres: The Alpine Study." *BMJ Open* 9 (2019): e025627.

Qi, Ling-Yu, Jing-Wen Yang, Shi-Yan Yan et al. "Acupuncture for the Treatment of Diarrhea-Predominant Irritable Bowel Syndrome: A Pilot Randomized Clinical Trial." *JAMA Network Open* 5, no. 12 (2022): e2248817.

Staudacher, H. M., K. Whelan, P. M. Irving, and M. C. E. Lomer. "Comparison of Symptoms Response Following Advice for a Diet Low in Fermentable Carbohydrates (FODMAPS) Versus Standard Dietary Advice in Patients with Irritable Bowel Syndrome." *Journal of Human Nutrition and Dietetics* 24, no. 5 (October 2011): 487–489.

LACTOSE INTOLERANCE

INTRODUCTION

Lactose intolerance occurs when people lack sufficient amounts of lactase, an enzyme needed to break down lactose, the sugar in milk and other dairy products. When these people consume milk or milk-containing products, they have a host of different digestive problems. During childhood, almost everyone produces this enzyme in their small intestine. As people mature, all too often the small intestine loses the ability to make adequate amounts of lactase. Everyone with lactose intolerance has lactose malabsorption; they are unable to properly absorb dairy products.

Normally, lactase turns milk sugar into two simple sugars—glucose and galactose—which are absorbed into the bloodstream through the intestinal lining. When people are lactase deficient, the lactose in the food is not properly absorbed and it moves into the colon (large intestine), where normal bacteria interact with undigested lactose, causing uncomfortable symptoms.

There are four main types of lactose intolerance. Primary lactose intolerance is caused by the reduction of lactase production by the small intestine; secondary lactose intolerance is caused by an injury or disease that affects the small intestine. Congenital lactose intolerance is caused by a lactase deficiency at birth, and developmental lactose intolerance is caused by premature birth, when the small intestine is not fully developed.

Unless it has been removed, lactose is found in most dairy products, such as cow's milk and goat's milk. Some dairy products have more lactose than others. For example, fresh milk and cream have high amounts of lactose, while hard cheese has less. Many people who are lactose intolerant are able to eat hard cheeses, such as parmesan. At the same time, others are sensitive to even small amounts of lactose. People who are sensitive should read labels carefully. Lactose is often found in processed foods, such as bread, lunch meats, coffee creamers, cake and cookie mixes, cereal, soups, salad dressings, and snacks. In addition, it may be added to prescription and over-the-counter medications and to supplements.

It is important to note that an intolerance to a specific food is not the same as an allergy. People who have an intolerance experience a host of different uncomfortable symptoms, but these symptoms are not life-threatening. People who have an allergic reaction to foods may have milder symptoms, such as a rash or hives, but they may also have trouble breathing or even die from tiny amounts of the offending food.

Lactose intolerance was first described by Hippocrates around 400 BC. During the past fifty years, this medical problem has gained a good deal more recognition.[1] And, selling products to those who are lactose intolerant has become a huge market. The global lactose-free dairy market size was valued at $11.45 billion in 2021 and is projected to reach $24.36 billion by 2031.[2]

SYMPTOMS, RISKS, AND COMPLICATIONS

There are several symptoms associated with lactose intolerance. They tend to begin between thirty minutes and two hours after consuming dairy products. These include a bloated stomach, intestinal gas, nausea and vomiting, stomach pain and cramping, stomach gurgling or rumbling, and diarrhea. As noted, these symptoms are caused by undigested lactose in the large intestine. Other less common symptoms associated with lactose intolerance include headaches, an inability to concentrate, fatigue, joint and muscle pain, and mouth ulcers.

It is well known that genetics play a role in lactose intolerance. But, certain groups of people also have higher rates of lactose intolerance. These groups include Asians, Native Americans, Hispanics, and people from or originally from Northern Europe, Africa, and the Middle East. People are more likely to have lactose intolerance if they have irritable bowel syndrome, visceral hypersensitivity, or small intestinal bacterial overgrowth (SIBO). Other factors that place people at increased risk include aging, injury, surgery, infections, or chronic diseases that may damage the cells that produce lactase, such as radiation therapy, small bowel resection, cystic fibrosis, inflammatory bowel disease, celiac disease, and enterocolitis. Once the small intestine loses the ability to produce lactase, the situation may well be permanent. Occasionally, however, the small intestine spontaneously starts to re-produce lactase.

While there are no serious complications directly associated with lactose intolerance, over time, people who totally avoid dairy products and do not take sufficient calcium and vitamin D supplementation may compromise their bones, muscles, and nervous system. Though the intake of adequate amounts of calcium and vitamin D is important for everyone, it is particularly crucial for growing children.

PREVALENCE

The prevalence of lactose intolerance varies by country and ethnic groups. In the United States, the prevalence is reported to be about 15 percent among Caucasians, 53 percent among Hispanics, and 80 percent among people of African ancestry. In South America, Africa, and Asia, rates of lactose intolerance tend to be more than 50 percent.[3]

DIAGNOSIS AND TREATMENT OPTIONS

It is not uncommon for people to self-diagnose lactose intolerance, especially when they repeatedly have uncomfortable gastrointestinal symptoms when they eat dairy products and foods that contain dairy products. But, there are also a few tests that are used to diagnose this medical problem. One of the most frequently used is the hydrogen breath test, which measures the amount of hydrogen and methane gases that are produced in the colon and exhaled in the breath. After ingesting lactose, people with lactose intolerance have higher levels of these gases. If this test is inconclusive, a medical provider may recommend a blood sugar test, which measures the sugar content in blood before and after the ingestion of lactose. If the blood sugar does not rise, then the sugar is not digested. Medical providers who suspect lactose intolerance in children may recommend a stool acidity test. After feeding a child lactose, the stool will be analyzed to determine if the lactose is absorbed.

Since people who are lactose intolerant do not have sufficient amounts of lactase, when they consume dairy products, they should consider taking lactase supplementation. Normally, lactase supplements, which are taken before the dairy product is consumed, are sold in capsules, tablets, and liquids. People often have different degrees of lactose intolerance. While some people cannot consume any dairy products, even with lactase supplements, many people are able to consume small amounts of dairy in certain foods. It is a good idea to begin by eliminating all dairy products from the diet, and then slowly reintroduce some. Researchers have found that certain people with lactose intolerance may tolerate up to 12 g of lactose, which is a cup of milk or a scoop of ice cream, at one time, or twice that amount over the course of a day.[4] It may help to consume the dairy-containing food with other foods or as part of a meal. There are also lactose-reduced and lactose-free dairy products sold in the refrigerator and freezer sections of food stores. Sometimes, these are fortified with calcium, vitamin D, vitamin A, vitamin B12, and/or riboflavin. An article in the journal *Nutrients* emphasized that lactose-free dairy products are an excellent source of dairy products for people with lactose intolerance.[5]

RESEARCH FINDINGS

Many Who Perceive They Are Lactose Intolerant Alter Their Behavior

In a study published in the journal *Applied Physiology, Nutrition, and Metabolism*, a researcher from British Columbia, Canada, examined input from Canadians who believed they were lactose intolerant and reviewed how that belief influenced their behavior. The researcher conducted a web-based survey of a population-representative sample of 2,251 Canadians who were nineteen years or older; 16.3 percent of the sample self-reported that they were lactose intolerant. The researchers learned that the belief that one was lactose intolerant was more frequently noted among women and nonwhites and less commonly in those who were older than fifty years and in those who completed the survey in French. When asked why they assumed that they were lactose intolerant, about 84 percent noted symptoms such as gas, bloating, cramps, and diarrhea after consuming milk products. Around 32 percent said that a health professional had told them that they were lactose intolerant, and about 20 percent said that a family member was lactose intolerant. Smaller percentages observed that they learned about lactose intolerance from the media or from friends. Not surprisingly, the respondents indicated that they had changed their dietary habits. Although only 5 percent completely excluded all dairy foods, the majority noted that they "reduced or eliminated" dairy products. More than 20 percent continued to use milk products, often switching to lactose-free milk or using lactase capsules. Other responses were cited by almost 10 percent. In most cases, this included a combination of actions, such as switching to lactose-free products and reducing the amount of milk consumed. The researchers learned that the people who self-reported lactose intolerance consumed significantly lower amounts of milk, cheese, and yogurt and greater amounts of a fortified soy beverage. As a result, they had lower intakes of calcium and vitamin D and were more likely to take calcium and vitamin D supplements. Yet, they still had significantly lower calcium intakes from the combination of milk products, alternatives, and supplements. The researcher concluded that "it is important that health professionals advise those with either diagnosed or self-reported lactose intolerance about how to avoid associated nutrient shortfalls though consuming milk products in a way that does not lead to symptoms and (or) using alternative products or supplements in amounts appropriate to meet their needs."[6]

People Who Believe They Are Lactose Intolerant May Have an Impaired Health-Related Quality of Life

In a three-year, prospective, cross-sectional trial published in the *European Journal of Clinical Nutrition*, researchers from Spain studied the association between self-perceived lactose intolerance and issues related to quality of life. The cohort consisted of 580 patients who were referred for a lactose hydrogen breath test; they had a median age of thirty years and 419 (72 percent) were female. Most were non-smokers or former smokers with a higher education. As part of their evaluation, the patients completed a questionnaire. When asked if they considered themselves tolerant or intolerant to dairy consumption, 255 patients (44 percent) thought they were tolerant, and 324 (56 percent) considered themselves intolerant. The researchers determined that those patients who believed they were lactose intolerant had more symptoms, restrictions on dairy consumption, and a worse quality of life. The researchers concluded that "subjective perception of lactose intolerance affects the decision to avoid dairy even more than objective malabsorption. However, both self-perception of lactose intolerance and objective lactose malabsorption are associated with poorer perceived quality of life."[7]

Lactase Supplementation Is Useful for People with Lactose Intolerance

In a randomized, double-blind, crossover, placebo-controlled trial published in the journal *JGH Open*, researchers from India assessed the effect of the intake of lactase chewable tablets on the clinical symptoms during a hydrogen breath test in people with lactose intolerance. The cohort consisted of forty-seven patients, thirty males and seventeen females, with a mean age of 33.6 years, with lactose intolerance, which was proven by an initial hydrogen breath test. The patients were divided into two groups; one group had twenty-three patients and the other had twenty-four. There were no statistically significant differences in the clinical symptoms of the patients in both groups; their symptoms included abdominal pain, bloating, gas, rumbling and gurgling, and diarrhea. Before undergoing a hydrogen breath test, half of the patients received lactase supplement chewable tablets and half had a placebo. Both tablets were identical in shape, size, color, and smell. After a one-week washout period, the patients had the alternative treatment. The researchers determined that after the patients took lactase supplements, they had statistically significant lower levels of breath test results and statistically significant fewer clinical symptoms. So, the lactase supplement improved the test results and the uncomfortable digestive symptoms. The researchers concluded that "clinical symptoms like bloating, abdominal pain, diarrhea, flatulence, and borborygmi improved and hydrogen breath levels were reduced in lactose-intolerant patients when they were given the lactose supplement."[8]

Probiotics May or May Not Help People with Lactose Intolerance

In a systematic review published in the *Journal of Family Practice*, researchers based in Pittsburgh, Pennsylvania, wanted to learn if adding probiotics to nonfermented dairy products during a breath hydrogen test would decrease the symptoms of lactose intolerance. They located ten randomized, placebo-controlled trials that met their inclusion criteria. Sample sizes ranged from five to twenty. Probiotic arms varied in subtype, strain, and concentration. Nine of the studies used the *Lactobacillus acidophilus* subtype as the intervention. Four trials examined probiotics other than or in addition to *L. acidophilus*. Four of the ten trials were crossover in design, while the remaining six varied in randomized designs. Of the nine studies that measured the disease-oriented outcome of breath hydrogen, three were positive, three were negative, and three had both positive and negative (mixed) results. Of the seven studies that measured the patient-oriented outcome of symptoms, one yielded positive results, five were negative, and one had mixed outcomes. The researchers concluded that probiotics were generally not effective at reducing the symptoms of lactose intolerance in adults. At the same time, there is some evidence that certain strains, concentrations, and preparations may be useful. "There were enough positive treatment arms to suggest there may be individuals who respond to probiotics." The researchers underscored the need for more crossover randomized double-blind research studies of selected probiotic strains and concentrations.[9]

Higher Milk Consumption Is Associated with a Lower Risk of Diabetes Mellitus

In a case-control trial published in the online journal *PLoS ONE*, researchers from Thailand examined the association between the consumption of milk and the risk of diabetes mellitus. The cohort consisted of 4,136 participants in the National Health Examination Survey, which was conducted in 2020; 1,756 had diabetes and 2,380 were controls; 62.2 percent were female and 98 percent were older than thirty years. When compared to controls, those with diabetes mellitus were more likely to be males who were older, had less education and higher BMI, were less active, and had been diagnosed with hypertension and metabolic syndrome. And, they consumed very little milk. In fact, 76 percent consumed less than one portion of milk per month. The people of Thailand seem to have very high rates of genetic-based lactose intolerance. That is probably why only 24 percent of the study population consumed milk products at least once a month. Yet, at the same time, it was quite evident that higher milk consumption was associated with a lower risk of diabetes mellitus. The researchers underscored the need for more research on this association.[10]

Lower Dairy Consumption among University Students Is Associated with an Increased Risk of Hypertension

In a study published in the journal *Diabetes, Metabolic Syndrome and Obesity: Targets and Therapy*, researchers from Iran assessed the association between dairy consumption and hypertension among a large population of university students. The cohort consisted of 67,011 university students who were part of the Mental and Physical Health Assessment of University Student project. Included in the information collected about these students were data on their dairy consumption and systolic and diastolic blood pressure. A systolic and diastolic blood pressure of 140/90 mmHg or higher was considered hypertension. The researchers found that 6.9 percent of the students had hypertension. There was a significant inverse association between dairy consumption and the odds of hypertension; the students with the highest levels of dairy consumption had an 85 percent lower risk for hypertension. "Such an inverse association was also found in males, females, normal-weight individuals, those with overweight or obesity and participants with and without a family history of hypertension."[11]

Self-Perceived Lactose Intolerance Appears Associated with Lower Intakes of Calcium and Diary Foods and Increased Risk for Hypertension and Diabetes

In a cross-sectional study published in the *American Journal of Clinical Nutrition*, researchers from Houston, Texas, and Birmingham, Alabama, investigated the effects of self-perceived lactose intolerance as it relates to calcium intake and related health problems. The cohort consisted of a national sample of 3,452 adults; 12.3 percent of these people considered themselves to be lactose intolerant. The age-adjusted prevalence of self-perceived lactose intolerance was 7.8 percent for non-Hispanic whites, 20.1 percent for non-Hispanic Blacks, and 8.8 percent for Hispanic individuals. Significantly more women perceived themselves to be lactose intolerant than men. Yet, men had significantly lower average daily calcium intakes from dairy foods and significantly higher average daily calcium intakes from nondairy foods. Significantly more non-Hispanic Blacks than non-Hispanic whites and Hispanic individuals thought they were lactose intolerant. However, the percentage of self-perceived lactose intolerance was similar for non-Hispanic whites and Hispanic individuals. Subjects who perceived themselves to be lactose intolerant had significantly lower average daily intake of calcium from dairy foods than did those without this belief. Further, a significantly higher percentage of subjects with self-perceived lactose intolerance reported having physician-diagnosed diabetes and hypertension. Interestingly, the odds of physician-diagnosed diabetes or hypertension decreased by factors of 0.70 and 0.60, respectively, for a 1,000 mg increase in calcium intake from dairy foods per day. The researchers noted that "the dairy food group is an important contributor of many nutrients lacking in America's diet, including calcium, potassium, and vitamin D, and limiting dairy food intake may have adverse effects."[12]

Lactose-Tolerant Premenopausal African American Women Consume More Calcium than Their Lactose-Intolerant Counterparts

In a trial published in the *Journal of the American College of Nutrition*, researchers from Tennessee investigated the effect of lactose intolerance on the intake of calcium in premenopausal African American women. The cohort consisted of fifty premenopausal women; twenty-six were lactose intolerant and twenty-four were lactose tolerant. A dietitian taught each of the participants how to keep a seven-day dietary intake record. While neither group reached the recommended intake of 1,000 mg per day of calcium, the intake was significantly less among the lactose-intolerant women (388 mg per day) than among the lactose-tolerant women (780 mg per day). Moreover, in addition to consuming less calcium, these women are probably absorbing less calcium. The major source of dietary calcium in the lactose-tolerant women was milk and other dairy products (45 percent) and mixed foods and calcium from nondairy sources (30 percent). In the lactose-intolerant women, 46 percent of calcium was from mixed foods and only 12 percent was from milk and dairy products. Though the women consumed similar amounts of energy, the lactose-intolerant women were heavier and had a higher BMI than lactose-tolerant women, and calcium was negatively associated with BMI. The researchers concluded that "lactose intolerance is associated with low levels of calcium intake." There is at least the possibility that it is associated with an "increased BMI in this population."[13]

There Seems to Be an Association between the Childhood Consumption of Non-Cow Beverages and Childhood Height

In a cross-sectional, observational study published in the *American Journal of Clinical Nutrition*, researchers from Ontario, Canada, assessed the association between the childhood consumption of non-cow beverages and childhood height. The cohort consisted of 5,034 healthy Canadian children between the ages of twenty-four and seventy-two months who were enrolled in the Applied Research Group for Kids. This group is a partnership between child health researchers and primary care physicians from the University of Toronto. Maternal ethnicity was primarily European, and the families tended to have middle to higher incomes. The researchers determined that there was a dose-dependent relationship between higher non-cow milk consumption and lower height. For each daily cup of non-cow milk that was consumed, the children were 0.4 cm shorter. The researchers commented that future research needs to focus on "which noncow milk beverages are most responsible for this association as well as understanding the causal relations between noncow milk consumption and childhood height."[14]

Fortified Soymilk Does Not Support Bone Health as Much as Cow's Milk

In an open-label, randomized, controlled trial published in the journal *Osteoporosis International*, researchers from China and Baltimore, Maryland, compared the bone-supporting properties of fortified cow's milk to fortified soymilk. The cohort consisted of 141 Chinese women without osteoporosis between the ages of forty-five and sixty-five years. All of the women had been postmenopausal for at least two years. For eighteen months, the women consumed either cow's milk with 250 mg calcium per day, soymilk with 250 mg calcium per day, or neither cow's milk nor soymilk. At baseline, the women had similar body measurements and demographic characteristics. The women had bone mineral density testing at baseline, six months, twelve months, and eighteen months. Ninety-eight women completed the entire trial. By the end of the trial, the women in the cow's milk group had significantly better bone mineral density than the women in the other two groups. Unfortunately, even though it was fortified, the soymilk appeared to have no notable impact on bone density. The researchers commented that "further long-term studies are required to explore a more long-term effect for bone mass maintenance in postmenopausal Chinese women."[15]

Children Who Avoid Drinking Cow Milk Have Low Dietary Calcium Intake and Poorer Bone Health

In a trial published in the *American Journal of Clinical Nutrition*, researchers from New Zealand wanted to learn more about the bone health of children who avoid drinking cow's milk, a somewhat common practice in their country. The researchers recruited thirty girls and twenty boys, between the ages of three and ten years, who avoid drinking milk. There were three main reasons for avoiding milk. Forty percent were intolerant, 42 percent indicated that it had a bad taste, and 18 percent noted that it was a life choice. They measured their current calcium intakes with a food frequency questionnaire, and they measured bone mineral densities with a dual-energy X-ray absorptiometry and compared the results to 200 milk-drinking control children—100 boys and 100 girls. Among the milk avoiders, dietary calcium intakes tended to be low, 443 mg calcium per day, and only a few children consumed substitute calcium-rich drinks or mineral supplements. They did tend to eat small amounts of some dairy products, such as cheese, yogurt, and ice cream. Fifteen of the milk avoiders were overweight; of these, nine had obesity. Only one of the avoiders had a low BMI. Twenty-three had a history of allergy, six of eczema, four of otitis media, and seventeen of asthma. They tended to be shorter, with smaller skeletons and lower bone mineral contents. The researchers advised that children who avoid milk should have a full dietary assessment "to help identify possible nutritional deficiencies and excesses."[16]

But, Children May Benefit from Soymilk

In a study published in the journal *Nutrition Today*, researchers from Washington, California, Missouri, and Texas compared the nutritional value of milks made from soy, rice, almonds, coconuts, and cashews to cow's milk. Focusing on the 2015 Dietary Guidelines for Americans, they reviewed amounts of potassium, dietary fiber, choline, magnesium, calcium, and vitamins A, D, E, and C, as well as sugars, saturated fats, and sodium. When nondairy milk alternatives were fortified with vitamins A, D, and calcium, they tended to have a nutrient profile similar to cow's milk; when non-fortified alternative milks were reviewed, soy was the only one that had a nutrient profile similar to cow's milk. Fat-free cow's milk and soymilk provided similar amounts of protein, 8 and 7 g respectively. Rice, almond, coconut, and cashew milks had approximately 1 g or less of protein per serving. Unfortified skim milk contained seven nutrients with more than 10 percent of the daily value, including protein, calcium, vitamin B12, riboflavin, niacin, phosphorus, and pantothenic acid. Unfortified soymilk had two nutrients greater than the 10 percent—calcium and protein. On the other hand, unfortified rice, almond, coconut, and cashew milks did not have any nutrients greater than 10 percent of the daily value. The researchers concluded that only soymilk was a good substitute for cow's milk for children.

If the reason for consuming a cow's milk alternative is to provide a lactose-free beverage that is nutritionally similar to cow's milk, then only soymilk met those requirements. Except for soymilk, the other milk alternatives that were reviewed "are not nutritionally similar to cow's milk and are not a good substitute when the goal is to provide a beverage nutritionally similar to cow's milk for growing children."[17]

Still, Another Study Failed to See the Value of Soymilk

In a study published in the *Journal of Pediatric Gastroenterology and Nutrition*, researchers from Buffalo, New York, and Springfield, Massachusetts, compared the nutritional value of cow's milk to the nutritional value of almond, cashew, coconut, hazelnut, hemp, oat, rice, and soy milks. The researchers examined nutrient information about the nondairy beverages sold on the shelves of stores in Buffalo and compared them to the nutrient content of cow's milk. The nutrient content of the nondairy beverages and cow's milk was also compared to the RDA figures for toddlers and young children. The researchers determined that cow's milk had a higher protein content and quality than most of the beverages, and they expressed concern that the inappropriate substitution of cow's milk for these beverages may lead to nutritional deficiencies. While substitutions are necessary for children who are actually allergic to cow's milk, that is only true for about 2–3 percent of children in developed countries. According to the researchers, it has long been established that cow's milk is a rich source of a host of different vitamins, including riboflavin, vitamin E, vitamin A, folate, thiamin, niacin, vitamin B6, and vitamin B12. And fortified milk is an excellent source of vitamin D. Though they are perceived as healthy, nondairy beverages vary greatly in their nutritional profiles and tend to have low protein, mineral, and vitamin content; the quality of the protein tends to be less than cow's milk. The researchers concluded that "cow's milk should not be removed from the diets of young children unless there is a medical indication to do so." And, in those instances, the child's entire diet should be carefully reviewed by a dietician.[18]

REFERENCES AND FURTHER READING

Baijal, Rajiv and Rakesh K. Tandon. "Effect of Lactase on Symptoms and Hydrogen Breath Levels in Lactose Intolerance: A Crossover Placebo-Controlled Study." *JGH Open* 5 (2021): 143–148.

Barr, Susan I. "Perceived Lactose Intolerance in Adult Canadians: A National Survey." *Applied Physiology, Nutrition, and Metabolism* 38 (2013): 830–835.

Black, Ruth E., Sheila M. Williams, Ianthe E. Jones, and Ailsa Goulding. "Children Who Avoid Drinking Cow Milk Have Low Dietary Calcium Intakes and Poor Bone Health." *American Journal of Clinical Nutrition* 76 (2002): 675–680.

Buchowski, M. S., J. Semenya, and A. O. Johnson. "Dietary Calcium Intake in Lactose Maldigesting Intolerant and Tolerant African-American Women." *Journal of the American College of Nutrition* 21, no. 1 (2002): 47–54.

Cassellas, F., A. Aparici, M. J. Pérez, and P. Rodríguez. "Perception of Lactose Intolerance Impairs Health-Related Quality of Life." *European Journal of Clinical Nutrition* 70 (2016): 1068–1072.

Dekker, P., D. Koenders, and M. Bruins. "Lactose-Free Dairy Products: Market Developments, Production, Nutrition and Health Benefits." *Nutrients* 11 (2019): 551.

Gui, J.-C., J. R. Brašić, X.-D. Liu et al. "Bone Mineral Density in Postmenopausal Chinese Women Treated with Calcium Fortification in Soymilk and Cow's Milk." *Osteoporosis International* 23 (2012): 1563–1570.

Levri, Kara M., Kari Ketvertis, Mark Deramo et al. "Do Probiotics Reduce Adult Lactose Intolerance? A Systematic Review." *Journal of Family Practice* 54, no. 7 (July 2005): 613–620.

Mansouri, M. , N. Pahlavani, F. Sharifi et al. "Dairy Consumption in Relation to Hypertension Among a Large Population of University Students: The MEPHASOUS Study." *Diabetes, Metabolic Syndrome and Obesity: Targets and Therapy* 13 (2020): 1633–1642.

Morency, Marie-Elssa, Catherine S. Birken, Gerald Lebovic et al. "Association Between Noncow Milk Beverage Consumption and Childhood Height." *American Journal of Clinical Nutrition* 106, no. 2 (August 2017): 597–602.

Nicklas, Theresa A., Haiyan Qu, Sheryl O. Hughes et al. "Self-Perceived Lactose Intolerance Results in Lower Intakes of Calcium and Dairy Foods and Is Associated with Hypertension and Diabetes." *American Journal of Clinical Nutrition* 94 (2011): 191–198.

Robles, Luelle and Ronny Priefer. "Lactose Intolerance: What Your Breath Can Tell You." *Diagnostics* 10 (2020): 412.

Schuster, Margaret J., Xinyue Wang, Tiffany Hawkins, and James E. Painter. "Comparison of the Nutrient Content of Cow's Milk and Nondairy Milk Alternatives: What's the Difference?" *Nutrition Today* 53, no. 4 (July/August 2018): 153–159.

Singhal, Sarita, Robert D. Baker, and Susan S. Baker. "A Comparison of the Nutritional Value of Cow's Milk and Nondairy Beverages." *Journal of Pediatric Gastroenterology and Nutrition* 64, no. 5 (May 2017): 799–805.

Tanpowpong, P., W. Aekplakorn, S. Chariyalertsak et al. "Higher Milk Consumption Is Associated with a Lower Risk of Diabetes Mellitus: A Case-Control Study." *PLoS One* 18, no. 8 (2023): e0289762

METABOLIC DYSFUNCTION-ASSOCIATED STEATOTIC LIVER DISEASE

INTRODUCTION

Previously known as nonalcoholic fatty liver disease (NAFLD), metabolic dysfunction-associated steatotic liver disease (MASLD) is the infiltration of fat into liver cells that is caused by factors other than alcohol. Some fat in the liver is normal. But, when the amount of fat is more than 10 percent of the weight of the liver, the liver may begin to have problems.

While the exact cause is not completely understood, it is known that MASLD occurs with other metabolic disorders, such as high cholesterol, high levels of triglycerides, obesity, diabetes, and hypertension. It also seems that a diet high in fructose, a sugar commonly used in high-fructose corn syrup, increases the risk. In addition, there may well be a genetic predisposition for this disorder.

Compared to many other medical problems, MASLD has only been identified for a few decades. The terms nonalcoholic fatty liver disease and nonalcoholic steatohepatitis were proposed in the 1980s.

SYMPTOMS, RISKS, AND COMPLICATIONS

People normally do not experience symptoms of MASLD until it has progressed to metabolic dysfunction-associated steatohepatitis (MASH). Still, some do have symptoms such as right upper quadrant abdominal discomfort and fatigue. Up to 20 percent of people with MASLD may develop MASH, a state of chronic liver inflammation that begins with the symptoms of inflammation, such as pain and swelling in the upper right abdomen, the location of the liver. Other symptoms include the build-up of fluid in the legs or abdomen and bleeding. Children may have patchy, dark discoloration of the skin over the neck and under the arms. Over time, there may be progressive liver damage, eventually causing the scarring or cirrhosis of the liver.

Certain people have an increased risk of MASLD. These include people with obesity and high cholesterol, as well as people with diabetes, high levels of triglycerides, metabolic syndrome, hypertension, and those who are middle aged. People with these risk factors should have annual liver blood tests. And, people with MASLD, who do not already have heart disease or diabetes, are at increased risk for those medical problems. People with MASH have an increased risk for hepatocellular carcinoma and/or end-stage liver disease, both of which impact a person's quality of life and life expectancy. In some cases, these people may require a liver transplant.

Women with MASLD who are pregnant have an increased risk of complications for both the woman and the growing fetus. In particular, pregnant women are three to four times more likely to have high blood pressure-related problems, such as preeclampsia.

PREVALENCE

Worldwide, up to 25 percent of people have MASLD. In the United States, that figure is even higher. Up to 30 percent may have this disorder. That means that about one hundred million adults have MASLD. It has been estimated that about two-thirds of adults with obesity and half of the children with obesity may have a fatty liver. Since they do not have any symptoms or their symptoms may be mild and mimic other problems, the overwhelming majority do not realize they have this disorder. Though more common in people of Hispanic descent and less common in Black people, MASLD may affect anyone, including all ages and races. About two to 5 percent of American adults and up to 20 percent of those with obesity may have MASH. The number of children with MASH is unknown.

DIAGNOSIS AND TREATMENT OPTIONS

If routine blood tests show high levels of certain liver enzymes or the liver appeared enlarged, a healthcare provider may recommend further blood tests. Imaging tests may also be advised. These may include a transabdominal ultrasound, which shows images of the abdomen, a CT scan, which takes many horizontal views of the body and provides detailed images, and/or a MRI scan, which uses a huge magnet to provide detailed images. A liver biopsy, in which tissue samples of the liver are analyzed, may also be used. During this procedure, a needle is inserted into the liver. Before a definitive diagnosis of MASLD is made, other factors which may caused elevated liver fats should be ruled out. These include drinking excess amounts of alcohol, certain medications, and other liver diseases. Why is this important? Because different liver diseases may have similar symptoms, and it is important to have a definitive diagnosis to obtain the best treatment.

At present, there is no medication that is able to reverse fatty liver disease. But, the disease may be slowed, stopped, or sometimes reversed if people make lifestyle changes, such as losing weight, eating a healthier diet, reducing portion sizes, drinking lots of water, avoiding foods with added sugars, significantly limiting processed snacks, participating in regular exercise such as walking about 10,000 steps each day, and lowering cholesterol, triglycerides, blood pressure, and levels of blood sugar. However, once MASLD has progressed to MASH and there is liver scarring, the damage may be permanent. In March 2024, the US Department of Food and Drug Administration approved the drug resmetirom for the treatment of MASH. This medication should be combined with lifestyle changes. It is important to note that people should attempt to lose an average of a pound or two a week. More rapid weight loss may make MASLD even worse. And, people who have been fairly sedentary should slowly increase exercise to at least thirty minutes each day. It is better to adhere to a regular thirty- to sixty-minute exercise program than to overexercise one day and then fail to exercise for several days.

RESEARCH FINDINGS

Devoting More Time to Moderate to Vigorous Exercise Appears to Result in Greater Improvements of MASLD

In a retrospective trial published in the journal *Hepatology*, researchers from Japan wanted to learn more about the beneficial effects that moderate to vigorous physical activity has for people with MASLD. The cohort consisted of 169 middle-aged men with obesity and MASLD. They were all enrolled in a twelve-week restrictive caloric weight reduction program that also included varying levels of exercise. Forty of the men performed moderate to vigorous exercise for less than 150 minutes per week; forty-two performed moderate to vigorous exercise for 150 to 250 minutes per week; and eighty-seven performed moderate to vigorous exercise for more than 250 minutes per week. The groups were similar in several demographics including age, BMI, smoking, and alcohol intake, and they had similar dietary intake, body adiposity, and blood test results. The researchers learned that compared to those who exercised less than 250 minutes per week, those who exercised more had significant improvements in their levels of liver fat. And, this improvement was likely independent of their weight reduction. The researchers concluded that their findings demonstrate "the beneficial effects of increasing the volume of MVPA [moderate to vigorous physical activity] combined with dietary restriction on managing NAFLD [nonalcoholic fatty liver disease] in middle-aged men."[1]

Still, People with MASLD May Have Different Barriers to Exercise

In a trial published in the *Journal of Clinical Medicine Research*, researchers from Australia noted that while adequate physical exercise is an "essential component" of treatment for MASLD, the majority of people with this disease appear to lead a sedentary life and engage in insufficient exercise. The researchers wanted to identify some of the barriers that limit the amount of exercise in people with MASLD. They recruited 81 subjects, 57 percent female, with a mean age of 55.3 years, from a hepatology outpatient clinic. The patients had a mean body mass index of 33.8. Levels of MASLD were assessed, and an online questionnaire was administered to determine patterns of exercise, barriers to exercise, and knowledge of the effectiveness of different types of exercise for MASLD. While 83 percent of the subjects considered MASLD to be a serious health concern, 73 percent did not achieve the recommended exercise levels of 150 minutes or more of moderate-intensity exercise per week or seventy-five minutes of vigorous exercise per week, and 54 percent were unsure about the role of exercise in the treatment of MASLD. When asked about their daily step count, 64 percent did not take at least 10,000 steps per day.

Twenty-one percent said that they did not monitor their step counts. Frequently reported barriers to exercise included physical and mental health issues (57 percent), a lack of time (43 percent), a lack of enjoyment in exercising (31 percent), fatigue from exercise (24 percent), and other (25 percent). Other exercise barriers included depression, laziness, lack of motivation, lack of energy to exercise after work, joint pain from osteoarthritis, lack of companionship, and other commitments taking precedence. Interestingly, the severity of disease did not significantly affect exercise behaviors, and the subjects who did not meet the exercise guidelines came from varied socioeconomic and educational backgrounds, as well as different occupations. There is, according to these researchers, a widespread problem of insufficient exercise among people with MASLD. Yet, people with MASLD who fail to exercise may well see their disease worsen. The researchers concluded that their subjects were aware of the serious health consequences of MASLD "but lacked awareness of the significance of exercise in its treatment." And, they had a host of different reasons for not exercising. "Developing personalized training programs tailored to individual fitness levels and patient preferences can promote long-term adherence and sustainability."[2]

Consumption of a Mediterranean Diet Seems to Improve Fat Liver Levels in People with MASLD

In a randomized, crossover intervention trial published in the *Journal of Hepatology*, researchers from Australia wanted to determine if the consumption of a Mediterranean diet would improve the levels of liver fat in people with MASLD. The cohort consisted of six female and six male subjects with biopsy-proven MASLD. All of the subjects ate both a six-week Mediterranean diet and a six-week low-fat, high-carbohydrate diet in random order, with a six-week washout period in between the diets. At baseline, there were no differences in physical activity between the subjects, their characteristics were similar, and they all had abdominal obesity. The researchers learned that the people on both diets had small weight losses, which were not significant, but they had significant reductions in liver fat on the Mediterranean diet and a much smaller reduction on the low-fat, high-carbohydrate diet, which is often recommended for MASLD. The researchers commented that their findings "present strong evidence that the MD [Mediterranean diet] may become the backbone of NAFLD therapy: however, larger longer-term studies are needed to explore the durability of the benefits of the MD."[3]

In a prospective, randomized, controlled, open-label, single-center, pilot trial published in the journal *Pediatric Obesity*, researchers from India compared the use of an Indo-Mediterranean diet to a calorie-restricted diet for treating overweight children or children with obesity who also have MASLD. The initial cohort consisted of thirty-nine consecutive biopsy-proven children with MASLD who were between the ages of eight and eighteen years. For 180 days, they ate either an Indian-style Mediterranean diet or a calorie-restricted diet that was about 500 fewer calories per day than would normally be recommended for a child of a specific age and sex. All of the children were instructed to restrict saturated fat intake and avoid eating certain foods such as processed products, candy, sugary drinks, ice cream, cream biscuits, cake, noodles, sweets, and instant beverages, and they were told to participate in both high and low-intensity exercises for specified periods of time several times per week. Thirty-four subjects completed the study. Eighteen subjects were in the Mediterranean diet group and sixteen were in the calorie-restricted group. They had a median age of 13.6 years, and 84 percent were male. There was a family history of MASLD in 49 percent, liver disease in 5 percent, diabetes in 28 percent, and hypertension in 26 percent. While the children in both groups improved significantly, those in the Mediterranean group had greater reductions in liver fat, weight, and BMI. The researchers underscored the need for more randomized controlled trials, with longer follow-up time periods, in order to verify their results.[4]

People Who Smoke Have an Increased Risk of MASLD

In a systematic review and meta-analysis published in the journal *SAGE Open Medicine*, researchers from Iran evaluated the association between cigarette smoking and MASLD. The researchers studied data from twenty observational studies—nine cross-sectional, six case-control, four cohort, and one retrospective cohort. The studies, which included a total population of 92,125 and 20,149 subjects, focused on measuring the prevalence of smoking in patients with and without MASLD. It is important to note that the classification of smoker varied from study to study. After the researchers conducted a meta-analysis on twelve of these studies—seven cross-sectional, three case-control, and two cohort, they observed a significant association between smoking and MASLD; this association was stronger in current smokers. The researchers concluded that "further studies are needed to compare the effects of passive and active smoking on non-alcoholic fatty liver disease."[5]

There Seems to Be an Association between High Consumption of Red and Processed Meat and MASLD

In a cross-sectional study published in the *Journal of Hepatology*, researchers from Israel investigated the relationship between the consumption of high amounts of red and processed meats and MASLD. The cohort consisted of people between the ages of forty and seventy years who had screening colonoscopies during a two-year period of time at the Department of Gastroenterology and Hepatology at the Tel Aviv Medical Center in Tel Aviv, Israel. They also had a series of tests that included fasting blood tests and a liver ultrasound. A total of 789 subjects completed a food frequency questionnaire and 357 of those subjects completed a meat questionnaire. To avoid reporting bias, the subjects did not learn the results of their blood and liver tests until they completed their questionnaires. Slightly over half of the subjects were male, and they had a mean age of 58.83 years, with a mean BMI of 28.54. The meat sub-sample had similar characteristics. MASLD was diagnosed in 38.70 percent of the subjects. High-meat eaters were slightly younger, were more likely to be men, and had a higher BMI and caloric intake, as well as a metabolic profile in need of improvement. And, the people in the meat sub-sample were more likely to have MASLD. On the other hand, the high-meat eaters did not have significantly worse lifestyle habits, and they had similar levels of physical activity, smoking, and sugared drink consumption. But, they did have a higher consumption of alcohol and, as might be expected, a higher consumption of foods with saturated fat and cholesterol. The researchers concluded that a higher intake of red meat and processed meat was independently associated with higher odds of having MASLD, and the higher the intake, the greater the risk.[6]

Certain Factors Increase the Risk of Adolescents Developing MASLD

In a systematic review published in the journal *Clinical Nutrition ESPEN*, researchers from Malaysia, Indonesia, and the UK wanted to determine which factors increase the risk that adolescents will develop MASLD. The researchers identified six studies that met their criteria; these studies included a total of 19,800 adolescents. The studies, which were conducted in the United States, Taiwan, Australia, and China, were published between January 1, 2002, and June 30, 2022, and written in English. Five were considered high quality, and one was moderate quality. The researchers learned that the prevalence of MASLD ranged from 8 percent in a study of 5,586 adolescents aged twelve to nineteen to 16 percent in a survey of 1,724 adolescents between the ages of twelve and thirteen. Two factors—dietary intake and physical activity—appeared to play a crucial role in determining which adolescents developed MASLD. Thus, while a healthy Chinese food diet, which included a high intake of whole grains, tubers, vegetables, fresh fruits, salted/ preserved eggs, soybeans, beans, tea, and fruit or vegetable juice, appeared to reduce the risk of MASLD, a Western diet, with higher intakes of red meat, processed or preserved meat, western fast food, dairy products, fish and shrimp, snack food, carbonated beverages, alcoholic beverages, and coffee, appeared to increase the risk. Two of the studies examined the association between physical exercise and MASLD. The physical activity level was categorized as low (less than one time per week), moderate (one to three times per week), and high (more than four times per week). Both studies found an inverse association between exercise and MASLD. The lack of physical exercise increased the risk of MASLD; teens who exercised lowered their risk of MASLD. Only a small number of the teens were smokers, and no pattern between smoking and MASLD was observed. The researchers concluded that "a healthier lifestyle (dietary pattern and physical activity) was associated with minimizing the risk of developing NAFLD among adolescents."[7]

Weight Loss May Well Benefit People with Nonalcoholic Steatohepatitis

In a randomized, controlled trial published in the journal *Hepatology*, researchers from Providence, Rhode Island; Bethesda, Maryland; and Whitewater, Wisconsin wanted to learn if a 7–10 percent weight loss and increased exercise would improve the symptoms of nonalcoholic steatohepatitis. The initial cohort consisted of thirty-one people with biopsy-proven nonalcoholic steatohepatitis who were overweight or living with obesity. They had a mean age of forty-eight years and a mean BMI of 34. Seventy-one percent were men. Twenty-six subjects were white, four were Hispanic, and one was American Indian/ Alaskan Native. Slightly less than half had type 2 diabetes, and 74 percent fulfilled the diagnostic criteria for metabolic syndrome. For forty-eight weeks, they received either an intensive lifestyle intervention, which focused on changing eating habits and participating in regular exercise, or structured education (control), which offered small group education sessions every twelve weeks. Thirty subjects completed the trial. The subjects in the lifestyle intervention group lost an average of 9.3 percent of their weight; the subjects in the control group lost only 0.2 percent. The subjects in the intervention group also had far greater improvements in their nonalcoholic steatohepatitis than those in the control group. The researchers commented that lifestyle modifications that focus on diet, exercise, and behavioral changes may result in dramatic improvements in nonalcoholic steatohepatitis. In fact, by the end of the trial, 67 percent of the subjects in the intervention group no longer met the minimal histologic criteria for nonalcoholic steatohepatitis. That figure was a much lower 20 percent for those in the control group. "Given the additional benefit of weight loss on cardiovascular risk factors, lifestyle intervention with the goal of at least 7 percent weight reduction represents an attractive therapy for this increasingly common disease."[8]

Certain Exercises Seem Better than Others for People with MASLD

In a systematic review and meta-analysis published in the journal *Scientific Reports*, researchers from China compared the usefulness of different types of exercise for people with MASLD. They located forty-three studies with 2,070 subjects with MASLD that met their criteria. Of these, twenty-two were in English and twenty-one were in Chinese. Intervention groups had 1,194 subjects and 876 subjects were in control groups. Study duration ranged from eight to twenty-four weeks. In these studies, 779 subjects participated in aerobic exercise, 159 in resistance training, 160 in high-intensity interval training, and ninety-six in aerobic exercise and resistance training. The researchers determined that the combination of aerobic exercise and resistance training was the best exercise for people with MASLD. Ideally, according to the researchers' findings, the most productive exercise program included ten weeks of combination exercises. Each week included three fifty-minute sessions.[9]

But Resistance Training Alone, Even without Weight Loss, Reduces Liver Fat

In a trial published in the journal *Gut*, researchers from the UK noted that therapies for MASLD tend to focus on weight loss. But, the weight loss achieved during trials is often not sustained over time. So, they wanted to learn if resistance training, which may well be better maintained, would be useful for a fatty liver. The cohort consisted of nineteen sedentary adults with clinically defined non-advanced MASLD. Eleven of the adults were assigned to eight weeks of resistance training—with a total of twenty-four sessions—and eight were assigned to "continued normal treatment" (control). The two groups were well matched for weight, BMI, and waist/hip circumference, but the exercise group was younger. The researchers learned that while the eight weeks of resistance training resulted in a 13 percent reduction in liver lipids, the resistance training had no effect on body weight, visceral adipose tissue volume, or whole body fat mass. The researchers concluded that "the absolute effect of resistance exercise studies in isolation was modest but similar to that of aerobic exercise."[10]

Before Bariatric Surgery, People with MASLD May Benefit from a Low-Carbohydrate Diet

In a trial published in the journal *Surgical Endoscopy*, researchers from Israel and Houston, Texas, wanted to learn if people with MASLD would benefit from eating a very low-carbohydrate diet before having major surgery to lose weight. Why is this important? It is known that bariatric surgery may be made more challenging by the enlargement of the liver, especially of the left lobe, which is caused by MASLD. The cohort consisted of fourteen subjects with MASLD; there were nine women and five men between the ages of twenty-four and forty-five years. Their mean BMI was 45.9. For four weeks before bariatric surgery, they were placed on a very low-carbohydrate diet. CT scans were performed both before and at the end of the diet period. When the diet ended, the subjects had significant decreases in their body weight, BMI, and HDL cholesterol. The researchers determined that four weeks of a very low-carbohydrate diet reduced the fat content and size of the liver, particularly of the left lobe. The researchers commented that the reduction in liver volume made the surgical procedure more manageable, and it "facilitated access to the region of the gastroesophageal junction, with no difficulty encountered during the necessary retraction." And, the researchers concluded that a short-term low-carbohydrate diet may prove to be an effective component in the treatment of MASLD.[11]

Smartphones May Not Provide a Significant Amount of Assistance to People with MASLD Who Want to Make Lifestyle Changes

In a randomized, double-blind, controlled trial published in *Scientific Reports*, researchers from southern Thailand wanted to learn if providing patients with MASLD additional information on lifestyle interventions on their phones would improve outcomes. The initial cohort consisted of 122 patients with MASLD; they were between the ages of eighteen and sixty-five years, with a median age of fifty-three years. Their median BMI was 27.3, and 64.7 percent were female. All of the patients were placed in either the intervention group or the control group. Both groups had sixty-one patients. While all of the patients received the same lifestyle intervention advice, those in the intervention group received additional information and lifestyle reminders every three to seven days on their phones. These messages included information on diet, physical activity, and exercise. The patients were instructed not to discuss the information they received with other patients. At the end of the twenty-four-week trial, 106 patients were included in the final analyses. Both groups had improvements in weight, fat mass, and liver parameters. While the improvements in the intervention group tended to be better, the differences between the two groups were not significant. And, only 21.3 percent of the intervention group and 18 percent of the control group achieved a weight loss of 5 percent or more. The people in the intervention group did have a significant improvement in liver stiffness, a sign of possible scarring, an improvement that was not observed in the control group. As a result, it may be useful to incorporate smartphone technology into the treatments for MASLD.[12]

Vitamin E May or May Not Be Useful for People with MASLD

In a randomized, placebo-controlled, open-label prospective trial published in the *Open Journal of Gastroenterology*, researchers from New York City wanted to learn if vitamin E and alpha-lipoic acid supplementation would be useful for people with MASLD or nonalcoholic steatohepatitis. The cohort consisted of 155 people with nonalcoholic fatty liver disease. For six months, forty people took 700 IU of vitamin E or 300 mg of alpha-lipoic acid or both vitamin E and alpha-lipoic acid. During the same time, thirty-five subjects took a placebo. The subjects were allowed to consume 1600 calories per day and to participate in moderate exercise—walking 150 minutes per week at the rate of one hundred steps per minute. A number of different tests and liver assessment tests were administered at baseline and at the end of the trial. The researchers learned that vitamin E alone or in combination with alpha-lipoic acid was an effective treatment for MASLD and nonalcoholic steatohepatitis and improved a number of clinical variables. According to the researchers, there is a need for more studies that are conducted for longer periods of time.[13]

In another study, published in *JAMA*, researchers from several locations in the United States but based in New York City compared the use of vitamin E and metformin, an antidiabetic agent, for treating children and adolescents with nonalcoholic fatty liver disease. This randomized, double-blind, placebo-controlled clinical trial was conducted at ten university clinical research centers. Initially, there were a total of 173 patients between the ages of eight and seventeen years—mean age of 13.1 years—with nonalcoholic fatty liver disease. Eighty-one percent were male, and 61 percent were Hispanic. Most of the patients had obesity and were insulin resistant. All of the patients were provided standard-of-care advice on diet and exercise. For ninety-six weeks, fifty-eight patients took daily doses of 800 IU vitamin E, fifty-seven patients took daily doses of 1,000 mg metformin, and fifty-eight patients took a placebo. The three groups of patients had similar demographic characteristics. During the course of the trial, the subjects had periodic medical visits that included medical evaluations and a host of additional tests, and a follow-up visit was held twenty-four weeks after the trial ended. Eighty-seven percent of the patients completed the entire trial. The subjects in all three groups had similar improvements in their fatty liver values. So, neither vitamin E nor metformin provided any notable significant benefits. "Neither vitamin E nor metformin was superior to placebo in attaining the primary outcome of sustained reduction in ALT level [enzyme in liver cells that is an indicator of MASLD] in patients with pediatric NAFLD."[14]

REFERENCES AND FURTHER READING

Akhavan Rezayat, Arash, Malihe Dadgar Moghadam, Mohammad Ghasemi Nour et al. "Association Between Smoking and Non-Alcoholic Fatty Liver Disease: A Systematic Review and Meta-Analysis." *SAGE Open Medicine* 6 (2018): NA.

Basu, Patrick P., Niraj J. Shah, Mark M. Aloysius, and Robert S. Brown Jr. "Effects of Vitamin E and Alpha Lipoic Acid in Nonalcoholic Fatty Liver Disease: A Randomized, Placebo-Controlled, Open-Label, Prospective Clinical Trial (VAIN Trial)." *Open Journal of Gastroenterology* 4, no. 5 (2014): 199–207.

Benjaminov, O., N. Beglaibter, L. Gindy et al. "The Effect of a Low-Carbohydrate Diet on the Nonalcoholic Fatty Liver in Morbidly Obese Patients. Before Bariatric Surgery." *Surgical Endoscopy* 21 (2007): 1423–1427.

Deshmukh, Aniket, Vikrant Sood, Bikrant Bihari Lal et al. "Effect of Indo-Mediterranean Diet Versus Calories-Restricted Diet in Children with Non-Alcoholic Fatty Liver Disease: A Pilot Randomized Control Trial." *Pediatric Obesity* 19, no. 11 (November 2024): e13163.

Deshpande, K., J. Olynyk, O. Ayonrinde, and K. Nosaka. "Barriers to Exercise in Patients with Metabolic Dysfunction-Associated Steatotic Liver Disease: A Patient Survey." *Journal of Clinical Medicine Research* 16, no. 2–3 (2024): 94–105.

Hallworth, Kate, Gulnar Fattakhova, Kieren G. Hollingsworth et al. "Resistance Exercise Reduces Liver Fat and Its Mediators in Non-Alcoholic Fatty Liver Disease Independent of Weight Loss." *Gut* 60 (2011): 1278–1283.

Kaewdech, A., S. Assawasuwannakit, C. Churuangsuk et al. "Effect of Smartphone-Assisted Lifestyle Intervention in MASLD Patients: A Randomized Controlled Trial. *Scientific Reports* 14 (2024): 13961.

Lavine, Joel E., Jeffrey B. Schwimmer, Mark L. Van Natta et al. "Effect of Vitamin E or Metformin for Treatment of Nonalcoholic Fatty Liver Disease in Children and Adolescents." *JAMA* 305, no. 16 (April 27, 2011): 1659–1668

Oh, Sechang, Takashi Shida, Kazumasa Yamagishi et al. Moderate to Vigorous Physical Activity Volume Is An Important Factor for Managing Nonalcoholic Fatty Liver Disease: A Retrospective Study." *Hepatology* 61, no. 4 (April 2015): 1205–1215.

Promrat, K., D. E. Kleiner, H. M. Niemeier et al. "Randomized Controlled Trial Testing the Effects of Weight Loss on Nonalcoholic Steatohepatitis (NASH)." *Hepatology* 51, no. 1 (January 2010): 121–129.

Raj, S. V., M. Ismail, W. K. Chan, and H. A. Majid. "A Systematic Review on Factors Associated with Non-Alcoholic Fatty Liver Disease (NAFLD) Among Adolescents." *Clinical Nutrition ESPEN* 57 (2023): 131–137.

Ryan, Marno C., Catherine Itsiopoulos, Tania Thodis el al. "The Mediterranean Diet Improves Hepatic Steatosis and Insulin Sensitivity in Individuals with Non-Alcoholic Fatty Liver Disease." *Journal of Hepatology* 59, no. 1 (July 2013): 138–143.

Xue, Yaqi, Yang Peng, Litian Zhang et al. "Effect of Different Exercise Modalities on Nonalcohlic Fatty Liver Disease: A Systematic Review and Network Meta-Analysis." *Scientific Reports* 14 (2024): 6212.

Zelber-Sagi, Shira, Dana Ivancovsky-Wajcman, Naomi Fliss Isakov et al. "High Red and Processed Meat Consumption Is Associated with Non-Alcoholic Fatty Liver Disease and Insulin Resistance." *Journal of Hepatology* 68 (2018): 1239–1246.

MICROSCOPIC COLITIS

INTRODUCTION

Microscopic colitis is a condition in which the lining of the colon is irritated and swollen or inflamed. In fact, the word colitis means inflammation of the colon. As a result, people dealing with this condition have chronic, non-bloody watery diarrhea. For some people, this diarrhea is part of their daily lives; for others, it is more sporadic. It may flare up in response to certain conditions, such as anxiety or the consumption of certain foods, or may appear for no apparent or obvious reason. Flares may last for a few days or for extended periods of time. While the tissue of the colon appears to be normal on colonoscopy, upon a closer look under the microscope, it becomes apparent that it is obviously abnormal in appearance, hence the name microscopic colitis.

There are two subtypes of microscopic colitis. With collagenous colitis, an abnormally thick layer of protein called collagen grows in colon tissue. This thickened connective tissue is similar to other connective tissue diseases in which collagen and elastin become inflamed, such as rheumatoid arthritis. And, with lymphocytic colitis, the surface layer of the colon has an abnormally high number of lymphocytes or white blood cells. In some cases, a person may have features of both types. Still, the two types have similar symptoms and the same treatment.

Researchers are uncertain about what causes microscopic colitis. Still, they believe that the causes may include some medications that cause inflammation of the colon, bile acid that is not absorbed, bacteria that produce toxins or viruses, or autoimmune diseases, such as rheumatoid arthritis, celiac disease, or psoriasis, that occur when the body's immune system attacks healthy tissue. There also appears to be a genetic link.

The features of collagenous colitis were first described by Clas G. Lindström, a Swedish pathologist, in 1976. That was followed by A. J. Lazenby and colleagues at the Johns Hopkins School of Medicine Department of Pathology, who outlined the details of lymphocytic colitis in 1989.

SYMPTOMS, RISKS, AND COMPLICATIONS

There are several symptoms associated with microscopic colitis. These include non-bloody watery diarrhea, abdominal pain, cramps or bloating, weight loss, nausea, vomiting, the inability to control bowel movements, a noisy digestive system, gluten sensitivity, fatigue, muscle cramps, muscle pain, joint pain and stiffness, headaches, migraines, mouth sores, skin rashes, acid reflux, swollen lymph nodes, thyroid and/or neurological problems, and dehydration. The watery diarrhea usually occurs about five to ten times per day, though some people have far less and some far more.

Certain factors place people at increased risk for microscopic colitis. Among these are age. People over the age of fifty have an increased risk. The median age at diagnosis is sixty-five years. Women have greater risk than men. This is especially true for postmenopausal women. Smokers have a higher risk than non-smokers, and there may well be a genetic link. Further, people with a family history of irritable bowel syndrome have a higher risk. And, people with an autoimmune disease, such as celiac disease, appear to have an increased risk. The use of certain medicines has also been linked to microscopic colitis. These include pain relievers, such as nonsteroidal anti-inflammatory agents like ibuprofen and naproxen sodium, proton pump inhibitors, such as lansoprazole and omeprazole, and selective serotonin reuptake inhibitors, such as sertraline and paroxetine.

Dehydration is the most common complication associated with microscopic colitis. Other complications include weight loss and, sometimes, malnutrition.

PREVALENCE

It has been estimated that in North America and Europe there are 4.9 cases of collagenous colitis and five cases of lymphocytic colitis for every 100,000 people. However, since many people with microscopic colitis probably do not realize they actually have a medical problem and simply accept the fact that they have chronic watery diarrhea, these figures may well underestimate the exact prevalence.

DIAGNOSIS AND TREATMENT OPTIONS

People with the symptoms associated with microscopic colitis will likely be referred to a gastroenterologist. That physician may order laboratory tests, a stool test, and imaging tests such as a CT scan, which takes numerous horizontal images of the body, and an MRI scan, which uses a huge magnet to take images of the body. If these are inconclusive, the gastroenterologist may proceed with a colonoscopy. During this procedure, the physician slides a long, flexible instrument known as a colonoscope into the rectum and colon and tissue samples are taken.

Treatments for microscopic colitis range from dietary lifestyle changes to over-the-counter and prescription medications. Patients may well be asked to eliminate certain foods and beverages from their diet. Some of the most common products that patients consider to trigger symptoms include alcohol, caffeine, and foods with gluten, dairy, sugar, and artificial sweeteners. It is also a good idea to try an elimination diet to determine which foods may be causing flare-ups. It is known that the Mediterranean diet, which is anti-inflammatory, may reduce symptoms. When flare-ups do occur, clinicians tend to recommend a soft diet comprised of low-fiber and low-fat foods. Frequently recommended medications include bulking agents such as psyllium, anti-diarrheals such as loperamide and diphenoxylate, bismuth subsalicylate (Pepto Bismol), budesonide, a corticosteroid that is absorbed in the colon, mesalamine, and bile acid sequestrants such as colesevelam and colestipol. For people who do not respond to these medications, other medications may be advised. These include immunosuppressants, TNF inhibitors, cromolyn sodium, and low-dose naltrexone.

RESEARCH FINDINGS

Budesonide Seems to Be Useful for Collagenous Colitis

In a placebo-controlled trial published in the *International Journal of Colorectal Disease*, researchers from Germany tested the efficacy of oral budesonide, a corticosteroid, for the improvement of quality of life issues for people with collagenous colitis. For six weeks, twenty-nine patients with collagenous colitis were placed on either 9 mg per day of budesonide (n = 17) or a placebo (n = 12). There were no demographic differences between the two groups. Quality of life issues were measured at baseline and at the end of the trial with the Gastroïntestinal Quality of Life Index. Scores ranged from zero to 144, with higher scores indicating a better quality of life. At baseline, the quality of life scores had a mean of 76. The patients randomized to the intervention group had a lower score than those in the placebo group. After six weeks of treatment, the mean scores increased significantly in the treatment group but remained unchanged in the placebo group. Compared with the placebo group, the mean scores of the emotional functioning and physical functioning in the intervention group increased significantly. A significantly larger proportion of the patients in the treatment group experienced improved stool consistency and stool frequency. The researchers commented that "budesonide is so far the only therapeutic intervention for which strong evidence of clinical and histological improvement in collagenous colitis exists."[1]

In a prospective, double-blind, placebo-controlled trial published in the journal *Gastroenterology*, researchers based in Belgium also evaluated the use of budesonide for collagenous colitis. The cohort consisted of twenty-eight patients—twenty females—with collagenous colitis. For eight weeks, fourteen were randomly assigned to take 9 mg per day of budesonide and fourteen took a placebo. Both groups had similar baseline characteristics of age, sex, median duration of disease, medication use, and associated autoimmune conditions. The patients were evaluated clinically and biopsy specimens were taken at baseline and week eight. Clinical response was defined as a decrease of at least 50 percent in the number of bowel movements in the previous seven days. At week eight, non-responders received open-label budesonide for eight weeks; the treatment of responders was discontinued. Three patients discontinued the trial prematurely. Eight of the patients in the budesonide group and three in the placebo group improved clinically. These effects were observed within the first two weeks and were maintained throughout the study. There did not appear to be any significant budesonide-related treatment toxicity. The researchers concluded that "budesonide is efficacious at inducing short-term clinical and histologic responses in patients with CC [collagenous colitis]."[2]

In a randomized, double-blind, placebo-controlled, thirty-eight center trial also published in *Gastroenterology*, researchers from Germany noted that while people tend to improve on budesonide during treatment, they often relapse when treatment ends. That is why they wanted to determine if budesonide may be used for longer periods of time. The cohort consisted of forty-six patients with collagenous colitis; they had a mean age of slightly under fifty-seven years and had suffered from diarrhea for over two years before diagnosis. For six months, they were placed on either 6 mg per day of budesonide or a placebo; there were twenty-three in each group. During the trial, additional medications for the treatment of collagenous colitis were not permitted. The researchers learned that compared to the placebo, budesonide was associated with a significantly lower cumulative rate of relapse, and there was a high correlation between clinical remission and histologic improvement. Further, a significantly higher proportion of patients treated with budesonide maintained clinical remission at months two, four, and six. The treatment also resulted in notable improvements of health-related quality of living. And, though four patients discontinued therapy because of adverse events, none of these were serious. The researchers commented that their findings demonstrated that "oral budesonide is efficacious and well tolerated for long-term maintenance if clinical remission (prevention of relapse) in patients with collagenous colitis."[3]

There Appears to Be an Association between Microscopic Colitis and Celiac Disease

In a systematic review and meta-analysis published in the *Annals of Gastroenterology*, researchers from several locations but based in Detroit, Michigan, examined the association between microscopic colitis and celiac disease. (See entry on celiac disease.) The researchers identified twenty-six studies with a total of 22,802 patients with microscopic colitis that met their criteria. There were six cross-sectional studies, fifteen cohort studies, and five case-control studies. They were published between 1997 and 2021. Seven were conducted in the United States, four in Sweden, three in Canada, three in the UK, three in the Netherlands, and one each in Finland, Hungary, Italy, Ireland, Denmark, and Spain. The case-control study from Denmark had the largest number of cases, more than 15,500. The researchers found a significant association between microscopic colitis and celiac disease, and celiac disease was prevalent in both types of microscopic colitis. The pooled event rate for microscopic colitis in patients with celiac disease was 6.7 percent, and the pooled event rate for celiac disease in patients with microscopic colitis was 7.7 percent. Yet, the underlying mechanism in this association remained "unclarified." It is known that both diseases are associated with elevated levels of certain inflammatory markers. But, there may well be other causes. For example, they are both immune-related illnesses. And, even though the studies were conducted on different populations from diverse countries, the association between microscopic colitis and celiac disease remained strong. In addition, a subset of patients with these illnesses continued to have symptoms even when they were treated. "Thus, establishing an association between [microscopic colitis] and CD [celiac disease] might be practice-changing and even life-changing."[4]

People with Microscopic Colitis Appear to Have a Higher Intake of Calcium than Other People with Diarrhea

In a case-control trial published in the journal *Clinical and Translational Gastroenterology*, researchers from Chapel Hill, North Carolina, conducted a hospital-based study of patients who had elective colonoscopies for chronic diarrhea. The researchers determined that 106 patients had either type of microscopic colitis and 215 did not have microscopic colitis; the latter group were considered controls. All of the patients were asked to complete questionnaires either online or by phone. The questionnaire asked a wide variety of questions, including inquiries about demographics, smoking, medical history, medications taken in the last year, microscopic colitis activity, and irritable bowel and bloating. The researchers found that the patients with microscopic colitis were more likely to be female, and they were older and better educated. They tended to have a lower BMI and had often lost weight. The people with microscopic colitis consumed less sugar-sweetened drinks. On the other hand, the controls were more likely to smoke cigarettes. The researchers learned that the subjects with the highest quartile of dietary calcium had a lower risk of microscopic colitis. According to the researchers, this suggests that calcium may play a protective role in preventing the development of microscopic colitis. The researchers commented that their results were "limited" because of the lack of diversity of the population and relatively small sample size. Still, the researchers noted, their findings warranted further investigation.[5]

Yet, People with Microscopic Colitis May or May Not Have an Increased Risk for Low Bone Density

In a trial published in the journal *BMC Gastroenterology*, researchers based in Hungary evaluated the association between microscopic colitis and low bone mass. The cohort consisted of fourteen patients with microscopic colitis, twenty-eight patients with Crohn's disease, and twenty-eight healthy persons. All of the subjects had their bone density measured with dual X-ray absorptiometry at the lumbar spine, femoral neck, and radius. In addition, measurements were made of serum bone formation and bone resorption markers. The researchers determined that 57.14 percent of the patients with microscopic colitis had low bone mass. That figure was more than the 46 percent in the Crohn's patients and 10.7 percent in the healthy controls. The difference between the microscopic colitis patients and the healthy controls was significant. One of the fourteen patients with microscopic colitis had osteoporosis and seven had osteopenia. Five patients with Crohn's disease had osteoporosis and twelve had osteopenia. Three of the healthy controls had osteopenia. In people with microscopic colitis, the bone mass was especially lower in the femoral neck and non-dominant radius than in the lumbar spine. The researchers noted that it is apparent that low bone mass is a common occurrence in people with microscopic colitis. Apparently, many of the cases are undiagnosed. The researchers concluded that their findings demonstrated that "bone loss can be an important problem in MC."[6]

In a systematic review and meta-analysis published in the journal *Therapeutic Advances in Gastroenterology*, researchers from Hungary reviewed the association between microscopic colitis and low bone density. They identified three full-text articles and one conference abstract that met their criteria. The articles were observational in design and used age- and sex-matched controls to evaluate the occurrence of low bone mass among people with microscopic colitis. The subjects were over the age of thirty-five years and the vast majority were female. The mean disease duration was 4.33 years. The researchers learned that people with microscopic colitis were twice as likely to have low bone mass; the odds of osteopenia were 2.4 times as likely, and osteoporosis were 1.4 times as likely. Two-thirds of the people with microscopic colitis had decreases in their bone density. Half of them had osteopenia, and one in ten had osteoporosis. As a result of their findings, the researchers advised that people with microscopic colitis be screened for bone mineral density "at the moment of diagnosis."[7]

In a prospective cohort trial published in the journal *Postgraduate Medicine*, researchers from Denmark addressed the association between microscopic colitis and bone mineral status. The cohort consisted of fifty consecutive patients with microscopic colitis, of whom forty-four were women. Ages ranged from forty-five to ninety-three years. The median disease duration was twenty-eight months. The majority of the patients had comorbidities, such as essential hypertension, obstructive lung disease, thyroid disease, diabetes mellitus, and previous breast cancer. The trial also included forty-nine age and sex-matched controls. All of the controls were volunteers without symptoms of intestinal disease, past gastrointestinal disease, or resections. Their demographic data and medical history were recorded, and their bone mineral status was evaluated with dual-energy X-ray absorptiometry and other tests. Smoking was far more prevalent among the patients than the controls. None of the participants had experienced a major osteoporotic fracture. In contrast to the previous two studies, the researchers determined that their patients with microscopic colitis did not have an increased risk for osteopenia or osteoporosis. While the researchers commented that they were unable to recommend routine screening for osteoporosis for patients with microscopic colitis, they did acknowledge that patients with a number of risk factors, such as smoking and treatment with budesonide, may have bone mineral health problems. And, in those instances, screening may be advised.[8]

People with Microscopic Colitis Appear to Have a Higher Risk for Major Adverse Cardiovascular Events

In a study published in the journal *Clinical Gastroenterology and Hepatology*, researchers from Sweden, Boston, Massachusetts, and New York City investigated the relationship between microscopic colitis and major adverse cardiovascular events. The study included Swedish adults with biopsy-proven microscopic colitis without previous cardiovascular disease, a cohort that consisted of 11,018 people. These patients were matched for age, sex, calendar year, and country with up to five individuals without microscopic colitis or cardiovascular disease. This second cohort had 48,371 people. At the start of the follow-up, the median age of the people with microscopic colitis was sixty years, and the group was 75.3 percent female. Comorbidities, such as diabetes, obesity, hypertension, dyslipidemia, chronic kidney disease, and celiac disease, were more prevalent in the microscopic colitis group than in the group of other Swedish adults. Over a median of 6.6 years of follow-up, there were 2,181 or 19.8 percent incident cases of major adverse cardiovascular events in the microscopic colitis patients and 6,661 or 13.8 percent in the second cohort. Thus, patients with microscopic colitis had a 77 percent higher risk of a major adverse cardiovascular event. The researchers theorized that at least some of this risk may be related to the inflammatory properties of microscopic colitis. "Given the high prevalence of CVD [cardiovascular disease] morbidity and mortality in the general population, the increased risk of MACE [major adverse cardiovascular events] in MC [microscopic colitis] patients underscores the need for awareness of CVD risk factors among patients and clinicians."[9]

Many People with Microscopic Colitis Also Have the Symptoms of IBS

In a cross-sectional trial reported in the journal *Therapeutic Advances in Gastroenterology*, researchers from the UK evaluated the hypothesis that many people with microscopic colitis also have irritable bowel syndrome. The cohort consisted of 151 individuals with newly diagnosed microscopic colitis who were seen at the Leeds Teaching Hospitals in northern England. During a six-year period of study, they completed questionnaires that included inquiries about demographics, physical functioning, role limitations due to physical health, role limitations due to emotional health, energy or fatigue, emotional well-being, social functioning, pain, and general health. Of the 151 subjects, 51.7 percent had collagenous colitis and 39.1 percent had lymphocytic colitis. Slightly less than 10 percent were placed in another category. About three-quarters of the cohort was female, and the cohort had a mean age of sixty-eight years. Fifty-two of the cohort reported irritable bowel syndrome symptoms. So, a third of the people in this study with microscopic colitis also have the symptoms of irritable bowel syndrome. The individuals with irritable bowel syndrome symptoms had significantly higher levels of anxiety, depression, and psychosomatic disorders. As a result, they had a significantly reduced quality of life in all of the areas studied except physical functioning. Rates of irritable bowel syndrome tended to be higher among patients who were treated for microscopic colitis, but their therapies were ineffective or made their symptoms worse. The researchers concluded that "further research is required to determine the relationship between MC and IBS-type symptoms, especially in terms of identifying methods to distinguish symptoms of genuine IBS from those of MC at the time of initial presentation, as well as those related to recurrent active MC, or potential coexistent functional GI problems, which may require alternative treatment strategies."[10]

Psychiatric Disorders Tend to Be More Common in People with Microscopic Colitis

In a study published in the *American Journal of Gastroenterology*, researchers from several locations but based in Sweden examined the association between microscopic colitis and psychiatric disorders. Using 2006 to 2017 data obtained from a nationwide Swedish histopathology database, the researchers identified 5,816 patients with colorectal biopsy-confirmed microscopic colitis who had no previous record of a psychiatric disorder; the median age at diagnosis was 64.4 years. Almost all of the patients had a Nordic origin, and a third had a college or university education. These patients were matched to 21,509 individuals from the general population and 5,051 of their siblings without microscopic colitis. From 2006 to 2021, 519 or 8.9 percent of the 5,816 patients with microscopic colitis were diagnosed with a psychiatric disorder. The corresponding figure for the general population was 6.1 percent and for the siblings was 5.4 percent. This equates to about one extra case of a psychiatric disorder for every twenty-nine patients with microscopic colitis followed for ten years. And, after ten years, the risks appeared to increase even more for unipolar depression, anxiety disorders, stress-related disorders, substance abuse, and suicide attempts. This was especially true for older people. The researchers concluded that "patients with MC are at increased risk of psychiatric disorders compared to the general population."[11]

People with Microscopic Colitis Seem to Have an Increased Risk of Psoriasis

In a study published in the journal *Clinical Epidemiology*, researchers from Sweden and New York City examined the association between microscopic colitis and psoriasis. Using a Swedish, nationwide, population-based cohort, the researchers identified 8,404 patients with biopsy-verified microscopic colitis, 37,033 other individuals from the general population without microscopic colitis or psoriasis, and 8,381 of their siblings who did not have microscopic colitis. About 70 percent of the patients with microscopic colitis were women, and the median age at diagnosis was 62.8 years. During a median follow-up of 9.2 years, 179 patients, 440 other individuals, and 115 siblings were diagnosed with psoriasis. The researchers observed that patients with microscopic colitis had almost double the risk of psoriasis as people in the general population, a finding that is supported by the fact that they are both "immune mediated diseases, with known associations to several autoimmune disorders." And compared to their siblings, their adjusted hazard ratio was 1.85. So, even though the patients in the microscopic colitis group shared a genetic make-up similar to their siblings, they had a higher risk for psoriasis. The researchers concluded that their findings "add to the knowledge of extraintestinal inflammatory conditions in MC and underscore the importance to study the mechanisms involved."[12]

Fatigue Is a Common Symptom in People with Microscopic Colitis

In a cross-sectional survey published in the journal *Therapeutic Advances in Gastroenterology*, researchers from the UK noted that fatigue is often seen in patients with irritable bowel syndrome and inflammatory bowel disease. That is why they wanted to learn if fatigue was also common in people with microscopic colitis. The cohort consisted of 129 patients with newly diagnosed microscopic colitis. Only a few of these patients reported having already been diagnosed with an autoimmune disease, such as celiac disease, thyroid disease, and rheumatoid arthritis. No one reported type 1 diabetes, autoimmune liver disease, or psoriasis. Using the Inflammatory Bowel Disease Fatigue Assessment Scale, the researchers collected data on levels of fatigue and the impact of the fatigue. Mean scores were compared against various patient characteristics, and they were correlated with anxiety, depression, somatization, and quality of life scores. Anxiety and depression were measured using the Hospital Anxiety and Depression Scale questionnaire, which includes seven questions on anxiety and seven on depression. Somatization was evaluated with the Patient Health Questionnaire 15, and health-related quality of life was assessed with the thirty-six item Short Form (SF-36). The researchers found that the patients indicated high levels of fatigue, and the patients with abnormal anxiety and depression scores and high levels of somatization had even higher levels of fatigue, which had a greater impact on their daily lives. Fatigue severity was also significantly higher among patients with IBS-type symptoms, but not among those with ongoing gastrointestinal symptoms they considered to be part of their microscopic colitis diagnosis. Not surprisingly, higher fatigue tended to lower quality of life scores. According to the researchers, "it is clear that, regardless of the aetiology of fatigue in patients with a prior diagnosis of MMC, coexistent anxiety, depression or somatization are associated with higher levels of fatigue severity, with a significant impact on patients' lives and detrimental effects on quality of life."[13]

There Does Not Appear to Be an Association between Microscopic Colitis and Vitamin D

In a trial published in the *Scandinavian Journal of Gastroenterology*, researchers from Sweden analyzed the association between microscopic colitis and levels of serum vitamin D. Because of the shortage of daylight in Sweden in the winter months, some people have speculated that vitamin D deficiency may trigger some disorders, such as microscopic colitis. Did people with microscopic colitis have higher rates of vitamin D deficiency than the general population? The initial cohort consisted of 133 patients with microscopic colitis who agreed to supply blood samples. A population-based group of 202 women who left blood samples during the same time period served as controls. The patients with microscopic colitis were older than the controls. The researchers found no difference in vitamin D levels between the patients with microscopic colitis and the controls. Thus, the researchers commented, vitamin D does not appear to influence the disease activity of microscopic colitis.[14]

There May Not Be an Association between Specific Dietary Components, Lifestyle Factors and Microscopic Colitis

In a long-term population-based study published in the *European Journal of Clinical Nutrition*, researchers from Sweden assessed the association between specific dietary components and microscopic colitis. Data were obtained from the Malmö Diet and Cancer Study of 28,095 individuals, in which information on dietary habits, lifestyle factors, and other issues of concern was collected. Of the total cohort, 11,062 (39 percent) were men and 17,033 (61 percent) were women; they had a mean age of fifty-eight years. During a twenty-two-year period of time, 135 people were diagnosed with microscopic colitis. Of these, twenty were men, with a mean age of sixty-one, and 115 were women, with a mean age of fifty-eight years. Intakes of protein, carbohydrates, sucrose, saturated fat, monounsaturated fat, polyunsaturated fat, omega-3 and omega-6 fatty acids, fiber, and zinc were calculated. None of these were found to be associated with the risk of microscopic colitis. "A diet quality index based on adherence to dietary recommendations failed to reveal any differences between cases and non-cases." Also not associated with the risk of microscopic colitis were BMI, physical activity, and education. On the other hand, smoking in females and the high consumption of alcohol were associated with microscopic colitis. "The aetiological mechanisms behind the positive impact of smoking and alcohol on MC risk should be investigated."[15]

The Use of Proton Pump Inhibitors Appears to Increase the Risk of Microscopic Colitis

In a study published in the journal *Alimentary Pharmacology & Therapeutics*, researchers from Denmark examined the association between microscopic colitis and the use of proton pump inhibitors. Over a ten-year period of time, the researchers identified 10,652 patients with a first-time diagnosis of microscopic colitis, including 6,254 (59 percent) with collagenous colitis and 4,398 (41 percent) with lymphocytic colitis. At the time of diagnosis, patients with collagenous colitis had an average age of sixty-eight years, and patients with lymphocytic colitis had an average age of sixty-six years. All of the cases were histologically confirmed in the Danish Pathology Register. Information on proton pump inhibitor use was obtained from the Danish Prescription Register. The researchers found a strong association between the use of proton pump inhibitors and both types of colitis. The strongest association was found with the recent and current use of lansoprazole. Patients who had the highest risk tended to develop microscopic colitis early and stopped proton pump inhibitor treatments, while patients who tolerated proton pump inhibitors well were likely to remain on them. The researchers added that it is currently unknown whether proton pump inhibitor-induced microscopic colitis is reversible.[16]

Bismuth Subsalicylate Is a Useful Treatment for Microscopic Colitis

In a trial published in *Gastroenterology*, researchers from Dallas, Texas, investigated the use of bismuth subsalicylate (Pepto Bismol) for treating microscopic colitis. The cohort consisted of thirteen patients with microscopic colitis; twelve were women. For eight weeks, they were treated with eight chewable 262 mg tablets of bismuth subsalicylate per day. They took three in the morning, two at midday, and three in the evening. During this time, every day, patients recorded the frequency of their bowel movements. Forty-eight hour stool collections and flexible sigmoidoscopies with twenty-four biopsies were performed on each patient before and after treatment. Twelve patients completed the trial; one patient discontinued treatment because of hives. Eleven of the twelve patients experienced a resolution of their diarrhea and a reduction in fecal weight. On average, it took about two weeks to respond. In nine patients, the microscopic colitis resolved. The mean frequency of bowel movements from all patients decreased from 5.3 to 1.6 per day. Posttreatment follow-up, which continued for seven to twenty-eight months, found that nine patients remained well and had no further treatment; two were well but required retreatment, and one continued to have diarrhea. The researchers commented that "bismuth subsalicylate significantly improved fecal consistency, decreased frequency of defecation in fecal weight in eighty-five percent of patients, and resolved histological colitis in seventy-five percent of patients." In addition, "after an eight-week course of treatment, clinical remission of diarrhea occurred for as long as twenty-eight months without further treatment."[17]

REFERENCES AND FURTHER READING

Baert, Filip, Alain Schmit, Geert D'Haens et al. "Budesonide in Collagenous Colitis: A Double-Blind Placebo-Controlled Trial with Histologic Follow-Up." *Gastroenterology* 122 (2002): 20–25.

Bergman, David, Bjorn Roelstraete, Jiangwei Sun et al. "Microscopic Colitis and Risk of Incident Psoriasis: A Nationwide Population-Based Matched Cohort Study." *Clinical Epidemiology* 16 (2024a): 213–225.

Bergman, David, Bjorn Roelstraete, Jiangwei Sun et al. "Psychiatric Disorders Among 5,800 Patients with Microscopic Colitis: A Nationwide Population-Based Matched Cohort Study." *American Journal of Gastroenterology* 19, no. 12 (December 2024): 2516-2525.

Bonderup, Ole K., Gunnar L. Nielsen, Michael Dall et al. "Significant Association Between the Use of Different Proton Pump Inhibitors and Microscopic Colitis: A Nationwide Danish Case-Control Study." *Alimentary Pharmacology & Therapeutics* 48, no. 6 (September 2018): 618–625.

Fine, Kenneth D. and Edward L. Lee. "Efficacy of Open-Label Bismuth Subsalicylate for the Treatment of Microscopic Colitis." *Gastroenterology* 114 (1998): 29–36.

Forss, Anders, David Bergman, Bjorn Roelstraete et al. "Patients with Microscopic Colitis Are at High Risk of Major Adverse Cardiovascular Events: A Matched Cohort Study." *Clinical Gastroenterology and Hepatology* 21 (2023): 3356–3364.

Kane, John S., Andrew J. Irvine, Yannick Derwa, and Alexander C. Ford. "Fatigue and Its Associated Factors in Microscopic Colitis." *Therapeutic Advances in Gastroenterology* 11 (September 13, 2018): NA.

Kane, John S., Andrew J. Irvine, Yannick Derwa et al. "High Prevalence of Irritable Bowel Syndrome-Type Symptoms in Microscopic Colitis: Implications for Treatment." *Therapeutic Advances in Gastroenterology* 11 (2018): NA.

Larsson, J. K., E. Sonestedt, B. Ohlsson et al. "The Association Between the Intake of Specific Dietary Components and Lifestyle Factors and Microscopic Colitis." *European Journal of Clinical Nutrition* 70 (2016): 1309–1317.

Lorinczy, Katalin, Gábor Lakatos, Katalin Müllner et al. "Low Bone Mass in Microscopic Colitis." *BMC Gastroenterology* 11 (2011): 58.

Madisch, Ahmed, Peter Heymer, Claudia Voss et al. "Oral Budesonide Therapy Improves Quality of Life in Patients with Collagenous Colitis." *International Journal of Colorectal Disease* 20 (2005): 312–316.

Mehlke, Stephan, Ahmed Madisch, Birgit Bethke et al. "Oral Budesonide for Maintenance Treatment of Collagenous Colitis: A Randomized, Double-Blind, Placebo-Controlled Trial." *Gastroenterology* 135 (2008): 15`0–1516.

Nimri, Faisal M., Adel Muhanna, Zain Almonani et al. "The Association Between Microscopic Colitis and Celiac Disease: A Systematic Review and Meta-Analysis." *Annals of Gastroenterology* 35 (2022): 281–289.

Rancz, Anett, Brigitta Teutsch, Marie Anne Engh et al. "Microscopic Colitis Is a Risk Factor for Low Bone Density: A Systematic Review and Meta-Analysis." *Therapeutic Advances in Gastroenterology* 16 (June 15, 2023): NA.

Sandler, Robert S., Shan Sun, Temitope O. Keku et al. "Dietary Calcium and Risk of Microscopic Colitis." *Clinical and Translational Gastroenterology* 16, no. 6 (February 24, 2023): e00569.

Sjöberg, Klas, Lina Vigren, Bodil Roth et al. "Vitamin D Levels in Microscopic Colitis." *Scandinavian Journal of Gastroenterology* 48 (2013): 987–988.

Wildt, Signe, Lars K. Munck, Sabine Becker et al. "Risk of Osteoporosis in Microscopic Colitis." *Postgraduate Medicine* 130, no. 3 (2018): 348–354.

PANCREATITIS

INTRODUCTION

Pancreatitis is the inflammation of the pancreas, which is an organ that is behind the stomach on the left side of the body. It is about the size and shape of a person's hand. The pancreas has two primary functions. It produces digestive enzymes (like amylase and lipase) and sends them via the pancreatic duct to the small intestine, where they break down proteins and fats. In addition, the pancreas makes the hormones insulin and glucagon, which enter the bloodstream and control the levels of blood sugar in the body.

There are two types of pancreatitis—acute and chronic. Acute pancreatitis develops quickly and lasts for a relatively short period of time. Though healing usually comes fairly quickly, attacks may be quite severe, requiring treatment in an intensive care unit (ICU). In some cases, people die from this illness. Mild acute pancreatitis has a mortality of less than 1 percent. The mortality of severe acute pancreatitis may be as high as 10–13 percent.[1] Repeat attacks of acute pancreatitis may lead to chronic pancreatitis, which may cause permanent damage and scarring to the pancreas. In some cases, the pancreas may stop making enzymes and/or insulin. The ten-year survival rate for patients who have had surgery for chronic pancreatitis is 63.2 percent.[2]

An article published in the journal *Pancreas* noted that a clinical description of acute pancreatitis was first presented in 1652 by the Dutch anatomist Nicholas Tulp,[3] and an article in the journal *Gastroenterología y Hepatología* said that in 1803, Antoine Portal, a physician to Louis XVIII and Charles X, and founding president of the *Académie Nationale de Médecine* in France, reported the clinical signs of chronic pancreatitis.[4]

SYMPTOMS, RISKS, AND COMPLICATIONS

Symptoms and signs of pancreatitis may vary from person to person, but they include moderate to severe abdominal pain that may spread to the chest or the back, abdominal tenderness, rapid heart rate, stomach upset, shortness of breath, nausea, vomiting, fever, lowered blood pressure, and yellowing of the skin and the eyes. The pain associated with acute pancreatitis tends to be more severe than that of the chronic form, which may vary in intensity. The pain of both acute and chronic pancreatitis may be worse when people lie flat, cough, exercise, and eat larger portions; the pain may subside when people sit upright, lean forward, curl in a fetal position, and eat smaller portions.

The most common causes of pancreatitis are alcohol abuse and gallstones that block the pancreatic duct, preventing enzymes from leaving the pancreas. These two causes represent about 80 percent of the cases. Other causes include abdominal surgery or injury, high triglyceride levels in the blood, high levels of calcium in the blood, certain medicines that irritate the pancreas, such as estrogens, steroids, and thiazide diuretics, and infections, such as mumps, hepatitis A or B, and salmonella; cystic fibrosis, reduced blood supply (ischemia); tumors; some genetic problems; congenital abnormalities of the pancreas; and cigarette smoking.

People with acute pancreatitis tend to recover quickly, within three to five days. Sometimes, small amounts of fluid collect around the pancreas and need to be drained. Still, there are more serious complications associated with acute pancreatitis. These include kidney and respiratory failure, as well as pancreatic infections. People with chronic pancreatitis are far more likely to have ongoing complications. These include chronic pain, diarrhea, weight loss, low vitamin levels from malabsorption, abdominal pain that is worse after eating, diabetes, oily, odorous stools, fluid around the pancreas, breathing problems, bile duct blockages, permanent pancreatic damage, such as scarring of the tissues (fibrosis), and pancreatic cancer. Over time, the pancreas produces fewer of the enzymes and hormones that the body needs. The reduction in enzymes causes malabsorption problems in the small intestine, especially fats and fat-soluble vitamins. Excess fat is expelled in the stool, resulting in chronic diarrhea. The reduction in hormones eventually results in the development of diabetes. Both acute and chronic pancreatitis are associated with pseudocysts or collections of fluid and debris that may rupture and cause internal bleeding, infection, and malnutrition.

PREVALENCE

In the United States, acute pancreatitis accounts for about 275,000 annual hospital admissions. Eighty percent of the patients have mild disease and are able to be discharged in a few days. Overall, the mortality rate of acute pancreatitis is about 2 percent. The relapse rate of acute pancreatitis is between 0.6 percent and 5.6 percent. The prevalence of chronic pancreatitis is 50 per 100,000 people. The most common age group is thirty to forty years, and it occurs more often in men than women.[5]

DIAGNOSIS AND TREATMENT OPTIONS

A medical provider may tentatively diagnose pancreatitis as a result of a medical history and examination. But, further testing will usually be performed. These tests may begin with blood, stool, and urine tests, which may be followed by imaging such as an abdominal X-ray and/or ultrasound. Other tests may include an endoscopic ultrasound, in which a flexible tube is inserted into the mouth, down the esophagus, and into the stomach and pancreas to obtain better ultrasound views, and endoscopic retrograde cholangiopancreatography, which uses an inserted flexible tube and dye to obtain better views of the liver, gallbladder, bile ducts, upper portion of the small intestine, and pancreas. For better images of the pancreas and its surrounding areas, a computed tomography (CT scan) and/or magnetic resonance cholangiopancreatography (a type of magnetic resonance imaging test or MRI) may be ordered. To enhance the images, a dye may be used.

Treatment for acute pancreatitis focuses on enabling the pancreas to rest and heal. Most people are hospitalized for a few days and given intravenous fluids and pain medications. Some are prescribed antibiotics. People who continuously vomit may require the insertion of a nasogastric tube. It is used to remove fluid and air and to slowly allow liquid nutrients into the stomach. The previously noted endoscopic retrograde cholangiopancreatography may be used to remove fluids, blockages, and gallstones or to insert stents to keep ducts open.

Similar treatments are used for chronic pancreatitis. However, a few additional treatments may be added. Thus, people who have alcohol-related pancreatitis may be advised to stop drinking, and those who have smoking-related pancreatitis may be told to stop smoking. People with chronic pancreatitis may require enzyme supplementation to enhance digestion and/or insulin to regulate blood sugar. Medical providers may counsel them to eat smaller meals with more protein and less fat and to keep hydrated. People who experience ongoing pain may require daily pain medication and/or treatment from a pain management specialist, and surgery may be needed to remove damaged portions of the pancreas, the entire pancreas (total pancreatectomy), gallstones, or the entire gallbladder. The entire gallbladder may usually be removed through minimally invasive laparoscopic surgery. The procedure is known as a laparoscopic cholecystectomy. Recovery from this type of surgery is relatively quick. In certain instances, traditional open surgery may be required. The recovery from traditional open surgery is more painful and requires more time. It may be best to prepare for a few weeks of reduced activity.

RESEARCH FINDINGS

People with Chronic Pancreatitis May Well Have Micronutrient Deficiencies

In a cross-sectional study published in the *European Journal of Gastroenterology & Hepatology*, researchers from Denmark investigated the prevalence of micronutrient deficiencies in patients with chronic pancreatitis. The cohort consisted of 115 consecutive patients with chronic pancreatitis; they had a mean age of 57.9 years; 71 percent were male. In half of the patients, chronic pancreatitis was associated with the intake of alcohol. Micronutrient assessments included plasma levels of the fat-soluble vitamins A, D, and E and of the trace elements magnesium and zinc. The researchers determined that the most common deficit was vitamin D deficiency, which was seen in 22 percent of the patients. That was followed by zinc deficiency in 20 percent. Vitamin A and E deficiencies were only seen in patients with exocrine pancreatic insufficiency (EPI), which is the lack of sufficient pancreatic enzymes in the duodenum to maintain the normal digestion of fats, proteins, and carbohydrates. The levels of magnesium and zinc were significantly associated with plasma albumin levels, and magnesium levels were related to the presence of diabetes mellitus. The researchers commented that their findings underscore "the complexity of micronutrient assessment" in patients with chronic pancreatitis.[6]

In a systematic review and meta-analysis published in the journal *Pancreatology*, researchers from several European countries but based in Spain evaluated the risk for deficiencies in vitamins A, D, E, and K in people with chronic pancreatitis. The researchers identified twelve studies with 548 patients that met their criteria. There were seven case-control studies and five cross-sectional studies. Seven of the studies were conducted in Europe, two in India, and one each in the United States, South Africa, and Argentina. Two of the studies were multicenter. Seventy-three percent of the patients were male, with a mean age that ranged between thirty-one and fifty-seven years. The most frequent cause of chronic pancreatitis was alcohol. The researchers learned that the prevalence of a fat-soluble vitamin deficiency was 16.8 percent, 29.2 percent, and 57.6 percent, respectively, for vitamins A, E, and D. Only one study addressed vitamin K; so, the researchers could not perform a pooled analysis on that vitamin. The researchers concluded that clinicians treating patients with chronic pancreatitis "should be aware that the deficiency of fat-soluble vitamins in this setting is common and should be actively considered as a factor potentially impairing the quality of life and comorbidities of CP [chronic pancreatitis] patients."[7]

People Who Eat More Fish Seems to Have Lower Rates of Acute Pancreatitis

In a study published in the *American Journal of Clinical Nutrition*, researchers based in Sweden wanted to determine if there was an association between the consumption of fish and the risk of non-gallstone-related acute pancreatitis. They used data obtained from two prospective cohorts, the Cohort of Swedish Men and the Swedish Mammography Cohort, which included 39,267 men and 32,191 women who were aged forty-five to eighty-four years at the start of a thirteen-year follow-up period. Fish consumption was assessed using a food frequency questionnaire at baseline, and cases of incident non-gallstone-related acute pancreatitis were identified with the Swedish National Patient Register. During the follow-up years, there were 320 cases of incident non-gallstone-related acute pancreatitis; 209 cases in men and 111 cases in women. Compared to the participants with the lowest fish consumption, those with the highest fish consumption were more likely to be older and well-educated, to have ever used fish oil supplements, and to consume more vegetables. They were less likely to be current smokers, but they tended to consume more alcohol and to have a higher prevalence of diabetes and hyperlipidemia. The researchers found an inverse association between total fish consumption and risk of non-gallstone-related acute pancreatitis. The lowest risk was seen in those consuming 2.4 servings per week. The results were similar for both fatty and lean fish. These results are notable. Consuming only a few servings of fish per week may significantly reduce the risk of acute pancreatitis and its related problems. These guidelines are similar to those often espoused by governmental health agencies. "Fish consumption of two to three servings per week is recommended in dietary guidelines of many countries."[8]

There Appears to Be an Association between Certain Dietary Factors and the Risk of Acute Pancreatitis

In a study published in the journal *Clinical Gastroenterology and Hepatology*, researchers from Los Angeles, Honolulu, and New York City evaluated the association between dietary factors and the risk of acute pancreatitis. The cohort consisted of 145,886 African Americans, Native Hawaiians, Japanese Americans, Latinos, and white individuals. At baseline, they were between the ages of forty-five and seventy-five years. The majority were female and aged fifty-five and older; 15.9 percent were current smokers, 12 percent had diabetes, and 48.8 percent drank alcohol. About one-fifth were dealing with obesity. The patients were classified as having gallstone-related acute pancreatitis (n = 1,210), acute pancreatitis that was not related to gallstones (1,222), or recurrent acute pancreatitis or suspected chronic pancreatitis (n = 378). Diet information was obtained from an administered questionnaire. The researchers found that diet and nutrient intake varied according to ethnic groups. African Americans had the highest intake of cholesterol, and Japanese Americans had the lowest. African Americans had the lowest intake of vegetables and coffee, and US-born Latinos and African Americans had the highest intake of saturated fat. The highest intake of red meat was seen in US-born Latinos and Native Hawaiians. Non-US-born Latinos had the highest intakes of dietary fiber and vegetables, and whites had the highest intake of vitamin D. The researchers learned that dietary intakes of saturated fat, cholesterol, and their food sources, including red meat and eggs, were positively associated with gallstone-related acute pancreatitis. On the other hand, fiber intake and vitamin D (primarily from milk) were inversely associated with gallstone-related acute pancreatitis. Interestingly, coffee consumption seemed to protect against acute pancreatitis. According to the researchers, "given the lack of an effective treatment of pancreatitis, studies to determine the effectiveness of dietary factor interventions are warranted."[9]

Electroacupuncture May Not Ease Abdominal Pain in People with Acute Pancreatitis

In a randomized, controlled, three-arm, parallel group, and multicenter study published in the *Journal of Integrative Medicine*, researchers from the South Korea wanted to learn if electroacupuncture would ease the abdominal pain associated with acute pancreatitis. The cohort consisted of eighty-eight patients with acute pancreatitis, who had a mean age of 47.3 years; there were sixty-one males. The patients were placed in one of three groups—patients who received local electroacupuncture (n = 30), patients who received local and distal electroacupuncture (n = 29), and patients who were controls (n = 29). The patients receiving electroacupuncture had one session each day for four days or until the pain was resolved or the patient discharged. The researchers learned that on day five there were no significant differences in levels of pain between the three groups. And, while the electroacupuncture did not appear to provide any pain relief, it did not cause any significant adverse effects. On the other hand, the patients having electroacupuncture were able to consume food significantly sooner than the controls. The researchers commented that "additional studies are required to establish procedures involving effective acupoints that can be used in clinical practice."[10]

People with Chronic Pancreatitis Tend to Be Less Physically Active than Matched Controls

In a study published in the journal *Digestive Surgery*, researchers from Dublin, Ireland, compared the overall physical activity levels of people with chronic pancreatitis to those without this disorder. The cohort consisted of seventeen people with chronic pancreatitis and fifteen controls, who were matched for age, sex, and body mass index. There were significantly more smokers in the chronic pancreatitis group and fewer current drinkers. The participants were interviewed and received ActiGraph accelerometers and activity diaries. Only one participant with chronic pancreatitis failed to complete the entire protocol. The researchers learned that the participants with chronic pancreatitis spent significantly less time participating in light, moderate, and moderately vigorous activity than those in the control group. However, there was no significant difference between the groups in vigorous or sedentary activity. While only two participants in the chronic pancreatitis group met the WHO guidelines for moderate activity, six of those in the control group met this benchmark. Most of those in both groups participated in no vigorous activity; such activity was "notably poor in both groups." According to the researchers, this lack of physical activity in people with chronic pancreatitis "could conceivably contribute to sarcopenia [loss of muscle tissue], poor functional capacity, and poor clinical outcomes." Unfortunately, "research in this area is lacking, both in the measurement of habitual activity, as well as in determining the effects of exercise interventions. Further investigation of this chronic illness population is strongly recommended."[11]

Osteoporosis and Sarcopenia Are Common and Insufficiently Diagnosed in People with Chronic Pancreatitis

In a trial published in the journal *BMC Gastroenterology*, researchers from Finland examined the prevalence of osteoporosis and sarcopenia in people with chronic pancreatitis. The cohort consisted of thirty-three patients with chronic pancreatitis; the median age was sixty-two years, and 61 percent were male. The median disease duration was six years. The cause of 49 percent of the diagnoses was alcohol. Thirty-six percent of the patients were active smokers, and 64 percent had a history of smoking. Sixty-six percent of the patients were overweight, and 24 percent had obesity. None of the patients had been diagnosed with osteoporosis, sarcopenia, or vitamin deficiency. The researchers learned that 45 percent of the males and 58 percent of the females had abnormal bone density. Osteoporosis was diagnosed in 20 percent and osteopenia in 23 percent. Possible sarcopenia was found in 48 percent of the patients in which it was measured. Patients were more likely to have this problem if their disease was of longer duration and/or they had pancreatic exocrine insufficiency (the failure of the pancreas to produce sufficient amounts of enzymes). The researchers concluded that their findings "open opportunities for interventional prospective studies with interventions for clinicians to gain a better understanding of how to treat CP [chronic pancreatitis] and PEI [pancreatic exocrine insufficiency] and to prevent or delay the progression of osteoporosis and sarcopenia in CP patients."[12]

In a systematic review and meta-analysis published in the journal *Clinical Nutrition*, researchers from the UK evaluated the risk of osteopenia, osteoporosis, and osteoporotic fractures in patients with chronic pancreatitis. The researchers identified nineteen studies that met their criteria; they had a total of 20,460 patients with chronic pancreatitis and 2,007,304 controls. All of the studies were published between 2000 and 2022. The mean ages of the patients ranged from thirty-one to fifty-nine years. Ten studies were from Europe, five from the United States, and four were from Asia. Fifteen were single-center studies and four were population-based. Eleven of the studies had the primary cause of chronic pancreatitis to be alcohol. The researchers determined that the pooled prevalence of osteoporosis was 19 percent. When compared to those in the control group, people with chronic pancreatitis were almost twice as likely to have osteoporosis. The prevalence of osteopenia and fractures in people with chronic pancreatitis was 37 percent and 14 percent, respectively. The researchers concluded that osteopenia and osteoporosis were very common in people with chronic pancreatitis. "Further large population-based studies need to be conducted to evaluate the disease burden of osteoporotic fractures, including the associated mortality in patients with chronic pancreatitis."[13]

Malnutrition Is Very Common in People with Chronic Pancreatitis

In a trial published in the journal *Frontiers in Nutrition*, researchers from Germany and Vietnam evaluated the prevalence of malnutrition in patients with chronic pancreatitis. The cohort consisted of sixty-six patients with a mean age of fifty-six years; fifty-one of the patients were males. There were an equal number of age and sex-matched controls. The researchers determined that forty-two patients (64 percent) were malnourished, with twenty-eight (42 percent) having severe malnutrition and fourteen (21 percent) having moderate malnutrition. Thus, almost two-thirds of the patients had malnutrition, and most often the condition was severe. Nutritional status was independent of age, sex, or any etiologic risk factor. The researchers noted that this impaired nutritional status appeared to be a result of "acute episodes of reduced food intake and exacerbations of systemic inflammation." Malnutrition was more often seen in patients who had their initial diagnosis within the previous year or who had higher grades on the Chronic Pancreatitis Prognosis Score, a validated scoring system that predicts the short-term prognosis in people with chronic pancreatitis. Interestingly, despite their poor nutritional status, the patients who were malnourished tended to have a higher activity level than those who were not malnourished. Patients who were moderately malnourished reported the highest level of physical activity, which was significantly higher than the controls. Although statistically non-significant, ongoing nicotine abuse tended to be more common in patients who were malnourished, especially in those with a severe grade of malnourishment. The researchers concluded that it is evident that malnutrition is a frequent component of chronic pancreatitis, and it results in "the loss of skeletal muscle mass but rarely concomitant functional impairment." However, in the more advanced stage of malnutrition, "regular testing for altered body composition is recommended."[14]

Dietary Counseling and Dietary Supplementation Are Both Useful for Malnutrition in Chronic Pancreatitis

In a randomized, controlled trial published in the journal *Clinical Gastroenterology and Hepatology*, researchers from India compared the efficacy of dietary counseling to enriched commercial dietary supplements for people with chronic pancreatitis-related malnutrition. The cohort consisted of sixty patients with chronic pancreatitis and malnourishment who were treated at a tertiary care hospital. For three months, they received either dietary counseling on consuming regular homemade food (n = 29), or they took a commercial medium-chain triglyceride-enriched commercial dietary supplement (n = 31). The vast majority of the patients were male; the mean age of the counseling group was thirty-two, and the mean age of the supplement group was twenty-eight. All of the patients also received the standard management of their chronic pancreatitis, including pancreatic enzyme supplements. The researchers determined that the patients in both groups had similar increases in their BMIs. During the trial, there were comparable improvements in tricep skinfold thickness, dietary intake, fecal fat, and pain. There was no evidence of any adverse effects in the patients in either group. The researchers concluded "that dietary counseling for a balanced homemade diet is as good as commercial food supplements in improving malnutrition in patients with CP [chronic pancreatitis]."[15]

High-Dose Vitamin C Seems to Be Useful for Acute Pancreatitis

In a trial published in the *World Journal of Gastroenterology*, researchers from China wanted to learn if high doses of vitamin C would be useful for patients dealing with acute pancreatitis. The cohort consisted of eighty-four patients with acute pancreatitis. The patients in the treatment group were given 10 g per day of intravenous vitamin C for five days, and the patients in the control group were given 1 g per day of intravenous vitamin C, also for five days. The patients were monitored for symptoms, physical signs, duration of hospitalization, complications, and mortality. Laboratory tests measured levels of vitamin C and other factors. In addition to significant improvement in a host of different laboratory tests, the patients taking the high-dose vitamin C had a higher cure rate, a lower complication rate, and a shorter hospital stay than those on the low dose. The researchers concluded that "high dose vitamin C has therapeutic efficacy on acute pancreatitis." Moreover, "the therapeutic efficacy of high dose vitamin C was much better than that of low dose vitamin C."[16]

People with Severe Acute Pancreatitis Do Not Appear to Benefit from the Administration of a Combination of Three Intravenous Antioxidants—N-Acetylcysteine, Selenium, and Vitamin C. And, There Is the Possibility That People May Be Harmed by This Treatment

In a randomized, double-blind, placebo-controlled trial published in the journal *Gut*, researchers based in the UK wanted to learn if patients with severe acute pancreatitis would benefit from an intravenous solution of the antioxidants N-acetylcysteine, selenium, and vitamin C. The cohort consisted of forty-three patients from three different hospitals; there were twenty-two in the antioxidant group and twenty-one in the placebo group. The average days of treatment in the antioxidant group was 4.1, and it was 4.7 in the placebo group. Relative serum levels of antioxidants rose and markers of oxidative stress fell in the active treatment group. Still, while there were no adverse effects that were directly attributable to the antioxidant therapy, the four deaths that occurred were all in the treatment group. No deaths occurred in the placebo group. As a result of these findings, the study was suspended. The researchers noted that the primary finding of their study was "that although antioxidant supplementation avoided the fall in antioxidant levels seen in the placebo group there is no evidence to support the use of intravenous antioxidants in patients with severe acute pancreatitis in terms of organ dysfunction, patient outcomes or reduced length of stay." Furthermore, "this study provides no evidence to justify continued use of n-acetylcysteine, selenium, vitamin C based antioxidant therapy in severe acute pancreatitis."[17]

Levels of Serum Vitamin D May Play a Role in the Severity of Acute Pancreatitis

In a prospective trial published in the *United European Gastroenterology Journal*, researchers from the South Korea wanted to learn more about the association between levels of serum vitamin D and the severity of acute pancreatitis. The initial cohort consisted of 242 patients with acute pancreatitis; there were 162 males and eighty females. The mean age was 58.8 years. Serum levels of vitamin D were assessed shortly after diagnosis. These levels were classified as normal, insufficient, or deficient. The severity of acute pancreatitis was also determined, and these were classified as mild, moderately severe, or severe. Mild acute pancreatitis was defined by the absence of organ failure and local or systemic complications. Moderately severe acute pancreatitis was described as transient organ failure that resolves within forty-eight hours. And, severe acute pancreatitis is persistent organ failure. According to this classification, 162 patients had mild acute pancreatitis, sixty-three had moderately severe, and seventeen had severe. The median hospital stay was five days, and thirty-six patients were admitted to the ICU. The etiology of the illness included gallstones (52.5 percent), alcohol consumption (36 percent), hypertriglyceridemia (5 percent), and idiopathic (6.6 percent). There were four mortalities. While thirty-seven patients had normal levels of vitamin D, sixty-nine had insufficient levels, and 136 were deficient. The researchers found that levels of serum vitamin D were inversely associated with the severity of acute pancreatitis. Further, lower serum vitamin D levels placed patients at increased risk of being admitted to the ICU; this association was independent of other traditional factors for severe acute pancreatitis. The researchers concluded that their findings suggest that vitamin D levels at admission may be useful to help predict the course of acute pancreatitis. According to the researchers, "this is the first study to reveal an independent association between vitamin D status and severity of AP [acute pancreatitis]."[18]

In a similar study, published a few years later in *Pancreatology*, researchers from Turkey addressed the association between levels of serum vitamin D and the severity of acute pancreatitis. The trial was conducted between June 2021 and August 2022 and had a total of 315 patients; the mean age of the patients was 57.7 years, and there were almost the same number of males and females. Gallstones were the cause of 74.3 percent of the cases of acute pancreatitis. That was followed by 7.9 percent for alcohol and 4.8 percent for drug intake. While 14.3 percent of the patients were smokers, 37.8 percent had hypertension, and 26 percent were diabetic. Blood samples were taken upon admission. Vitamin D levels were described as sufficient, insufficient, or deficient. The researchers learned that serum levels of vitamin D were negatively correlated with the severity of acute pancreatitis. People with low levels of vitamin D had more severe illness. And, this association was statistically significant. But, levels of vitamin D did not appear to be related to admission to the ICU or mortality. The researchers speculated that vitamin D may prove to be "a new potential therapeutic agent in this mechanically complex, burdensome disorder."[19]

There Does Not Appear to Be Sufficient Evidence That Pancreatic Enzyme Supplements Relieve Abdominal Pain in People with Chronic Pancreatitis

In a systematic review and meta-analysis published in the *Canadian Journal of Gastroenterology and Hepatology*, researchers from Canada, Boston, Massachusetts, and Charleston, South Carolina examined the effectiveness of pancreatic enzyme supplements for the abdominal pain associated with chronic pancreatitis. The researchers located five studies that met their criteria. Four of the studies were crossover, double-blind randomized, and controlled trials and one was a parallel, double-blind randomized controlled trial. All of the studies had similar methodologies. While four of the studies that used enteric-coated pancreatic enzyme supplementation failed to show any improvement in pain as compared to the placebo, the only study that used non-enteric-coated enzymes did demonstrate a reduction in pain scores. In this study, ten of the nineteen patients had significant improvements in pain; nine did not. During the week of active treatment, fifteen patients reported subjective pain relief, as compared to the week of placebo. But, the researchers commented that this study was small and had a major methodological concern of possible selection bias, "since forty percent of the included patients had previously undergone surgery and the authors did not report subgroup data for those who had not had surgery." As a result, the researchers noted that their findings failed to show definitive evidence that proton pump inhibitors help manage the pain associated with chronic pancreatitis. The researchers concluded that "pancreatic enzyme supplements do not seem to relieve abdominal pain in patients with chronic pancreatitis and should not be prescribed solely for this purpose, given the significant cost and potential side effects."[20]

REFERENCES AND FURTHER READING

Du, Wei-Dong, Zu-Rong Yuan, Jian Sun et al. "Therapeutic Efficacy of High-Dose Vitamin C on Acute Pancreatitis and its Potential Mechanisms." *World Journal of Gastroenterology* 9, no. 11 (2003): 2565–2569.

Huh, Ji Hye, Jae Woo Kim, and Kyong Joo Lee. "Vitamin D Deficiency Predicts Severe Acute Pancreatitis." *United European Gastroenterology Journal* 7, no. 1 (February 2019): 90–95.

Jang, Dong Kee, Jun Kyu Lee, Chan Yung Jung et al. "Electroacupuncture for Abdominal Pain Relief in Patients with Acute Pancreatitis: A Three-Arm Randomized Controlled Trial." *Journal of Integrative Medicine* 21, no. 6 (November 2023): 537–542.

Jøker-Jensen, Henriette, Anne Sofie Mathiasen, Marianne Køhler et al. "Micronutrient Deficits in Patients with Chronic Pancreatitis: Prevalence, Risk Factors and Pitfalls." *European Journal of Gastroenterology & Hepatology* 32 (2020): 1328–1334.

Koh, Amanda, Olamide Oyende, David J. Humes, and Dileep N. Lobo. "Risk of Osteopenia, Osteoporosis and Osteoporotic Fractures in Patients with Chronic Pancreatitis: A Systematic Review and Meta-Analysis." *Clinical Nutrition* 42 (2023): 1086–1094.

Martínez-Moneo, Emma, Serena Stigliano, Aleksandra Hedström et al. "Deficiency of Fat-Soluble Vitamins in Chronic Pancreatitis: A Systematic Review and Meta-Analysis." *Pancreatology* 16 (2016): 988–994.

Monaghan, Brenda, Ann Monaghan, Qurat UI Ain et al. "Significantly Lower Physical Activity Participation in Individuals with Chronic Pancreatitis Compared to Controls: An Exploratory Study of Objectively Assessed Physical Activity Levels." *Digestive Surgery* 40 (2023): 69–75.

Navarro, Salvador. "Chronic Pancreatitis. Some Important Historical Aspects." *Gastroenterología y Hepatología* 41, no. 7 (August 2018): 474.e1–474.e8.

Ocal, Serkan, Kubra Cerci, Osman Cagin Buldukoglu et al. "Effect of Serum Vitamin D Levels on the Severity of Acute Pancreatitis: A Prospective Study." *Pancreatology* 24 (2024): 206–210.

Oskarsson, V., N. Orsini, O. Sadr-Azodi, and A. Wolk. "Fish Consumption and Risk of Non-Gallstone-Related Acute Pancreatitis: A Prospective Cohort Study." *American Journal of Clinical Nutrition* 101 (2015): 72–78.

Pannala, Rahul, Mark Kidd, and Irvin M. Modin. "Acute Pancreatitis: A Historical Perspective." *Pancreas* 38, no. 4 (May 2009): 355–366.

Parhiala, Mikael, Mika Ukkonen, Juhani Sand, and Johanna Laukkarinen. "Osteoporosis and Sarcopenia Are Common and Insufficiently Diagnosed Among Chronic Pancreatitis Patients." *BMC Gastroenterology* 23 (2023): 124.

Setiawan, Veronica Wendy, Stephen J. Pandol, Jacqueline Porcel et al. "Dietary Factors Reduce Risk of Acute Pancreatitis in a Large Multiethnic Cohort." *Clinical Gastroenterology and Hepatology* 15 (February 2017): 257–265.

Singh, S., S. Midha, N. Singh et al. "Dietary Counseling Versus Dietary Supplements for Malnutrition in Chronic Pancreatitis: A Randomized Controlled Trial." *Clinical Gastroenterology and Hepatology* 6 (2008): 353–359.

Siriwardena, Ajith K., James M. Mason, Srinivasan Balachandra et al. "Randomised, Double Blind, Placebo Controlled Trial of Intravenous Antioxidant (N-Acetylcysteine, Selenium, Vitamin C) Therapy in Severe Acute Pancreatitis." *Gut* 56 (2007): 1439–1444.

Wiese, Mats, Simone Gärtner, Nele von Essen et al. "Malnutrition Is Highly Prevalent in Patients with Chronic Pancreatitis and Characterized by Loss of Skeletal Muscle Mass but Absence of Impaired Physical Function." *Frontiers in Nutrition* 9 (June 2022): 889489.

Yaghoobi, M., J. McNabb-Baltar, R. Bijarchi, and P. B. Cotton. "Pancreatic Enzyme Supplements Are Not Effective for Relieving Abdominal Pain in Patients with Chronic Pancreatitis: Meta-Analysis and Systematic Review of Randomized Controlled Trials." *Canadian Journal of Gastroenterology and Hepatology* 2016 (2016): 8541839.

PEPTIC ULCER DISEASE

INTRODUCTION

Peptic ulcers are open sores in the inner lining of the stomach and the upper part of the small intestine, known as the duodenum. The word "peptic" means that it is related to digestion. The word is derived from pepsin, the major digestive enzyme that the stomach produces.

The gastrointestinal tract has a protective outer mucous lining that insulates it from the substances inside. But, in peptic ulcer disease, this protective lining fails, and digestive juices can leak through the lining into the deeper layers of the wall.

The most common causes of peptic ulcers are infections from the bacteria Helicobacter pylori (H. pylori) and the long-term use of nonsteroidal anti-inflammatory drugs (NSAIDs), such as ibuprofen, naproxen sodium, and aspirin. H. pylori may be spread from person to person through close contact or kissing and may also be contracted from contaminated food or water. NSAIDs irritate the lining of the stomach and intestine, especially when they are used for a longer period of time. Acetaminophen (Tylenol) does not cause peptic ulcers. Stress alone and spicy food also do not cause peptic ulcers.

There are two main types of peptic ulcers. Gastric stomach ulcers appear on the inside of the stomach, and duodenal ulcers appear on the inside of the upper portion of the small intestine. Almost 20 percent of peptic ulcers are gastric and almost 80 percent are duodenal. Though unusual, it is possible to have a peptic ulcer at other locations in the gastrointestinal tract. For example, chronic acid reflux may erode the mucous lining of the esophagus.

In the late twentieth century, two Australian physician researchers, Barry Marshall and Robin Warren, first identified H. pylori as a cause of peptic ulcers. They received the Nobel Prize for their discovery in 2005.

SYMPTOMS, RISKS, AND COMPLICATIONS

While 70 percent of people with peptic ulcers do not have any symptoms, the most common symptom is a dull or burning pain below the sternum or breastbone, which may worsen between meals and at night or after meals. A gastric ulcer tends to feel worse after eating a meal. A duodenal ulcer tends to feel better after eating, but abdominal pain may occur two to five hours after eating, especially between 11:00 p.m. and 2 a.m. It is not uncommon for the pain associated with duodenal ulcer to interrupt sleep. Other symptoms include the feeling of fullness or bloating, even after eating a relatively small amount of food, loss of appetite, weight loss, burping or belching, indigestion, heartburn, nausea, and vomiting. In some instances, peptic ulcers bleed. When this occurs, the symptoms may be vomiting red coffee grounds-colored blood, or stools that are dark or tarry. Due to blood loss, an individual may complain of dizziness or feeling faint. Symptoms of a gastrointestinal perforation or a hole through the entire wall, include sudden, sharp abdominal pain, abdominal swelling and tenderness to touch, fever, and chills. Symptoms of a gastrointestinal obstruction may include abdominal bloating, swelling, pain, nausea and vomiting, loss of appetite, and weight loss.

Certain factors place people at increased risk for peptic ulcers. These include aging; people over the age of sixty have a higher risk. Other risks include NSAID use and prior peptic ulcers.

Untreated peptic ulcers may result in complications. These include slow blood loss that may result in anemia or quickened blood loss that may require hospitalization and transfusion. Blood loss may result in black or bloody vomit and/or bloody stools. In addition, a peptic ulcer may cause a hole in the wall of the stomach or small intestine, which increases the risk of an infection of the abdomen known as peritonitis. Peptic ulcers may also prevent food from moving through the digestive tract, resulting in a blockage that triggers vomiting and weight loss. And, people infected with H. pylori are known to have an increased risk for stomach cancer. Other complications include dizziness, fainting, paleness, and rapid heart rate.

PREVALENCE

Peptic ulcer disease is a relatively common medical problem. Worldwide, between 5 and 10 percent of people develop peptic ulcers at some point in their lives. While people of any age may develop peptic ulcers, it is more common in middle-aged adults, and it is more common in people assigned male at birth than in people assigned female at birth.

DIAGNOSIS AND TREATMENT OPTIONS

The most accurate diagnostic tool for peptic ulcer disease is an upper endoscopy. Most people with the symptoms of peptic ulcer disease, who have an H. pylori infection or use NSAIDs, will have this procedure. During an upper endoscopy, a thin, lighted tube is inserted into the throat, down the esophagus, and into the stomach and duodenum. The medical provider looks for ulcers and takes tissue samples. If any of the ulcers are bleeding, they will be treated.

Sometimes, imaging tests, such as CT and MRI scans, will be conducted. Tests for the H. pylori infection include a urea breath test and/or a stool test.

Since they address the cause of peptic ulcer disease, medications are the main treatment for peptic ulcer disease. These include medications to reduce gastric acid and help protect and repair the tissues. People with H. pylori infection will also be prescribed antibiotics. Examples of these medications include cytoprotective agents that help coat and protect the gastrointestinal lining while it heals (sucralfate, misoprostol, bismuth subsalicylate), histamine receptor blockers (H2 blockers) that reduce stomach acid (famotidine, cimetidine, nizatidine), and PPIs that reduce stomach acid and coat and protect the mucous lining while it heals (esomeprazole, dexlansoprazole, lansoprazole, omeprazole, pantoprazole). Common antibiotics for H. pylori include doxycycline, metronidazole, clarithromycin, and amoxicillin/clavulanic acid.

RESEARCH FINDINGS

Proton Pump Inhibitors Appear to Be a Better Choice for Preventing and Treating Gastric Peptic Ulcers

In a systematic review and meta-analysis published in the journal *BMC Gastroenterology*, researchers from Concord, Massachusetts, and Montreal, Canada, compared the treatment of peptic ulcers with proton pump inhibitors, the histamine 2-receptor antagonist ranitidine, and a placebo. They located sixteen randomized, controlled clinical trials that included a proton pump inhibitor in at least one treatment arm. Four compared treatment with a proton pump inhibitor to a placebo, nine compared it to ranitidine, and three compared a newer proton pump inhibitor to omeprazole, an older treatment. The criteria for the diagnosis of gastric ulcers varied; the vast majority defined healing as the complete re-epithelization of the ulcer crater. The mean age of the patients was fifty-six years. The researchers learned that each of the trials found that the clinical symptoms improved better with a newer proton pump inhibitor (rabeprazole, pantoprazole, or lansoprazole) than ranitidine or omeprazole. This was especially true for pantoprazole and lansoprazole. Healing rates were consistently lower with the placebos; for the majority of the patients, placebos did not heal the ulcers. As a result of these findings, the researchers concluded "that the first-line drug therapy for patients diagnosed with gastric ulcer should be a PPI, in preference to an H2 antagonist." And, "compared with ranitidine the PPIs provide faster onset of action, greater relief of symptoms and increased healing rates."[1]

In a systematic review and meta-analysis published in the online journal *PLoS One*, researchers from China compared the use of proton pump inhibitors to H2 receptor antagonists for the prevention of upper gastrointestinal injury, such as ulcers, in people who use low-dose aspirin. It is well known that the long-term use of low-dose aspirin increases the risk of upper gastrointestinal injuries, such as gastric ulcers and bleeding. The researchers located nine randomized, controlled trials in English and Chinese that met their criteria. All of the studies were published in the United States or China. The number of participants in the experimental groups ranged from forty-two to 163, and the duration of follow-ups ranged from four to fifty-two weeks. The proton pump inhibitors studied were pantoprazole, rabeprazole, esomeprazole, omeprazole, and lansoprazole, at doses ranging from 10 to 40 mg per day. The H2 receptor antagonists included famotidine, 20–80 mg per day, and ranitidine, 300 mg per day. The patients' risk factors varied according to the study. The researchers determined that proton pump inhibitors were "superior" to H2 receptor antagonists for the prevention of low-dose aspirin-associated upper gastrointestinal ulcers and bleeding. However, it should be noted that among the nine included studies, six were from mainland China and had small samples and were "poorly reported." Moreover, "the bias of random sequence generation, allocation concealment, blinding method, incomplete outcome data, and other bias in most of the studies were not clear, which means that the results of our meta-analysis should be interpreted with caution."[2]

There Appears to Be a Strong Association between Gastric and Duodenal Ulcers and the H. pylori Infection

In a large prospective study published in the journal *Clinical Gastroenterology and Hepatology*, researchers from Germany evaluated the association between gastric and duodenal ulcers and the H. pylori infection. The researchers obtained their data from a population-based German cohort of 9,953 adults. At baseline, the adults were between the ages of fifty and seventy-four years, with a median age of sixty-two years. Fifty-five percent were female. The incidence of ulcers was determined by questionnaires sent to study participants and general practitioners two to five years later and was validated by medical records. A lifetime history of peptic ulcer disease was reported by 1,030 (11.8 percent) of the participants. According to serology, 4,420 (50.8 percent) participants were infected with H. pylori. The researchers determined that H. pylori was significantly associated with a lifetime history of peptic ulcer disease. Other associations with peptic ulcer disease included male sex, smoking, family history of peptic ulcer disease, and the daily use of analgesics. Still, the researchers cautioned that the participants were recruited during a voluntary health check-up and therefore do not represent a random sample of the German population. But, they added that the participants were similar to the German population with respect to major sociodemographic and socioeconomic factors. And, they concluded that their findings indicated that the proportion of peptic ulcer disease attributable to H. pylori may well be larger than was previously believed.[3]

There Does Not Appear to Be an Association between Peptic Ulcer Disease and Obesity and Metabolically Healthy Obesity

In a retrospective cohort study published in the journal *Nutrients*, researchers based in Korea assessed the association between peptic ulcer disease, obesity, and metabolically healthy obesity. The cohort consisted of 32,472 subjects without peptic ulcer disease at baseline. They had a mean age of 50.2 years. They all had repeated health examinations, were stratified by body mass index, and had a mean BMI of 23.6. The prevalence of obesity was 31.3 percent. Compared to subjects who did not have obesity, the subjects with obesity were more likely to be male, slightly older, current smokers, and heavy drinkers. They were more likely to exercise regularly, have higher levels of total cholesterol and LDL-cholesterol, and lower levels of HDL cholesterol. During 166,256.6 person-years of follow-up, there were 1,940 cases of peptic ulcer disease. The cumulative incidence rate of peptic ulcer disease and gastric ulcers was significantly higher in the obesity group than in the non-obesity group. But when adjusted for possible confounding factors, the association was no longer significant. At the same time, the cumulative incidence rate of duodenal ulcers was not significantly different between the two groups, and there was no significant association. Further, the risks of developing either type of peptic ulcer were not significantly associated with individuals with metabolically healthy obesity. The researchers concluded that their findings determined that "the risk of developing PUD [peptic ulcer disease] was not significantly increased in obese or MHO [metabolically healthy obese] individuals compared to normal weight individuals. . . . Previously reported association between obesity and PUD appears to be due to confounding factors including various lifestyle factors or metabolic syndrome."[4]

Smoking and Alcohol Seem to Be Risk Factors for Bleeding and Perforated Peptic Ulcers

In a prospective, population-based study published in the journal *Epidemiology*, researchers from Denmark examined the association between smoking and alcohol intake and bleeding and perforated peptic ulcers. The cohort consisted of 26,518 Danish subjects who were followed for an average of 13.4 years. During that time, there were 214 cases of incident bleeding and 107 cases of perforated ulcers. The researchers learned that compared to people who never smoked, people who smoked more than fifteen cigarettes per day had more than three times the risk of developing a perforated ulcer. The more people smoked and the longer they smoked, the greater the risk. And, compared to drinking less than one drink per week, those who drank more than forty-two drinks per week had four times the risk of a bleeding ulcer. Likewise, subjects who drank more than twenty-one drinks per week but drank no wine had a higher risk of a bleeding ulcer than drinkers of the same amount of alcohol but with more than 25 percent of their intake as wine. The researchers commented that "perforated and bleeding peptic ulcers have different risk factors, with smoking being associated with perforation and moderate to high drinking alcohol intake with bleeding."[5]

Even Secondhand Smoke Is Associated with Peptic Ulcer Disease

In a population-based study published in the journal *Frontiers in Public Health*, researchers from Taiwan investigated the association between exposure to secondhand smoke and peptic ulcer disease. The cohort consisted of 88,297 never smokers (18,595 male and 69,702 female), with a mean age of 50.1 years. The cohort consisted of people who had been exposed to secondhand smoke and those who had never been exposed to secondhand smoke. The researchers divided those who had been exposed to secondhand smoke into those exposed less than one hour per week and those exposed one hour or more per week. Of the entire cohort, 11,909 had peptic ulcer disease and 76,539 did not. Compared to the participants without peptic ulcer disease, those with peptic ulcer disease were older, predominantly male, had higher rates of diabetes mellitus, hypertension, alcohol use, and exercise. Their systolic blood pressure was higher, as was their fasting glucose, hemoglobin, triglyceride, fasting glucose, total cholesterol and LDL-cholesterol. The researchers determined that there was a significant association between exposure to secondhand smoke and peptic ulcer disease. In addition, those exposed to secondhand smoke one hour or more per week had an even higher risk. In fact, their risk was 1.23 times higher. The researchers concluded that secondhand smoke was significantly associated with peptic ulcer disease.[6]

Psychological Stress Increases the Risk of Peptic Ulcer Disease

In a prospective study published in the journal *Clinical Gastroenterology and Hepatology*, researchers from Italy and Denmark evaluated the association between psychological stress and peptic ulcer disease. The initial cohort consisted of 3,379 Danish adults without a history of peptic ulcer disease. A stress index scale was used to measure stress on the basis of concrete life stressors and perceived distress. Over the course of approximately eleven years, seventy-six subjects were diagnosed with ulcers. Thirty had gastric ulcers, thirty-nine had duodenal ulcers, and one had both. Six of the locations were unknown. In fifty-three cases, diagnosis was made by endoscopy, seventeen cases were made by contrast radiology, and six were made by surgery. On the basis of the stress index scale, ulcer incidence was significantly higher among the subjects in the highest group of stress scores (3.5 percent) than the lowest group (1.6 percent). The subjects in the middle group had a rate of 1.5 percent. So, those in the highest group had essentially twice the rate. Low socioeconomic status, H. pylori, smoking, and nonsteroidal anti-inflammatory drugs were each significantly associated with subsequent ulcer; lack of leisure time physical exercise was marginally significant. The researchers concluded that "life stress at baseline increased the risk of subsequent confirmed peptic ulcer in a population-based cohort without a history of ulcer at baseline." And that is why, "clinicians treating ulcer patients should investigate potential psychological stress among other risk factors."[7]

People with Peptic Ulcer Disease Are at Increased Risk for Mental Health Problems

In a population-based cross-sectional study published in the journal *Medicine*, researchers from Korea examined the association between peptic ulcer disease and mental health problems. The cohort consisted of 14,266 subjects who participated in the fourth annual Korea National Health and Nutrition Examination Survey. Among this cohort, 813 participants (5.7 percent) had self-reported peptic ulcer disease. Compared to the subjects without peptic ulcer disease, those with this disease had a higher percentage of males, more current smokers and heavy drinkers, lower education status, lower income, and a higher percentage of people with diabetes mellitus, hypertension, metabolic syndrome, and mental health problems, including severe stress, depressed mood, suicidal ideation, and history of psychological counseling. After adjustments for lifestyle, medical, and environmental factors, the researchers determined that people with mental health problems had a significantly higher risk for peptic ulcer disease. As a result, the researchers observed that they "found a close relationship between PUD [peptic ulcer disease] and mental health problems such as severe stress, depressive mood, and suicidal ideation." Thus, "the subjects with PUD were more likely to have psychological problems. Psychological problems were significantly associated with the history of PUD even after adjusting for other well-known risk factors such as age, gender, smoking, drinking, low socio-economic status, and metabolic diseases." And, they advised clinicians to be aware of this association.[8]

Generalized Anxiety Disorder, a Somewhat Common Mental Health Problem, Appears to Be Associated with Peptic Ulcer Disease in Adults

In a study published in the journal *Psychosomatic Medicine*, researchers from New York City and La Jolla, California, assessed the association between generalized anxiety disorder and peptic ulcer disease. Data were obtained from the National Comorbidity Survey, a representative household survey of the adult population of the United States; it included 8,098 participants. The researchers learned that after adjusting for differences in sociodemographic characteristics, comorbid mental disorders, and physical morbidity, generalized anxiety disorder significantly increased the risk of peptic ulcer disorder. Compared to patients without generalized anxiety disorder, generalized anxiety disorder was associated with an almost five-fold increase in the likelihood of peptic ulcer disease. And, there was a dose-response relationship between the number of generalized anxiety disorder symptoms and the increased risk for self-reported peptic ulcer disease. Each additional generalized anxiety disorder symptom was associated with a 20 percent increase in the odds of peptic ulcer disease. Interestingly, peptic ulcer disorder was the only physical illness associated with a statistically significant increase in the likelihood of generalized anxiety disorder. According to the researchers, while these findings are consistent with previous clinical and epidemiologic data, the mechanism of this association remains unknown. "From a clinical perspective, increased awareness of the likelihood that patients seeking help for PUD [peptic ulcer disease] may be at increased risk for concurrent GAD [generalized anxiety disorder] may improve rates of identification and treatment of this common yet frequently unrecognized anxiety disorder, especially in general medical settings, where it is most likely to be seen."[9]

The Number of Members of a Household Seems to Be Associated with the Risk of Peptic Ulcer Disease

In a cross-sectional study published in the journal *Scientific Reports*, researchers from Korea evaluated the association between the number of household members and the risk of peptic ulcer disease. Apparently, no previous studies on this potential association had ever been published. The researchers used data from the Korea National Health and Nutrition Examination Survey of the Korea Centers for Disease Control and Prevention. The researchers learned that the number of household members was associated with a wide number of factors, including peptic ulcer disease. Compared to men or women living alone, men with other household members had a higher risk of peptic ulcer disease. The opposite was true for women. Women who lived with other family members had a lower risk of peptic ulcer disease. Regardless of the number of household members, men consistently had higher rates of peptic ulcer disease than women.[10]

Smoking May Be a Causal Factor for Ulcer Perforation

In a trial published in the journal *Gut*, researchers based in Norway examined the association between smoking and ulcer perforation. The cohort consisted of 168 consecutive patients with gastric or duodenal ulcer perforation admitted to three surgical departments in western Norway, and 4,469 control subjects from a population-based health survey. One hundred and thirty-eight patients were interviewed in the hospital, and twenty-two were interviewed by telephone after discharge. In some cases, information on smoking was obtained from relatives. A total of 102 patients reported daily cigarette smoking, while seven patients smoked only a pipe or cigars. Patients noting that they did not smoke were asked if they had ever smoked. Smokers tended to be older individuals who had other medical problems. And, they frequently drank higher amounts of alcohol. Thirteen patients who were believed to have problems with alcohol were all current smokers. The researchers determined that smoking increased the risk for ulcer perforation by almost ten times in people ages fifteen to seventy-four years, and there was a highly significant dose-response relationship. The more people smoked, the greater their risk for ulcer perforation. The results were similar in men and women and for gastric and duodenal ulcer perforation. No increase in risk was noted for previous smokers. As a result of their findings, the researchers commented that it appears "that most ulcer perforations among persons aged less than seventy-five years are caused by smoking." Further, "the incidence of ulcer perforation can only be markedly reduced, on a population basis, by smoking prevention."[11]

Physical Activity May Reduce the Incidence of Duodenal Ulcers in Men

In a trial published in the *Western Journal of Medicine*, researchers from South Carolina, Georgia, and Texas examined the association between physical activity and the incidence of peptic ulcers. The cohort consisted of 8,529 men and 2,884 women who attended the Cooper Institute for Aerobics Research in Dallas, Texas, during a twenty-year period of time. While at the clinic, they had a clinical evaluation, including a physical examination, and completed a detailed questionnaire. Then, they were classified into one of three activity groups. Active participants walked or jogged ten or more miles per week; moderately active participants walked or ran less than ten miles per week or did another regular activity; and the third group had no regular physical activity. In a follow-up mail survey, the participants were asked if a physician had diagnosed the presence of a gastric or duodenal ulcer. The researchers learned that moderate and higher levels of physical activity appeared to have a possible protective effect on the development of duodenal ulcers in men, and the data suggested that the greater the amount of exercise, the better the effect. Apparently, no such effect was seen on gastric ulcers in men and on both type of ulcers in women. The researchers commented that "physical activity may prove to be a good candidate for nonpharmacologic intervention to prevent the development of duodenal ulcers among men."[12]

Consumption of Ultra-Processed Foods Seems to Increase the Risk of Peptic Ulcer Disease

In a prospective study published in the *European Journal of Nutrition*, researchers from Italy assessed the association between the consumption of ultra-processed foods and peptic ulcer disease. The cohort consisted of 18,066 participants; 62.9 percent were women. At baseline, they had a median age of thirty-five years and a median daily consumption of ultra-processed food of 260 g/day, contributing 28.9 percent of total energy intake. During a median follow-up of 12.2 years, the researchers noted 322 new cases of peptic ulcer disease (1.56 cases per one thousand person-years). When compared to the subjects in the lowest third of ultra-processed food consumption, subjects in the highest third had a 52 percent increased relative risk of peptic ulcer disease. For every 100 g per day of ultra-processed food consumption, there was a 7 percent increase in relative risk for peptic ulcer disease. After ten years of follow-up, the association was still statistically significant. These results remained consistent even when participants who took NSAIDs and aspirin and who had known H. pylori infection were excluded. However, since many H. pylori infections are asymptomatic, large numbers of people may well be unaware that they are infected. The researchers commented that the consumption of ultra-processed foods "could be an environmental factor that increases the risk of PUD [peptic ulcer disease]."[13]

Central Obesity and Other Factors Increase the Risk of Peptic Ulcer Disease

In a retrospective, cross-sectional study published in the *Journal of Personalized Medicine*, researchers from Taiwan reviewed the association between peptic ulcer disease, bone mineral density, and metabolic syndrome and their components in healthy populations. The cohort consisted of 5,102 subjects (2,159 females and 2,943 males) who had an assessment for metabolic factors, an upper gastrointestinal endoscopy, and a dual-energy X-ray absorptiometry scan. The subjects had a mean age of 52.4 years. Slightly more than one-quarter of the cohort had peptic ulcer disease. Eight hundred and eighty subjects had a gastric ulcer and 601 had a duodenal ulcer. Additionally, 31.8 percent of subjects were diagnosed with metabolic syndrome. The researchers found an association between larger waist circumference and peptic ulcer disease. At the same time, high triglycerides were associated with gastric ulcer, and low HDL and osteoporosis were associated with duodenal ulcer. The researchers concluded that "further prospective cohort studies are warranted to clarify the cause-and-effect relationships."[14]

Another Study Also Found an Association between Peptic Ulcer Disease and Osteoporosis

In a study published in *Medicine*, researchers from Taiwan investigated the risk of osteoporosis in people with peptic ulcer disease. The Taiwan National Health Insurance Research Database had 27,132 subjects nineteen years and older who were diagnosed with peptic ulcer disease. The control group had 27,132 randomly selected age and gender-matched subjects who did not have peptic ulcer disease. The largest age group was between fifty and fifty-nine years, followed by forty to forty-nine years. The subjects in the peptic ulcer group were far more likely to have hypertension, diabetes mellitus, hyperlipidemia, chronic kidney disease, chronic liver disease, chronic pulmonary disease, hyperthyroidism, and other medical problems. During a follow-up period, osteoporosis was diagnosed in 2,538 subjects in the peptic ulcer disease group and 2,259 in the non-peptic ulcer group. After adjusting for covariates, the researchers determined that compared to the subjects in the non-peptic ulcer group, the subjects with peptic ulcer disease had 1.85 times the risk of developing osteoporosis. The researchers concluded that peptic ulcer disease "may be an early predictor of osteoporosis." That is why, "physicians should be alerted to these associations so that patients at risk for osteoporosis can be identified at an early stage."[15]

The Incidence of Peptic Ulcers in Men May Be Inversely Correlated with Blood Pressure

In a study published in the *American Journal of Gastroenterology*, researchers from Japan evaluated the association between the incidence of peptic ulcers and blood pressure. The cohort consisted of 100,085 Japanese adults who had health screening examinations. There were 76,698 men and 23,387 women in their thirties, forties, fifties, and sixties. These individuals were found to have 769 endoscopic confirmed cases of gastric ulcers and 344 endoscopic confirmed cases of duodenal ulcers. The blood pressure in these patients was compared to that of 57,208 normal Japanese controls with no gastrointestinal abnormalities. The researchers learned that the blood pressure of the younger and middle-aged men with gastric and duodenal ulcers was lower than that of the male controls. Except for the diastolic blood pressure of women in their fifties, the blood pressure of women with peptic ulcers and the normal controls did not differ significantly. The researchers concluded that there was an inverse association between peptic ulcers in Japanese men and blood pressure levels. Men with peptic ulcers tended to have lower blood pressure levels. This relationship was not seen in women. The researchers hypothesized that "sex hormones may perhaps influence the inhibitory effect of the sympathetic nervous system on ulcer formation in patients with hypertension."[16]

People with Gastric Ulcers Have a Higher Risk of Gastric Cancer than Those with Duodenal Ulcers

In a trial published in the journal *Digestive and Liver Disease*, researchers from Japan compared the risks of developing gastric cancer from the two types of peptic ulcer disease. Over a four-decade period of time, 1,504 patients were diagnosed with peptic ulcer disease in a hospital in Japan. There were 978 patients with gastric ulcers and 444 patients with duodenal ulcers. The remaining patients had evidence of both types of ulcers. During the course of the study, thirty-two patients with gastric ulcers (3.3 percent) and three patients with duodenal ulcers (0.68 percent) developed gastric cancers. Clearly, the incidence of gastric cancer in the patients with duodenal ulcers was significantly less than the incidence of gastric cancer in the patients with gastric ulcers. The researchers concluded that "the risk for patients with duodenal ulcer to develop gastric cancer over the long term is significantly less than in those with gastric ulcer."[17]

REFERENCES AND FURTHER READING

Andersen Bak, Inger, Torben Jørgensen, Olaf Bonnevie et al. "Smoking and Alcohol Intake as Risk Factors for Bleeding and Perforated Peptic Ulcers: A Population-Based Cohort Study." *Epidemiology* 11, no. 4 (July 2000): 434–439.

Cheng, Y., C. A. Macera, D. R., Davis, and S. N. Blair. "Physical Activity and Peptic Ulcers." *Western Journal of Medicine* 173, no. 2 (August 2000): 101–107.

Goodwin, Renee D. and Murray B. Stein. "Generalized Anxiety Disorder and Peptic Ulcer Disease Among Adults in the United States." *Psychosomatic Medicine* 64 (2002): 862–866.

Lee, Young Bok, Jihan Yu, Hyun Ho Choi et al. "The Association Between Peptic Ulcer Diseases and Mental Health Problems." *Medicine* 96, no. 34 (August 2017): e7828.

Leone, Alessandro, Carmen De la Fuente-Arrillaga, Mariano Valdrés Mas et al. "Association Between the Consumption of Ultra-Processed Foods and the Incidence of Peptic Ulcer Disease in the SUN Project: A Spanish Prospective Cohort Study." *European Journal of Nutrition* 63 (2024): 2367–2378.

Levenstein, Susan, Steffan Rosenstock, Rikke Kart Jacobsen et al. "Psychological Stress Increases Risk for Peptic Ulcer, Regardless of *Helicobacter pylori* Infection of Use of Nonsteroidal Anti-Inflammatory Drugs." *Clinical Gastroenterology and Hepatology* 13 (2015): 498–506.

Loke, Song-Seng and Wen-Cheng Li. "Peptic Ulcer Disease Associated with Central Obesity." *Journal of Personalized Medicine* 12 (2022): 1968.

Mo, Chen, Gang Sun, Yan-Zhi Wang et al. "PPI versus Histamine H2 Preceptor Antagonists for Prevention of Upper Gastrointestinal Injury Associated with Low-Dose Aspirin: Systematic Review and Meta-Analysis." *PLoS ONE* 10, no. 7 (2015): e0131558.

Ogura, M., Y. Yamaji, Y. Hikiba et al. "Gastric Cancer Among Peptic Ulcer Patients: Retrospective, Long-Term Follow-Up." *Digestive and Liver Disease* 38 (2006): 811–814.

Pyo, J. H., H. Lee, J. E. Kim et al. "Obesity and Risk of Peptic Ulcer Disease: A Large-Scale Health Check-Up Cohort Study." *Nutrients* 11 (2019): 1288.

Salas, Maribel, Alexandra Ward, and Jaime Caro. "Are Proton Pump Inhibitors the First Choice for Acute Treatment of Gastric Ulcers? A Meta Analysis of Randomized Clinical Trials." *BMC Gastroenterology* 2 (July 15, 2002): 17.

Schöttker, Ben, Mariam A. Adamu, Melanie N. Weck, and Hermann Brenner. "Helicobacter Pylori Infection Is Strongly Associated with Gastric and Duodenal Ulcers in a Large Prospective Study." *Clinical Gastroenterology and Hepatology* 10, no. 5 (May 2012): 487–493.

Segawa, Kose, Yasumasa Niwa, Tomiyasu Arisawa et al. "Incidence of Peptic Ulcer in Men Is Inversely Correlated with Blood Pressure: Study in an Apparently Healthy Japanese Population." *American Journal of Gastroenterology* 90, no. 3 (1995): 399–402.

Svanes, C., J. A. Søreide, A. Skarstein et al. "Smoking and Ulcer Perforation." *Gut* 41 (1997): 177–180.

Wu, Chieh-Hsin, Yi-Ching Tung, Chee-Yin Chai et al. "Increased Risk of Osteoporosis in Patients with Peptic Ulcer Disease." *Medicine* 95, no. 16 (April 2016): e3309.

Yen, Pei-Chi, Jiun-Hung Geng, Pei-Yu Wu et al. "Secondhand Smoke Is Associated with Peptic Ulcer Disease and Gastroesophageal Reflux Disease in Non-Smoker in a Large Taiwanese Population Study." *Frontiers in Public Health* 12 (2024): 1450481.

Yim, M Hong, Keun Ho Kim, and Bum Ju Lee. "The Number of Household Members as a Risk Factor for Peptic Ulcer Disease." *Scientific Reports* 11 (2021): 5274.

ULCERATIVE COLITIS

INTRODUCTION

An inflammatory bowel disease, ulcerative colitis causes irritation and ulcers (open sores) in the large intestine. The severity of ulcerative colitis is dependent on the amount and location of the inflammation. Some people have more intense inflammation that is confined to a smaller area, while others have mild inflammation over a larger area. Usually, the inflammation begins in the rectum and spreads into the colon. When the inflammation is confined to the lower portion of the colon, it is called ulcerative proctitis; if the entire large colon is affected, it is called pancolitis; and if only the left side of the colon is involved, it is called limited or distal colitis.

In the United States, even before the Civil War began, there were reports of a disease with the symptoms of ulcerative colitis. But, ulcerative colitis was not named as a distinct disease until 1875. It was then that two English physicians noted that ulcerative colitis was different from diarrheal diseases caused by infectious agents.[1]

SYMPTOMS, RISKS, AND COMPLICATIONS

Ulcerative colitis often causes diarrhea with blood, cramping, and bowel movement urgency, symptoms that are so strong that they may awaken people in the middle of the night. Other symptoms may include fatigue, nausea, and weight loss. As time passes, more symptoms may emerge. These include blood, mucus, or pus in bowel movements, fever, skin rashes, mouth sores, joint pain, red, painful eyes, and loss of fluids and nutrients. In pediatric ulcerative colitis, there may be delayed or poor growth.

People with ulcerative colitis tend to have a pattern of flare-ups when they have active disease and the symptoms worsen. During times of remission, they may have few, if any symptoms. The goal of physicians treating patients with ulcerative colitis is to extend the remissions as long as possible. It is not uncommon for people with ulcerative colitis to have other medical problems, such as arthritis, inflammation of the eye, liver disease, and osteoporosis. It has been hypothesized that these problems may be caused by inflammation triggered by the immune system. Ulcerative colitis treatments tend to resolve these other medical problems.

It is known that certain factors increase the risk of flare-ups. Probably one of the main risk factors is emotional stress. To reduce the risk of emotional stress, it is important to get sufficient sleep, exercise regularly, and incorporate stress-reducing techniques, such as meditation, into everyday life. Some physicians recommend avoiding nonsteroidal anti-inflammatory drugs such as ibuprofen. Instead, they advise acetaminophen for pain and fever. As for diet, it is known that certain foods may exacerbate the symptoms in some people. These include greasy and high-fat foods, foods with high levels of sugar, carbonated beverages, salt, dairy products, and alcohol.

PREVALENCE

Ulcerative colitis is not uncommon. Together with Crohn's disease, another inflammatory bowel disease, it affects up to one in 250 people in North America and Europe. Though it may occur in people of any age and may start in a child as young as two years old, the first signs of ulcerative colitis normally begin between the ages of fifteen and thirty years, and it occurs less often in people between the ages of fifty and seventy years. It affects the sexes equally and seems to run in families; up to 20 percent of people with ulcerative colitis have a family member with ulcerative colitis or Crohn's disease. It is more common in Jewish people and in those who eat a high-fat diet; it also occurs more often in frequent users of nonsteroidal anti-inflammatory drugs.

DIAGNOSIS AND TREATMENT OPTIONS

A number of different tests may be used to diagnose ulcerative colitis. These include blood tests to look for an infection or anemia, stool samples that detect infections, parasites, and inflammation, an imaging test which shows pictures of the colon and rectum, and endoscopic tests, such as a sigmoidoscopy and colonoscopy, that determine the overall health of the rectum and colon.

While there are no cures for ulcerative colitis, medications prescribed for children, adolescents, and adults may calm the inflammation, reduce the pain and bouts of diarrhea, and help patients feel better and lead more normal lives. The treatment for ulcerative colitis is complicated based on the severity of the disease, its location in the colon, the patient's history of previous medication, as well as the patient's tolerance to using rectal or oral medications. Among the medications used for mild to moderate ulcerative colitis are aminosalicylates, including mesalamine and sulfasalazine. They come in both oral and topical forms, including enemas or suppositories. Steroids may be used topically in the colon or given orally. Various presentations of ulcerative colitis may require a corticosteroid, such as prednisone or budesonide in pill, enema, or suppository form. For an overactive immune system, a healthcare provider may recommend an immunomodulator, such as 6-mercaptopurine, azathioprine, or methotrexate. And, to quiet the immune system in moderate to severe ulcerative colitis, the healthcare provider might prescribe a biologic, such as infliximab, adalimumab, vedolizumab, or ustekinumab. For some individuals with moderate to severe ulcerative colitis that is not responding to these therapies, a rapidly acting, oral, small-molecule Janus kinase inhibitor such as tofacitinib may be used.

Even with all these medication options, some people with ulcerative colitis, such as those with ongoing bleeding or children with abnormal growth and those who do not respond to the medications, may require surgery. At some point, about 30 percent of people with ulcerative colitis have surgery; about 20 percent of children with ulcerative colitis need surgery during their childhood. The most common procedure for ulcerative colitis is the proctocolectomy and ileoanal pouch or J-pouch surgery. (A proctocolectomy removes the colon and rectum; a colectomy removes only the colon; and a proctectomy removes only the rectum.) In a surgery that normally requires more than one procedure, the surgeon begins by removing the colon and rectum and forms an ileoanal pouch, a bag made from a part of the small intestine, to create a rectum. While the body and pouch heal, the surgeon creates a temporary ileostomy or an opening or stoma in the lower belly. The small intestine is attached to the stoma. Waste from the small intestine is then removed from the body into an attached bag or ostomy bag. The bag should be changed as needed throughout the day. Once the ileoanal pouch has healed, the surgeon may remove the ileostomy, which allows waste to exit the body through the anus. But, there will be more frequent bowel movements, an average of four to eight each day. Still, the pain and cramping from the ulcerative colitis are gone. It should be noted that not everyone is able to have an ileoanal pouch. Some people require a permanent ileostomy.

RESEARCH FINDINGS

Vedolizumab Seems to Be More Effective than Adalimumab for Treating Moderate to Severe Ulcerative Colitis

In a double-blind, randomized trial published in the *New England Journal of Medicine*, researchers from different United States and European locations but based in New York City compared the usefulness of two biologic medicines, vedolizumab and adalimumab, for treating people with moderate to severe ulcerative colitis. Conducted at 245 centers in thirty-four countries, the trial included 383 patients who received at least one dose of vedolizumab and 386 patients who received at least one dose of adalimumab. The patients in both groups had similar demographic characteristics. Discontinuation of treatment because of lack of efficacy occurred in forty-one patients in the vedolizumab group and eighty-two patients in the adalimumab group. The researchers determined that clinical remission at week fifty-two occurred in 31.3 percent of the patients in the vedolizumab group and 22.5 percent of the patients in the adalimumab group. Also, at week fifty-two, endoscopic improvement was seen in 39.7 percent of the vedolizumab group and 27.7 percent of the adalimumab group. Of particular interest was the fact that at week fifty-two, slightly more than half of the patients in the vedolizumab group reported that they had an improved quality of life, as did slightly more than 40 percent of those in the adalimumab group. On the other hand, a corticosteroid-free clinical remission occurred in 12.6 percent of the patients in the vedolizumab group and in 21.8 percent of those in the adalimumab group. The researchers concluded that their findings showed "the superiority of vedolizumab over adalimumab in terms of clinical remission and endoscopic improvement but not of corticosteroid-free clinical remission."[2]

Tofacitinib Is a Newer Effective Agent Against Ulcerative Colitis

In a retrospective case-control study published in the journal *Clinical Gastroenterology and Hepatology*, researchers from Ann Arbor and Ypsilanti, Michigan examined the ability of tofacitinib to help patients hospitalized with acute severe ulcerative colitis. The patients were all over the age of eighteen years and were hospitalized between January 2014 and February 2021. The researchers focused on the ability of tofacitinib to prevent the failure of treatment and the need to perform a colectomy within ninety days of admission. The researchers noted that the current standard hospitalization treatment for acute severe ulcerative colitis is intravenous (IV) corticosteroids. However, 30 percent of patients do not respond to that treatment. Patients treated with tofacitinib and IV corticosteroids were matched randomly 1:3 with controls, who received only IV corticosteroids. The researchers located forty patients treated with tofacitinib that met their criteria, and 113 were in the control group. Tofacitinib was administered either at the standard dose of 10 mg twice daily for the duration of the hospitalization or at a high-intensity off-label dose of 10 mg three times daily for nine doses followed by 10 mg twice daily. While many of the demographic characteristics of the two groups were similar, the patients in the tofacitinib were more likely to have previously been treated with a biologic and they had a higher duration of prior corticosteroid use. Six patients (15 percent) of the tofacitinib group and twenty-three patients (20.4 percent) in the control group were forced to have a colectomy within ninety days of admission. So, the patients in the tofacitinib were significantly less likely to need that surgical procedure. Moreover, none of the six patients in the tofacitinib group and nine of the patients in the control group who had the colectomy had a post-surgery infection. Clearly, the patients on the combination therapy appeared to have better outcomes than those on IV corticosteroids alone. "Inpatient tofacitinib induction therapy, in addition to intravenous corticosteroids, was associated with a lower risk of colectomy at ninety days compared to controls." Furthermore, "this study represents the current best evidence for the use of tofacitinib in biologic-experienced patients with ASUC [acute severe ulcerative colitis]."[3]

Tofacitinib Induction Therapy Reduces Symptoms within Three Days for Patients with Ulcerative Colitis

In a study also published in *Clinical Gastroenterology and Hepatology*, researchers from several locations in the United States and abroad, but based in Evanston, Illinois, evaluated the use of tofacitinib for patients who had intolerances or poor responses to previous medications. For eight weeks, 905 patients took 10 mg of tofacitinib twice daily and 234 took a placebo. Patients were instructed on how to record their number of bowel movements per day and the presence of blood in the stools, if any. The researchers learned that the patients on tofacitinib had a significant improvement in stool frequency within three days. That was followed by additional improvement through day fifteen. Similar improvements were seen in rectal bleeding. And, the patients who did not achieve a response by day three or day seven were still able to receive efficacy by week eight. The researchers observed that "tofacitinib is the first agent to demonstrate rapid onset of action, along with robust induction and maintenance efficacy."[4]

Acupuncture May or May Not Be Useful for People with Ulcerative Colitis

In a systematic review and meta-analysis published in the journal *BMC Complementary Medicine and Therapies*, researchers from China investigated the usefulness of acupuncture for treating ulcerative colitis. They located thirteen randomized controlled studies with 515 subjects in the acupuncture groups and 515 subjects in the control groups that met their criteria. One trial tested head acupuncture; the other trials tested body acupuncture. Treatment durations ranged from fourteen to sixty days, and the participants were aged twenty to seventy-eight years old. There were 543 males and 487 females. Seven trials compared acupuncture to conventional medicine, and six compared acupuncture combined with conventional medicine to conventional medicine alone. All of the trials were conducted in China and were published in Chinese. Eight of the studies were considered to have a high risk of bias. The researchers determined that the clinical effect of acupuncture combined with mesalamine (an aminosalicylate) was better than that of mesalamine alone. The clinical effect of acupuncture alone was better than that of metronidazole combined with sulfasalazine. There was no significant difference in the clinical effect between acupuncture alone and mesalamine alone. And, there were no significant differences in the adverse effects between the acupuncture groups and the control groups. The researchers commented that "although it is undeniable that acupuncture may have potential effectiveness in treating UC, more high-quality trials are needed to prove it." As a result, they were unable to "draw firm conclusions based on the evidence of trials included in this review."[5]

Sulfasalazine May Be More Effective than Metronidazole for Active, Not Severe, Ulcerative Colitis

In a multicenter, double-blind, controlled trial published in the *Journal of Clinical Gastroenterology*, researchers from Israel compared the use of sulfasalazine and metronidazole for active, but not severe, ulcerative colitis. The cohort consisted of forty-two patients experiencing an acute attack of ulcerative colitis. For twenty-eight days, nineteen patients took 4.5 g per day of sulfasalazine, and twenty-three took 1.35 g per day of metronidazole. Information on the number of bowel movements, the presence of blood in the stool, nocturnal diarrhea, and incontinence were recorded on a daily chart and evaluated before and at one, two, and four weeks. Flexible sigmoidoscopies were conducted, and biopsies were taken. While thirteen of the nineteen (68 percent) of those taking sulfasalazine improved, only six of the twenty-three (26 percent) of those taking metronidazole improved. The difference between these findings is statistically significant. No patient had significant side effects; only a few patients reported minor gastrointestinal side effects, such as a bitter taste in the mouth or nausea. After a minimum of a one-month remission, four patients completed a crossover trial. One improved on both medications, two improved only on sulfasalazine, and one improved on metronidazole. The researchers concluded that metronidazole "proved ineffective in the therapy of the acute attack of UC."[6]

While Not Useful in the Therapy of an Acute Attack, Metronidazole May Be an Effective Medication to Help Maintain Remission in Patients with Ulcerative Colitis

In a double-blind, randomized trial published in the *Journal of Clinical Gastroenterology*, some of the same Israeli researchers from the previous trial, along with a few new ones, compared the ability of sulfasalazine and metronidazole to help patients with ulcerative colitis maintain remission and avoid future acute attacks. The trial began with forty patients who had all been in remission for between one to eleven months. For twelve months, they took either 2 g per day of sulfasalazine or 0.6 g per day of metronidazole. The two groups had similar demographic characteristics. Five patients dropped out early in the study. As in the previous trial, symptoms such as the number of bowel movements, the presence of blood in the stools, nocturnal diarrhea, and incontinence were periodically assessed. A sigmoidoscopy was conducted at baseline and at one year or if a recurrence occurred. By the end of the twelve months, only twelve patients were still in remission. Nine of them were treated with metronidazole and three were treated with sulfasalazine. The difference was statistically significant. No marked side effects were noted in any patient, but a few had minor gastrointestinal complaints. Following relapse, six patients performed a crossover trial and had a remission of their disease. Three of the six patients remained in remission for twelve months on metronidazole, and none of those on sulfasalazine remained in remission.[7]

Combination Therapy with Infliximab and Azathioprine Is Superior to Monotherapy with Either Agent for Ulcerative Colitis

In a randomized, double-blind trial published in the journal *Gastroenterology*, researchers from Canada, the UK, New Jersey, Italy, and Belgium wanted to learn if the combination of infliximab and azathioprine was better than monotherapy with either agent for moderate to severe ulcerative colitis. During the sixteen-week trial, which was performed at sixty-two centers, seventy-six patients received azathioprine monotherapy, seventy-seven received infliximab monotherapy, and seventy-eight received the combination therapy. At baseline, the three groups had similar demographic characteristics. Corticosteroid-free remission at week sixteen was achieved by 23.7 percent (eighteen of seventy-six) of those on azathioprine monotherapy, 22.1 percent (seventeen of seventy-seven) of those on infliximab monotherapy, and 39.7 percent (thirty-one of seventy-eight) of those on combination therapy. So about twice as many patients received good results with the combination therapy. Mucosal healing at week sixteen was achieved by 36.8 percent (twenty-eight of seventy-six) of those on azathioprine monotherapy, 54.6 percent (forty-two of seventy-seven) of those on infliximab, and 62.8 percent (forty-nine of seventy-eight) of those on combination therapy. Serious infections occurred in one patient on azathioprine monotherapy and one patient on infliximab monotherapy. The researchers concluded that the patients with moderate to severe ulcerative colitis who are treated with the combination therapy "were more likely to achieve corticosteroid-free remission at sixteen weeks than those receiving either monotherapy."[8]

The Combination of Corticosteroids and Mesalamine Does Not Work Any Better than Corticosteroids Alone for Acute Severe Ulcerative Colitis

In a randomized controlled trial published in *Clinical Gastroenterology and Hepatology*, researchers from many different countries but based in Israel wanted to determine if combining corticosteroids with mesalamine would be more effective than corticosteroids alone in treating acute severe ulcerative colitis. The trial was conducted in ten centers in seven countries—Israel, Serbia, Greece, China, France, Korea, and Italy. It included 149 patients who were hospitalized with acute severe ulcerative colitis. Of these, seventy-three patients received intravenous corticosteroids and mesalamine and seventy-six received intravenous corticosteroids alone. The demographic characteristics of the patients in each group were similar. In each center, the assessment of the patient clinical score and study outcomes was performed by a blinded investigator. During hospitalizations, several tests were performed; the primary end point was the percentage of patients who responded to the treatment by day seven. This end point was obtained by fifty-three patients in the corticosteroids and mesalamine group and fifty-eight in the corticosteroids alone group. The researchers found that adding mesalamine to the corticosteroid treatment of patients hospitalized with acute severe ulcerative colitis offered no benefit. "Continuing or starting mesalamine concomitantly with corticosteroids does not confer any additional clinical benefit compared with corticosteroids alone in patients hospitalized with ASUC [acute severe ulcerative colitis]."[9]

There Appears to Be An Association between Dietary Intake and the Risk of Developing Inflammatory Bowel Disease

In a systematic review published in the *American Journal of Gastroenterology*, researchers from Houston, Texas wanted to determine if there was an association between dietary intake and the subsequent risk of developing inflammatory bowel disease. The researchers located nineteen studies that included 1,340 patients with ulcerative colitis, 1,269 patients with Crohn's disease, and over 4,000 controls. Eighteen studies had a case-control design, and a cohort design was used in one study. Eighteen studies had only adults, and one study had only children. Dietary data were collected for nutrients and food groups, as well as total fat intake, saturated fat, monounsaturated fatty acids, total polyunsaturated fatty acids, omega-3 fatty acids, long-chain omega-3 fatty acids, and omega-6 fatty acids. Carbohydrate and protein intake were also categorized. The researchers determined that people who ate higher amounts of total fat, polyunsaturated fatty acids, omega-6 fatty acids, and meats had an increased risk of developing ulcerative colitis. There was no consistent association between total carbohydrate intake and the risk of inflammatory bowel disease, even in studies that reported intake of more than double the recommended daily intake. High vegetable intake was consistently associated with a decreased risk of developing ulcerative colitis. The researchers commented that they were unable to pool data from different studies because of heterogeneity in the study design, nutrient cutoffs, and study populations. The researchers underscored the need for more studies using prospectively collected data.[10]

People with Inflammatory Bowel Disease May Well Have Micronutrient Deficiencies

In a review published in the journal *Current Opinion in Clinical Nutrition & Metabolic Care*, researchers from Haifa, Israel, noted that malnutrition is present in up to 85 percent of patients with inflammatory bowel disease, during both the active stage of the disease and when it is in remission. The reasons for this problem include insufficient dietary intake, impaired absorption, abdominal pain, nausea, patient preferences, and the effects of medications. Some nutrient deficiencies are more likely to occur than others. The most common deficiency in people with inflammatory bowel disease is iron. Some studies have found that more than half of the patients with inflammatory bowel disease are anemic. The treatment for iron deficiency is oral or parenteral iron supplementation. Other common micronutrient deficiencies due to inflammatory bowel disease include vitamin B12, folic acid, vitamin A, vitamin D, vitamin K, selenium, zinc, and vitamin B1. The researchers concluded that when treating patients with inflammatory bowel diseases, there should be a "high suspicion of micronutrient deficiencies."[11]

In a meta-analysis published in the journal *Nutrients*, researchers from China performed a comprehensive literature search of studies published between 1970 and December 2016 on the association between inflammatory bowel diseases and deficiencies in folate and vitamin B12. The researchers located twelve studies with 2,570 participants that met their criteria; there were 1,086 people with inflammatory bowel disease and 1,484 controls. The researchers found that the serum folate concentration of patients with inflammatory bowel disease was lower than in healthy controls, and the difference was significant. However, no such significant differences were observed with levels of B12. The serum vitamin B12 concentrations were only lower in the Asian patients. Still, the researchers recommended the routine screening of inflammatory bowel disease patients for levels of folate and vitamin B12.[12]

In a multicenter, randomized, double-blind, placebo-controlled trial published in the *European Journal of Nutrition*, researchers from Iran wanted to learn if supplementation with selenium would benefit people with mild to moderate ulcerative colitis. The cohort consisted of one hundred people with mild to moderate ulcerative colitis. For ten weeks, fifty participants took 200 mcg per day of selenium and another fifty participants took a placebo. Disease activity was measured with the Simple Clinical Colitis Activity Index (SCCAI); the scoring for this index is based on certain clinical parameters—day and night defecation frequency, urgency of defecation, blood in stool, general well-being, and extra-colonic features. Forty-four patients in the selenium group and forty-five in the placebo group completed the trial. While there were no demographic differences in the two groups at baseline, by the end of the trial the patients in the selenium group had improved, and ten patients in the selenium group and two in the placebo group were in remission. The researchers concluded that 200 mg per day of selenium "supplementation could improve disease activity and induce clinical remission in mild-to-moderate UC patients."[13]

People with Ulcerative Colitis May Do Better on a Low-Fat, High-Fiber Diet

In a parallel group crossover study published in *Clinical Gastroenterology and Hepatology*, researchers from Miami, Florida, and St. Paul, Minnesota, examined the dietary intake of seventeen patients with ulcerative colitis who were in remission or had mild cases of the disorder. One-third of the patients were using biologics, and the others were on mesalamine or no medication. From February 25, 2015, until September 11, 2018, for four weeks, the participants were assigned to eat a low-fat, high-fiber diet. Then, after a two-week washout period, for another four weeks, they ate a standard American diet with higher quantities of fruits, vegetables, and fiber. The meals were catered and delivered to their homes. Serum and stool samples were collected at baseline and at the end of each diet. Before the study, the patients' diets were similar to the standard American diet. While the patients tolerated both experimental diets well, the low-fat, high-fiber diet decreased markers of inflammation and reduced intestinal dysbiosis in fecal samples. And, neither diet exacerbated the symptoms of ulcerative colitis. The researchers suggested that "future studies should address patients with moderate disease, longer diet interventions, and strategies to solidify long-term adherence to effective diets to increase the likelihood of maintaining remission."[14]

Pregnant Women with Inflammatory Bowel Disease Face Additional Challenges

In a retrospective cohort study of pregnant patients admitted to hospitals in the United States between the years 2016 and 2018, published in the *International Journal of Colorectal Disease*, researchers from several locations but based in Columbia, Missouri, wanted to determine the extra challenges faced by pregnant women with inflammatory bowel diseases. The researchers examined information on all the female patients above the age of fifteen years admitted with a primary diagnosis of pregnancy and a secondary diagnosis of inflammatory bowel disease. They collected information on more than eight million pregnancies; 14,129 of these women had inflammatory bowel disease. While the mean age of the women with inflammatory bowel disease was thirty years, the mean age of all the other women was twenty-eight years. The majority of the pregnant women were white, followed by Black and Hispanic individuals. More patients were admitted to large urban hospitals. The researchers determined that the pregnant women with inflammatory bowel disease had an increased risk for gestational diabetes/glucose intolerance, hypertensive complications, and pre-term delivery. They also had an increased risk for fetal growth restriction and fetal death, as well as longer hospital stays with increased costs. The researchers concluded that women with moderate to severe inflammatory bowel disease should seek medical advice before conceiving. Ideally, before becoming pregnant, they should achieve remission.[15]

REFERENCES AND FURTHER READING

Ben-Horin, Shomron, Ofir Har-Noy, Konstantinos H. Katsanos et al. "Corticosteroids and Mesalamine Versus Corticosteroids for Acute Severe Ulcerative Colitis: A Randomized Controlled Trial." *Clinical Gastroenterology and Hepatology* 20, no. 12 (December 2022): 2868–2875.

Berinstein, Jeffrey A., Jessica Sheehan, Michael Dias et al. "Tofacitinib for Biologic-Experienced Hospitalized Patients with Acute Severe Ulcerative Colitis: A Retrospective Case-Control Study." *Clinical Gastroenterology and Hepatology* 19, no. 10 (October 2021): 2112–2120.

Fritsch, Julia, Luis Garces, Maria A. Quintero et al. "Low-Fat, High-Fiber Diet Reduces Markers of Inflammation and Dysbiosis and Improves Quality of Life in Patients with Ulcerative Colitis." *Clinical Gastroenterology and Hepatology* 19 (2021): 1189–1199.

Gilat, T., A. Suissa, G. Leichtman et al. "A Comparative Study of Metronidazole and Sulfasalazine in Active, Not Severe, Ulcerative Colitis." *Journal of Clinical Gastroenterology* 9, no. 4 (1987): 415–417.

Gilat, T., G. Leichtman, G. Delpre et al. "A Comparison of Metronidazole and Sulfasalazine in the Maintenance of Remission in Patients with Ulcerative Colitis." *Journal of Clinical Gastroenterology* 11, no.4 (1989): 392–395.

Hanauer, Stephen, Remo Panaccione, Silvio Danese et al. "Tofacitinib Induction Therapy Reduces Symptoms Within Three Days for Patients with Ulcerative Colitis." *Clinical Gastroenterology and Hepatology* 17 (2019): 139–147.

Hou, Jason K., Bincy Abraham, Hashem El-Serag. "Dietary Intake and Risk of Developing Inflammatory Bowel Disease: A Systematic Review of the Literature." *American Journal of Gastroenterology* 106, no. 4 (April 2011): 563–573.

Khazdouz, Maryam, Naser Ebrahimi Daryani, Makan Cheraghpour et al. "The Effect of Selenium Supplementation on Disease Activity and Immune-Inflammatory Biomarkers in Patients with Mild-to-Moderate Ulcerative Colitis: A Randomized, Double-Blind, Placebo-Controlled Clinical Trial." *European Journal of Nutrition*. 62, no. 8 (December 2023): 3125–3134.

Pan, Yun, Ya Liu, Haizhuo Guo et al. "Associations Between Folate and Vitamin B12 Levels and Inflammatory Bowel Disease: A Meta-Analysis." *Nutrients* 9 (2017): 382.

Panaccione, Remo, Subrata Ghosh, Stephen Middleton et al. "Combination Therapy with Infliximab and Azathioprine Is Superior to Monotherapy with Either Agent in Ulcerative Colitis." *Gastroenterology* 146 (2014): 392–400.

Sands, Bruce W., Laurent Peyrin-Biroulet, Edward V. Loftus Jr. et al. "Vedolizumab verses Adalimumab for Moderate-to-Severe Ulcerative Colitis." *New England Journal of Medicine* 381 (2019): 1215–1226.

Tarar, Zahid Ijaz, Umer Farooq, Muhammad Usman Zafar et al. "A National Study of Pregnancy-Related Maternal and Fetal Outcomes in Women with Inflammatory Bowel Disease." *International Journal of Colorectal Disease* 37 (2022): 1535–1543.

Wang, Xiao, Nan-qi Zhao, Yu-xin Sun et al. "Acupuncture for Ulcerative Colitis: A Systematic Review and Meta-Analysis of Randomized Clinical Trials." *BMC Complementary Therapies and Medicine* 20 (2020): 309.

Weisshof, Roni and Irit Chermesh. "Micronutrient Deficiencies in Inflammatory Bowel Disease." *Current Opinion in Clinical Nutrition & Metabolic Care* 18, no. 6 (November 2015): 576–581.

NOTES

APPENDICITIS

1 https://columbiasurgery.org/news/2015/06/04/history-medicine-mysterious-appendix.

2 Adamidis, D., E. Roma-Giannikou, K. Karamolegou et al. "Fiber Intake and Childhood Appendicitis." *International Journal of Food Sciences and Nutrition* 51 (2000): 153–157.

3 Brender, Jean D., Noel S. Weiss, Thomas D. Koepsell, and Edgar K. Marcuse. "Fiber Intake and Childhood Appendicitis." *American Journal of Public Health* 75, no. 4 (1985): 399–400.

4 Nelson, M., J. Morris, D. J. P. Barker, and S. Simmonds. "A Case-Control Study of Acute Appendicitis and Diet in Children." *Journal of Epidemiology and Community Health* 41 (1986): 316–318.

5 Peeters, Toon, Bert Houben, Peter Cools et al. "An Observational Study on Lifestyle and Environmental Risk Factors in Patients with Acute Appendicitis." *Heliyon* 9 (2023): e15131.

6 Basson, Marc D., Daniel Persinger, and William P. Newman. "Association of Colonoscopy with Risk of Appendicitis." *JAMA Surgery* 153, no. 1 (January 1, 2018): 90–91.

7 Lee, Steven L., Rebecca Stark, Arezou Yaghoubian et al. "Does Age Affect the Outcomes and Management of Pediatric Appendicitis?" *Journal of Pediatric Surgery* 46 (2011): 2342–2345.

8 Putnam, Luke R., KuoJen Tsao, Hoang T. Nguyen et al. "The Impact of Socioeconomic Status on Appendiceal Perforation in Pediatric Appendicitis." *Journal of Pediatrics* 170 (March 2016): 156–160.e1.

9 Bayissa, Badhaasaa Beyene, Pufa Miressa, Adnan Abulkadir, and Gelana Fekadu. "Predictors of Complicated Appendicitis Among Patients Presented to Public Referral Hospitals in Harari, Eastern Ethiopia: A Case-Control Study." *Surgery in Practice and Science* 9 (2022): 100072.

10 Yeob, K. E., S. Y. Kim, J. E. Park, and J. H. Park. "Complicated Appendicitis Among Adults with and Without Disabilities: A Cross-Sectional Nationwide Study in South Korea." *Frontiers in Public Health* 10 (2022): 813608.

11 Flum, D. R., G. H. Davidson, S. E. Monsell et al. "A Randomized Trial Comparing Antibiotics with Appendectomy for Appendicitis." *New England Journal of Medicine* 383, no. 20 (November 12, 2020): 1907–1919.

12 Lunardi, Nicole, Melissa Thornton, Ben L. Zarzaur et al. "Potential Risks of Nonoperative Management of Appendicitis in High-Risk Patients." *Surgery* 176, no. 6 (December 2024): 1568–1575.

13 Sippola, Suvi, Jussi Haijanen, Lauri Viinikainen et al. "Quality of Life and Patient Satisfaction at Seven-Year Follow-Up of Antibiotics Therapy vs Appendectomy for Uncomplicated Acute Appendicitis." *JAMA Surgery* 155, no. 4 (February 19, 2020): 283–289.

14 St. Peter, Shawn D., Janelle R. Noel-MacDonnell, Nigel J. Hall et al. "Appendectomy versus Antibiotics for Acute Uncomplicated Appendicitis in Children: An Open-Label, International, Multicentre, Randomised, Non-Inferiority Trial." *Lancet* 405, no. 10474 (January 2025): 233–240.

15 Ghahramani, Leila, Reza Roshanravan, Shahin Khodaei et al. "Acute Appendicitis as Complication of Colon Transit Time Study: A Case Report." *Middle East Journal of Digestive Diseases* 7, no. 3 (July 2015): 185–188.

16 Kao, Li-Ting, Ming-Chieh Tsai, Herng-Ching, and Cha-Ze Lee. "Association Between Gastroesophageal Reflux Disease and Appendicitis: A Population-Based Case-Control Study." *Scientific Reports* 6, no. 1 (March 2016): 22430.

17 Kim, So Young, Hyung-Jong Kim, Hyun Lim et al. "Increased Risk of Appendectomy in Patients with Gastroesophageal Reflux Disease." *Medicine* 97, no. 52 (2018): e13700.

BARRETT'S ESOPHAGUS

1 Shalauta, Mark A., and Richard Saad. "Barrett's Esophagus." *American Family Physician* 69, no. 9 (May 1, 2004): 2113–2118.

2 Kubo, Ai, T. R. Levin, Gladys Block et al. "Dietary Antioxidants, Fruits and Vegetables, and the Risk of Barrett's Esophagus." *American Journal of Gastroenterology* 103, no. 7 (July 2008): 1614–1624.

3 Thompson, Olivia M., Shirley A. A. Beresford, Elizabeth A. Kirk, and Thomas I. Vaughan. "Vegetable and Fruit Intakes and Risk of Barrett's Esophagus in Men and Women." *American Journal of Clinical Nutrition* 89 (2009): 890–896.

4 Sun, Lingli, Zhizhong Zhang, Jian Xu et al. "Dietary Fiber Intake Reduces Risk for Barrett's Esophagus and Esophageal Cancer." *Critical Reviews in Food Science and Nutrition* 57, no. 13 (2017): 2749–2757.

5 Gashi, Zaim, Ljube Ivkovski, Ragip Shabani et al. "What Are Protective Factors for Developing of Barrett's Esophagus in Patients with GERD—Our Experience." *Acta Informatica Medica* 19, no. 3 (September 2011): 146–148.

6 O'Doherty, Mark G., Marie M. Cantwell, Liam J. Murray et al. "Dietary Fat and Meat Intakes and Risk of Reflux Esophagitis, Barrett's Esophagus and Esophageal Adenocarcinoma." *International Journal of Cancer* 129, no. 6 (September 15, 2011): 1493–1502.

7 Coleman, Helen G., Shivaram Bhat, Brian T. Johnston et al. "Tobacco Smoking Increases the Risk of High-Grade Dysplasia and Cancer Among Patients with Barrett's Esophagus." *Gastroenterology* 142 (2012): 233–240.

8 El-Serag, Hashem B., Peter Kvapil, Joan Hacken-Bitar, and Jennifer R. Kramer. "Abdominal Obesity and the Risk of Barrett's Esophagus." *American Journal of Gastroenterology* 100 (2005): 2151–2156.

9 Hilal, J., H. B. El-Serag, D. Ramsey et al. "Physical Activity and the Risk of Barrett's Esophagus." *Diseases of the Esophagus* 29 (2016): 248–254.

10 Lam, Stephen, Leo Alexandre, Robert Luben, and Andrew Hart. "The Association Between Physical Activity and the Risk of Symptomatic Barrett's Oesophagus: A UK Prospective Cohort Study." *European Journal of Gastroenterology & Hepatology* 30 (2018): 71–75.

11 Jankowski, J. A. Z., J. de Caestecker, S. B. Love et al. "Esomeprazole and Aspirin in Barrett's Oesophagus (AspECT): A Randomized Factorial Trial." *Lancet* 392 (2018): 400–408.

12 Jovani, M., Y. Cao, D. Feskanich et al. "Aspirin Use is Associated with Lower Risk of Barrett's Esophagus in Women." *Clinical and Translational Gastroenterology* 8, no. 12 (December 2017): e131.

13 Hu, Q., T. T. Sun, J. Hong et al. "Proton Pump Inhibitors Do Not Reduce the Risk of Esophageal Adenocarcinoma in Patients with Barrett's Esophagus: A Systematic Review and Meta-Analysis." *PLoS One* 12, no. 1 (2017): e0169691.

14 Karimian, M., M. Salamati, and M. Azami. "The Relationship Between Metabolic Syndrome and Increased Risk of Barrett's Esophagus: An Updated Systematic Review and Meta-Analysis." *BMC Gastroenterology* 20 (2020): 138.

15 Ren, Lin-Lin, Ting-Ting Yan, Zhen-Hua Wang et al. "Alcohol Consumption and the Risk of Barrett's Esophagus: A Comprehensive Meta-Analysis." *Scientific Reports* 5 (2015): 16048.

16 Sikkema, M., P. J. F. De Jonge, E. W. Steyerberg, and E. J. Kuipers. "Risk of Esophageal Adenocarcinoma and Mortality in Patients with Barrett's Esophagus: A Systematic Review and Meta-Analysis." *Clinical Gastroenterology and Hepatology* 8 (2010): 235–244.

CANCER, COLORECTAL

1 Schlussel, Andrew T., Ronald A. Gagliano Jr., Susan Seto-Donlon et al. "The Evolution of Colorectal Cancer Genetics—Part 1: From Discovery to Practice." *Journal of Gastrointestinal Oncology* 5, no. 5 (2014): 326–335.

2 https://www.cancer.org/cancer/types/colon-rectal-cancer/about/key-statistics.html.

3 Jin, D., Y. Lu, W. Wu et al. "Diet-Wide Association, Genetic Susceptibility and Colorectal Cancer Risk: A Prospective Cohort Study." *Nutrients* 15 (2023): 4801.

4 O'Sullivan, Dylan E., R. Liam Sutherland, Susanna Town et al. "Risk Factors for Early-Onset Colorectal Cancer: A Systematic Review and Meta-Analysis." *Clinical Gastroenterology and Hepatology* 20 (2022): 1229–1240.

5 Papadimitriou, N., E. Bouras, P. A. van den Brandt et al. "A Prospective Diet-Wide Association Study for Risk of Colorectal Cancer in EPIC." *Clinical Gastroenterology and Hepatology* 20, no. 4 (April 2022): 864–873.

6 Yang, Yunfan, Li Yang, Liping Zhou, and Siyuan Tang. "A Critical Review of the Effect of Dietary Fiber Intake on the Prevention of Colorectal Cancer in Eastern Asian Countries." *Journal of Healthcare Engineering* 2021 (2021): 6680698.

7 Chan, Doris S., Rosa Lau, Dagfinn Aune et al. "Red and Processed Meat and Colorectal Cancer Incidence: Meta-Analysis of Prospective Studies." *PLoS One* 6, no. 6 (June 2011): e20456.

8 Shroff, Jennifer, Nirav Thosani, Sachin Batra et al. "Reduced Incidence and Mortality from Colorectal Cancer with Flexible Sigmoidoscopy Screening: A Meta-Analysis." *World Journal of Gastroenterology* 20, no. 48 (December 28, 2014): 18466–18476.

9 Chierici, Andrea, Paolo Amoretti, Céline Drai et al. "Does Bariatric Surgery Reduce the Risk of Colorectal Cancer in Individuals with Morbid Obesity? A Systematic Review and Meta-Analysis." *Nutrients* 15 (2023): 467.

10 Derogar, Maryam, Mark A. Hull, Prashant Kant et al. "Increased Risk of Colorectal Cancer After Obesity Surgery." *Annals of Surgery* 258, no. 6 (December 2013): 983–988.

11 Jafari, F., S. Yarmand, M. Nouri et al. "Ultra-Processed Food Intake and Risk of Colorectal Cancer: A Matched Case-Control Study." *Nutrition and Cancer* 75, no. 2 2023): 532–541.

12 Leufkens, Anke M., Fränzel J. B. Van Duijnhoven, Peter D. Siersema et al. "Cigarette Smoking and Colorectal Cancer Risk in the European Prospective Investigation into Cancer and Nutrition Study." *Clinical Gastroenterology and Hepatology* 9 (2011): 137–144.

13 Boughanem, H., S. Canudas, P. Hernandez-Alonso et al. "Vitamin D Intake and the Risk of Colorectal Cancer: An Updated Meta-Analysis and Systematic Review of Case-Control and Prospective Cohort Studies." *Cancers* 13 (2021): 2814.

14 Gylling, B., R. Myte, J. Schneede et al. "Vitamin B-6 and Colorectal Cancer Risk: A Prospective Population-Based Study Using 3 Distinct Plasma Markers of Vitamin B-6 Status." *American Journal of Clinical Nutrition* 105 (2017): 897–904.

15 Huang, Chu-Yi, Alinuer Abulimiti, Xin Zhang et al. "Dietary B Vitamins and Methionine Intakes and Risk for Colorectal Cancer: A Case-Control Study in China." *British Journal of Nutrition* 123 (2020): 1277–1289.

16 Jacobs, Eric J., Cari J. Connell, Alpa V. Patel et al. "Vitamin C and Vitamin E Supplement Use and Colorectal Cancer Mortality in a Large American Cancer Society Cohort." *Cancer Epidemiology, Biomarkers & Prevention* 10 (January 2001): 17–23.

17 Wang, Yu, Jing-Wen Yang, Shi-Yan Yan et al. "Electroacupuncture vs Sham Electroacupuncture in the Treatment of Postoperative Ileus After Laparoscopic Surgery for Colorectal Cancer: A Multicenter, Randomized Clinical Trial." *JAMA Surgery* 158, no. 1 (2023): 20–27.

CANCER, ESOPHAGEAL

1 Eslick, Guy D. "Esophageal Cancer: A Historical Perspective." *Gastroenterology Clinics of North America* 38, no. 1 (2009): 1–15.

2 https://www.cancer.org/cancer/types/esophagus-cancer/about/key-statistics.html.

3 Zhang, Han-Ze, Guang-Fu Jin, and Hong-Bing Shen. "Epidemiologic Differences in Esophageal Cancer Between Asian and Western Populations." *Chinese Journal of Cancer* 31, no. 6 (2012): 281–286.

4 Oze, Isao, Keitaro Matsuo, Hidemi Ito et al. "Cigarette Smoking and Esophageal Cancer Risk: An Evaluation Based on a Systematic Review of Epidemiologic Evidence Among the Japanese Population." *Japanese Journal of Clinical Oncology* 42, no. 1 (2012): 63–73.

5 Wang, Qiao-Li, Shao-Hua Xie, Wen-Tao Li, and Jesper Lagergren. "Smoking Cessation and Risk of Esophageal Cancer by Histological Type: Systematic Review and Meta-Analysis." *JNCI Journal of the National Cancer Institute* 109, no. 12 (2017): djx115.

6 Kumagai, N., T. Wakai, K. Akazawa et al. "Heavy Alcohol Intake is a Risk Factor for Esophageal Squamous Cell Carcinoma Among Middle-Aged Men: A Case-Control and Simulation Study." *Molecular and Clinical Oncology* 1 (2013): 811–816.

7 Cho, Jae Ho, Cheol Min Shin, Kyung-Do Han et al. "Abdominal Obesity Increases Risk for Esophageal Cancer: A Nationwide Population-Based Cohort Study of South Korea." *Journal of Gastroenterology* 55 (2020): 307–316.

8 Luo, Hui and Hong Ge. "Hot Tea Consumption and Esophageal Cancer Risk: A Meta-Analysis of Observational Studies." *Frontiers in Nutrition* 9 (April 2022): 831567.

9 Engeland, Anders, Steinar Tretli, and Tone Bjørge. "Height and Body Mass Index in Relation to Esophageal Cancer; 23-Year Follow-Up of Two Million Norwegian Men and Women." *Cancer Causes and Control* 15 (2004): 837–843.

10 Keszei, A. P., L. J. Schouten, R. A. Goldbohm, and P. A. van den Brandt. "Red and Processed Meat Consumption and the Risk of Esophageal and Gastric Cancer Subtypes in The Netherlands Cohort Study." *Annals of Oncology* 23 (2012): 2319–2326.

11 Liu, Jun, Jian Wang, Ye Leng, and Changxing Lv. "Intake of Fruit and Vegetables and Risk of Esophageal Squamous Cell Carcinoma: A Meta-Analysis of Observational Studies." *International Journal of Cancer* 133 (2013): 473–486.

12 Tang, L., A. H. Lee, F. Xu et al. "Fruit and Vegetable Consumption and Risk of Esophageal Cancer: A Case-Control Study in North-West China." *Diseases of the Esophagus* 27 (2014): 777–782.

13 Wang, Lu, Cong Wang, Jiangfeng Wang et al. "Longitudinal, Observational Study on Associations Between Postoperative Nutritional Vitamin D Supplementation and Clinical Outcomes in Esophageal Cancer Patients Undergoing Esophagectomy." *Scientific Reports* 6 (2016): 38962.

14 Ma, Jun-Li, Yan Zhao, Chen-Yang Guo et al. "Dietary Vitamin B Intake and the Risk of Esophageal Cancer: A Meta-Analysis." *Cancer Management and Research* 10 (2018): 5395–5410.

15 Bo, Yacong, Yan Lu, Yan Zhao et al. "Association Between Dietary Vitamin C Intake and Risk of Esophageal Cancer: A Dose-Response Meta-Analysis." *International Journal of Cancer* 138 (2016): 1843–1850.

16 Cui, Lingling, Li Li, Yalan Tian et al. "Association Between Dietary Vitamin E Intake and Esophageal Cancer Risk: An Update Meta-Analysis." *Nutrients* 10 (2018): 801.

17 Hong, Seungcheol, Bongki Park, Hyeonseok Noh, and Dong-Jun Choi. "Herbal Medicine for Dumping Syndrome: A Systematic Review and Meta-Analysis." *Integrative Cancer Therapies* 18 (2019): NA.

18 Li, Honglin, Chunzheng Ma, Sisi Chang et al. "Traditional Chinese Medicine Decoctions Improve Longevity Following Diagnosis with Stage IV Esophageal Squamous Cell Carcinoma: A Retrospective Analysis." *International Journal of General Medicine* 15 (2022): 1665–1675.

CANCER, LIVER

1 https://www.aacr.org/blog/2020/10/19/how-two-nobel-prize-winning-discoveries-help-shape-liver-cancer-prevention/#:~:text=In%20the%201960s%2C%20while%20analyzing,HBV%20could%20cause%20liver%20cancer.

2 https://www.cancer.org/cancer/types/liver-cancer/about/what-is-key-statistics.html.

3 Zhang, Wei, Xiao-Ou Shu, Honglan Li et al. "Vitamin Intake and Liver Cancer Risk: A Report from Two Cohort Studies in China." *Journal of the National Cancer Institute* 104 (2012): 1173–1181.

4 Lee, Junga. "Associations Between Physical Activity and Liver Cancer Risks and Mortality: A Systematic Review and Meta-Analysis." *International Journal of Environmental Research and Public Health* 17 (2020): 8943.

5 Li, Juan, Qinqin Cheng, Xiangqian Zhu et al. "The Relationship of Exercise and Cancer-Related Fatigue in Patients with Advanced Liver Cancer: A Cross-Sectional Study." *Scientific Reports* 13 (2023): 17341.

6 Yi, Zhenghui, Linjie Wang, and Xiangqun Tu. "Effect of Vitamin D deficiency on Liver Cancer Risk: A Systematic Review and Meta-Analysis." *Asian Pacific Journal of Cancer Prevention* 22, no. 4 (April 2021): 991–997.

7 Koh, W.-P., K. Robien, R. Wang et al. "Smoking as an Independent Risk Factor for Hepatocellular Carcinoma: The Singapore Chinese Health Study." *British Journal of Cancer* 105 (2011): 1430–1435.

8 Wen, Q., K. H. Chan, K. Shi et al. "Tobacco Smoking and Solid Fuels for Cooking and Risk of Liver Cancer: A Prospective Cohort Study of 0.5 Million Chinese Adults." *International Journal of Cancer* 151 (2022): 181–190.

9 de Martel, C., D. Maucort-Boulch, M. Plummer, and S. Franceshi. "World-Wide Relative Contribution of Hepatitis B and C Viruses in Hepatocellular Carcinoma." *Hepatology* 62 (2015): 1190–1200.

10 Park, Hana, Seung Kak Shin, Ijin Joo et al. "Systematic Review and Meta-Analysis: Low-Level Alcohol Consumption and the Risk of Liver Cancer." *Gut and Liver* 14, no. 6 (2020): 792–807.

11 Okinaga, Hiroko, Hideo Yasunaga, Kiyoshi Hasegawa et al. "Short-Term Outcomes Following Hepatectomy in Elderly Patients with Hepatocellular Carcinoma: An Analysis of 10,805 Septuagenarians and 2,381 Octo- and Nonagenarians in Japan." *Liver Cancer* 7 (2018): 55–64.

12 Kim, Gyuri, Suk-Yong Jang, Chung Mo Nam, and Eun Seok Kang. "Statin Use and the Risk of Hepatocellular Carcinoma in Patients at High Risk: A Nationwide Nested Case-Control Study." *Journal of Hepatology* 68 (2018): 476–484.

13 Thrift, A. P., Y. Natarajan, Y. Liu, and H. B. El-Serag. "Statin Use After Diagnosis of Hepatocellular Carcinoma is Associated with Decreased Mortality." *Clinical Gastroenterology and Hepatology* 17 (2019): 2117–2125.

14 Zhang, Qiao, Rong Wan, and Changdan Liu. "The Impact of Intense Nursing Care in Improving Anxiety, Depression, and Quality of Life in Patients with Liver Cancer." *Medicine* 99 (2020): 34.

15 Peng, L., L. Xiang, Z. Xu et al. "Association Between Low-Fat Diet and Liver Cancer Risk in 98,455 Participants: Results from a Prospective Study." *Frontiers in Nutrition* 9 (2022): 1013643.

16 Lee, Chang-Hyeong, Byung-Seok Kim, Ji-Suk Kim et al. "The Effects of Acupuncture on the Insomnia, Anxiety and Depression of Liver Cancer Patients: Pilot Study." *Journal of Korean Oriental Medicine* 33, no. 2 (2012): 34–46.

CANCER, ORAL

1 Inchingolo, F., L. Santacroce, A. Ballini et al. "Oral Cancer: A Historical Review." *International Journal of Environmental Research and Public Health* 17, no. 9 (2020): 3168.

2 https://www.nidcr.nih.gov/health-info/oral-cancer.

3 Inchingolo, Santacroce, Ballini et al. "Oral Cancer: A Historical Review." *International Journal of Environmental Research and Public Health* 17 (2020); 3168.

4 Ou, Meijun, Guifen Wang, Yixia Yan et al. "Perioperative Symptoms Burden and Its Influencing Factors in Patients with Oral Cancer: A Longitudinal Study." *Asia-Pacific Journal of Oncology Nursing* 9 (2022): 100073.

5 Murariu, Alice, Elena-Raluca Baciu, Livia Bobu et al. "Knowledge, Practice, and Awareness of Oral Cancer and HPV Infection Among Dental Students and Residents: A Cross-Sectional Study." *Medicina* 58 (2022): 806.

6 Mariano, Lorena C., Saman Warnakulasuriya, Kurt Straif, and Luis Monteiro. "Secondhand Smoke Exposure and Oral Cancer Risk: A Systematic Review and Meta-Analysis." *Tobacco Control* 31, no. 5 (2022): 597–607.

7 Yoo, J. E., K. Han, D. W. Shin et al. "Association Between Changes in Alcohol Consumption and Cancer Risk." *JAMA Network Open* 5, no. 8 (2022): e2228544.

8 Shimpi, Neel, Monica Jethwani, Aditi Bharatkumar et al. "Patient Awareness/Knowledge Towards Oral Cancer: A Cross-Sectional Survey." *BMC Oral Health* 18 (2018): 86.

9 Gulve, N. D., P. R. Tripathi, S. D. Dahivelkar et al. "Evaluation of YouTube Videos as a Source of Information About Oral Self-Examination to Detect Oral Cancer and Precancerous Lesions." *Journal of International Society of Preventive and Community Dentistry* 12 (2022): 226–234.

10 Ndayisabye, H., A. Ndagijimana, E. Biracyaza, and A. Umubyeyi. "Factors Associated with Oral Cancer Adverse Outcome at the Rwanda Military Hospital, a Retrospective Cross-Sectional Study." *Frontiers in Oral Health* 3 (March 2022): 844254.

11 Mu, G., J. Wang, Z. Liu et al. "Association Between Smokeless Tobacco Use and Oral Cavity Cancer Risk in Women Compared with Men: A Systematic Review and Meta-Analysis." *BMC Cancer* 21 (2021): 960.

12 Khan, Z., S. Dreger, S. M. H. Shah et al. "Oral Cancer via the Bargain Bin: The Risk of Oral Cancer Associated with a Smokeless Tobacco Product (Naswar)." *PLoS One* 12, no. 7 (2017): e0180445.

13 Cameron, Alice, Hao Meng Yip, and Montey Garg. "E-Cigarettes and Oral Cancer: What Do We Know So Far?" *British Journal of Oral and Maxillofacial Surgery* 61 (2023): 380–382.

14 Nguyen, Hoang, Joseph P. Kitzmiller, Kieu Tho Nguyen et al. "Oral Carcinoma Associated with Chronic Use of Electronic Cigarettes." *Otolaryngology* 7, no. 2 (2017): 304.

15 Udeabor, Samuel E., Abdullah M. Albejadi, Waleed A. K. Al-Shehri et al. "Serum Levels of 25-Hydroxy-Vitamin D in Patients with Oral Squamous Cell Carcinoma: Making the Case for Chemoprevention." *Clinical and Experimental Dental Research* 6 (2020): 428–432.

16 Wang, Jing, Yi Fan, Jiawen Qian et al. "Relationship Between Dietary Fiber and Vitamin C Intake and Oral Cancer." *Frontiers in Public Health* 10 (2022): 880506.

CANCER, PANCREATIC

1 https://my.clevelandclinic.org/health/diseases/15806-pancreatic-cancer.

2 Griffin, James F., Katherine E. Poruk, and Christopher L. Wolfgang. "Pancreatic Cancer Surgery: Past, Present, and Future." *Chinese Journal of Cancer Research* 27, no. 4 (August 2015): 332–348.

3 https://my.clevelandclinic.org/health/diseases/15806-pancreatic-cancer.

4 https://www.cancer.org/cancer/types/pancreatic-cancer/about/key-statistics.html.

5 Jansen, Rick J., Dennis P. Robinson, Rachael Z. Stolzenberg-Solomon et al. "Nutrients from Fruits and Vegetable Consumption Reduce the Risk of Pancreatic Cancer." *Journal of Gastrointestinal Cancer* 44, no. 2 (June 2013): 152–161.

6 Larsson, Susanna C., Niclas Håkansson, Ingmar Näslund et al. "Fruit and Vegetable Consumption in Relation to Pancreatic Cancer Risk: A Prospective Study." *Cancer Epidemiology Biomarkers & Prevention* 15, no. 2 (February 2006): 301–305.

7 Bosetti, C., F. Turati, A. Dal Pont et al. "The Role of Mediterranean Diet on the Risk of Pancreatic Cancer." *British Journal of Cancer* 109 (2013): 1360–1366.

8 Nöthlings, Ute, Lynne R. Wilkens, Suzanne P. Murphy et al. "Meat and Fat Intake as Risk Factors for Pancreatic Cancer: The Multiethnic Cohort Study." *Journal of the National Cancer Institute* 97, no. 19 (October 5, 2005): 1458–1465.

9 Wolpin, Brian M., Kimmie Ng, Ying Bao et al. "Plasma 25-Hydroxyvitamin D and Risk of Pancreatic Cancer." *Cancer Epidemiology, Biomarkers & Prevention* 21, no. 1 (January 2012): 82–91.

10 Cho, May, Parvin F. Peddi, Kevin Ding et al. "Vitamin D Deficiency and Prognostics Among Patients with Pancreatic Adenocarcinoma." *Journal of Translational Medicine* 11 (2013): 206.

11 Fan, Hua, Jiantao Kou, Dongdong Han et al. "Association Between Vitamin C Intake and the Risk of Pancreatic Cancer: A Meta-Analysis of Observational Studies." *Scientific Reports* 5 (2015): 13973.

12 Wei, Dan-Hong and Qi-Qi Mao. "Vitamin B6, Vitamin B12 and Methionine and Risk of Pancreatic Cancer: A Meta-Analysis." *Nutrition Journal* 19 (2020): 111.

13 Rosebrock, Kim, Marianne Sinn, Faik G. Uzunoglu et al. "Effects of Exercise Training on Patient-Specific Outcomes in Pancreatic Cancer Patients: A Scoping Review." *Cancers* 15 (2023): 5899.

14 Wong, Wendy, Bing Zhong Chen, Allyson Kin Yan Lee et al. "Chinese Herbal Medicine Effectively Prolongs the Overall Survival of Pancreatic Cancer Patients: A Case Series." *Integrative Cancer Therapies* 18 (2019): NA.

15 Li, Bin, Run Gan, Quanjun Yang et al. "Chinese Herbal Medicines as an Adjunctive Therapy for Unresectable Pancreatic Cancer: A Systematic Review and Meta-Analysis." *Evidence-Based Complementary and Alternative Medicine* 2015 (2015): 350730.

16 Eggers, Christine, Elisabeth Olliges, Stefan Boeck et al. "Exploring Pain, Quality of Life, and Emotional Well-Being in Patients with Advanced Pancreatic Cancer Practicing Spiritual Meditation: A Pilot Study." *Complementary Medicine Research* 30 (2023): 289–298.

CANCER, STOMACH

1 https://www.uptodate.com/contents/epidemiology-of-gastric-cancer/print#:~:text=Gastric%20cancer%20has%20been%20described,most%20common%20and%20lethal%20cancer.

2 https://www.cancer.org/cancer/types/stomach-cancer/about/key-statistics.html.

3 https://www.uptodate.com/contents/epidemiology-of-gastric-cancer/print#:~:text=Gastric%20cancer%20has%20been%20described,most%20common%20and%20lethal%20cancer.

4 Shimazu, T., K. Wakai, A. Tamakoshi et al. "Association of Vegetable and Fruit Intake with Gastric Cancer Risk Among Japanese: A Pooled Analysis of Four Cohort Studies." *Annals of Oncology* 25 (2014): 1228–1233.

5 Wang, Q., Y. Chen, X. Wang et al. "Consumption of Fruit, But Not Vegetables, May Reduce Risk of Gastric Cancer: Results from a Meta-Analysis of Cohort Studies." *European Journal of Cancer* 50 (2014): 1498–1509.

6 Naemi Kermanshahi, M., E. Safaei, H. Tutunchi et al. "Fruit and Vegetable Intake in Relation to Gastric Cancer Risk: A Comprehensive and Updated Systematic Review and Dose-Response Meta-Analysis of Cohort Studies." *Frontiers in Nutrition* 10 (2023): 973171.

7 Zhu, Qin, Long Shu, Feng Zhou et al. "Adherence to the Mediterranean Diet and Risk of Gastric Cancer: A Systematic Review and Dose-Response Meta-Analysis." *Frontiers in Nutrition* 10 (September 8, 2023): 1259453.

8 Ladeiras-Lopes, Ricardo, Alexandra Kirchhofer Pereira, Amanda Nogueira et al. "Smoking and Gastric Cancer: Systematic Review and Meta-Analysis of Cohort Studies." *Cancer Causes & Control* 19 (2008): 689–701.

9 Vyas, Neil, Rafael Ching Companioni, Melik Tiba et al. "Association Between Serum Vitamin D Levels and Gastric Cancer: A Retrospective Chart Analysis." *World Journal of Gastrointestinal Oncology* 8, no. 9 (September 15, 2016): 688–694.

10 Hoang, B. V., J. Lee, I. J. Choi et al. "Effect of Dietary Vitamin C on Gastric Cancer Risk in the Korean Population." *World Journal of Gastroenterology* 22, no. 27 (July 21, 2016): 6257–6267.

11 He, J., H. Fu, C. Li et al. "Association Between Vitamin B12 and Risk of Gastric Cancer: A Systematic Review and Meta-Analysis of Epidemiological Studies." *Nutrition and Cancer* 74, no. 9 (2022): 3263–3273.

12 Khairan, Paramita, Tomotaka Sobue, Ehab Salah Eshak et al. "Association of B Vitamins and Methionine Intake with the Risk of Gastric Cancer: The Japan Public Health Center-Based Prospective Study." *Cancer Prevention Research* 15 (2022): 101–110.

13 Zhou, Y., W. Zhuang, W. Hu et al. "Consumption of Large Amounts of *Allium* Vegetables Reduces Risk for Gastric Cancer in a Meta-Analysis." Gastroenterology 141 (2011): 80–89.

14 Kim, Hanseul, NaNa Keum, Edward L. Giovannucci et al. "Garlic Intake and Gastric Cancer Risk: Results from Two Large Prospective US Cohort Studies." *International Journal of Cancer* 143, no. 5 (September 1, 2018): 1047–1053.

15 Zhao, Z., Z. Yin, and Q. Zhao. "Red and Processed Meat Consumption and Gastric Cancer Risk: A Systematic Review and Meta-Analysis." *Oncotarget* 8, no. 18 (2017): 30563–30575.

16 Zhu, H., X. Yang, C. Zhang et al. "Red and Processed Meat Intake is Associated with Higher Gastric Cancer Risk: A Meta-Analysis of Epidemiological Observational Studies." *PLoS One* 8, no. 8 (2013): e70955.

17 Wu, X., L. Chen, J. Cheng et al. "Effects of Dietary Salt Intake on Risk of Gastric Cancer: A Systematic Review and Meta-Analysis of Case-Control Studies." *Nutrients* 14 (2022): 4260.

18 Song, Minkyo, Ji-Yeob Chai, Jae Jeong Yang et al. "Obesity at Adolescence and Gastric Cancer Risk." *Cancer Causes & Control* 26 (2015): 247–256.

CELIAC DISEASE

1 https://www.beyondceliac.org/celiac-disease/celiac-history/.

2 Murray, J. A., T. Watson, B. Clearman, and F. Mitros. "Effect of a Gluten-Free Diet on Gastrointestinal Symptoms in Celiac Disease." *American Journal of Clinical Nutrition* 79 (2004): 669–673.

3 Wierdsma, Nicolette, Marian A. E. van Bokhorst-de van der Schueren, Marijke Beerkenpas et al. "Vitamin and Mineral Deficiencies are Highly Prevalent in Newly Diagnosed Celiac Disease Patients." *Nutrients* 5 (2013): 3975–3992.

4 Berry, Neha, Jahangeer Basha, Neelam Varma et al. "Anemia in Celiac Disease is Multifactorial in Etiology: A Prospective Study from India." *JGH Open* 2 (2018): 196–200.

5 Mosca, Caterina, Fanney Thorsteinsdottir, Bo Abrahamsen et al. "Newly Diagnosed Celiac Disease and Bone Health in Young Adults: A Systematic Literature Review." *Calcified Tissue International* 110 (2022): 641–648.

6 Fedewa, Michael V., JessicaL. Bentley, Simon Higgins et al. "Celiac Disease and Bone Health in Children and Adolescents: A Systematic Review and Meta-Analysis." *Journal of Clinical Densitometry* 23, no. 2 (2020): 200–211.

7 Ganji, Reza, Meysam Moghbeli, Ramin Sadeghi et al. "Prevalence of Osteoporosis and Osteopenia in Men and Premenopausal Women with Celiac Disease: A Systematic Review." *Nutrition Journal* 18 (2019): 9.

8 Kotze, Lorete M. S., Thelma Skare, Antonella Vinholi et al. "Impact of a Gluten-Free Diet on Bone Mineral Density in Celiac Patients." *Revista Espanõla de Enfermedades Digestivas* 108, no. 2 (2016): 84–88.

9 Shahbazkhani, B., N. Aletaha, A. Khonche et al. "Is It Necessary to Screen for Celiac Disease in Adult Idiopathic Osteoporosis?" *Gastroenterology and Hepatology from Bed to Bench* 8, no. 2 (2015): 140–145.

10 Costa, Allysson and Gleisson A. P. de Brito. "Aerobic Exercise Associated with Fish Oil Supplementation Decreases C-Reactive Protein and Interleukin-6 in Celiac Disease Patients." *Journal of Nutrition and Metabolism* 2022 (2022): 3908675.

11 Grode, L., B. H. Bech, O. Plana-Rippoll et al. "Reproductive Life in Women with Celiac Disease: A Nationwide, Population-Based Matched Cohort Study." *Human Reproduction* 33, no. 8 (2018): 1538–1547.

12 Ghadir, M., A. Iranikhah, M. Jandaghi et al. "Unexplained Infertility as Primary Presentation of Celiac Disease, a Case Report and Literature Review." *Iranian Journal of Reproductive Medicine* 9, no. 2 (Spring 2011): 135–140.

13 Ungprasert, Patompong, Karn Wijarnpreecha, and Pansakorn Tanratana. "Risk of Venous Thromboembolism in Patients with Celiac Disease: A Systematic Review and Meta-Analysis." *Journal of Gastroenterology and Hepatology* 31, no. 7 (July 2016): 1240–1245.

14 Riznik, Petra, Luigina De Leo, Jasmina Dolinsek et al. "The Knowledge About Celiac Disease Among Healthcare Professionals and Patients in Central Europe." *Journal of Pediatric Gastroenterology and Nutrition* 72, no. 4 (April 1, 2021): 552–557.

15 Lebwohl, Benjamin, Peter H. R. Green, Louise Emilsson et al. "Cancer Risk in 47,241 Individuals with Celiac Disease: A Nationwide Cohort Study." *Clinical Gastroenterology and Hepatology* 20 (2022): e111–e131.

16 Green, Peter H. R., Aaron T. Fleischauer, Govind Bhagat et al. "Risk of Malignancy in Patients with Celiac Disease." *American Journal of Medicine* 115, no. 3 (August 15, 2003): 191–195.

COLON POLYPS

1 Fliss-Isakov, Naomi, Revital Kariv, Muriel Webb et al. "Mediterranean Dietary Components are Inversely Associated with Advanced Colorectal Polyps: A Case-Control Study." *World Journal of Gastroenterology* 24, no. 24 (June 29, 2018): 2617–2627.

2 Tantamango, Y. M., S. F. Knutsen, L. Beeson et al. "Association Between Dietary Fiber and Incident Cases of Colon Polyps: The Adventist Health Study." *Gastrointestinal Cancer Research* 4 (2011): 161–167.

3 Sonnenberg, Amnon, Kevin O. Turner, and Robert M. Genta. "Increased Risk for Colon Polyps in Patients with Reflux Disease." *Digestive Diseases and Sciences* 63 (2018): 228–233.

4 Salimian, Sina, Maryam Habbi, Mojtaba Sehat, and Abbas Hajian. "Obesity and Incidence of Colorectal Polyps: A Case-Control Study." *Annals of Medicine & Surgery* 85 (2023): 306–310.

5 Kim, Hong-Bae, Yong-Jae Lee, Jae-Yong Shim, and Hye-Ree Lee. "The Association Between Coronary Calcification and Adenomatous Polyps of Colon in Korean Adults." *Clinics and Research in Hepatology and Gastroenterology* 38 (2014): 649–654.

6 Huang, Hsin-En, Yi-Ching Yang, Jin-Shang Wu et al. "The Relationship Between Different Glycemic Statuses and Colon Polyps in a Taiwanese Population." *Journal of Gastroenterology* 49 (2014): 1145–1151.

7 Song, Mingyang, I-Min Lee, JoAnn E. Manson et al. "No Association Between Vitamin D Supplementation and Risk of Colorectal Adenomas or Serrated Polyps in a Randomized Trial." *Clinical Gastroenterology and Hepatology* 19, no. 1 (January 2021): 128–135.

8 Sun, Manchun, Manyi Sun, Li Zhang et al. "Colorectal Polyp Risk is Linked to an Elevated Level of Homocysteine." *Bioscience Reports* 38, no. 2 (April 2018): BSR20171699.

9 Fliss-Isakov, Naomi, Shira Zelber-Sagi, Muriel Webb et al. "Smoking Habits Are Strongly Associated with Colorectal Polyps in a Population-Based Case Control Study." *Journal of Clinical Gastroenterology* 52, no. 9 (October 2018): 805–811.

10 Figueiredo, Jane C., Seth D. Crookett, Dale C. Snover et al. "Smoking-Associated Risks of Conventional Adenomas and Serrated Polyps in the Colorectum." *Cancer Causes & Control* 26 (2015): 377–386.

11 Carr, Prudence R., Bernd Holleczek, Christa Stegmaier et al. "Meat Intake and Risk of Colorectal Polyps: Results from a Large Population-Based Screening Study in Germany." *American Journal of Clinical Nutrition* 105 (2017): 1453–1461.

12 Dowswell, George, Angela Ryan, Aliki Taylor et al. "Designing an Intervention to Help People with Colorectal Adenomas Reduce Their Intake of Red and Processed Meat and Increase Their Levels of Physical Activity: A Qualitative Study." *BMC Cancer* 12 (2012): 255.

13 McKeown-Eyssen, Gail, Catherine Holloway, Vartouhi Jazmaji et al. "A Randomized Trial of Vitamins C and E in the Prevention of Recurrence of Colorectal Polyps." *Cancer Research* 48 (August 15, 1988): 4701–4705.

14 Crockett, Seth D., Elizabeth L. Barry, Leila A. Mott et al. "Calcium and Vitamin D Supplementation and Increased Risk of Serrated Polyps: Results from a Randomized Clinical Trial." *Gut* 68, no. 3 (March 2019): 475–486.

15 Baillie, Lesley, Maurice B. Loughrey, and Helen G. Coleman. "Lifestyle Risk Factors for Serrated Colorectal Polyps: A Systematic Review and Meta-Analysis." *Gastroenterology* 152 (2017): 92–104.

16 Tran, Fiona and Jenn Hian Koo. "Birthplace Is Not a Determinant of Colorectal Adenomas." *World Journal of Gastroenterology* 20, no. 26 (July 14, 2014): 8606–8611.

CROHN'S DISEASE

1 https://www.crohnscolitisfoundation.org/about/our-beginning.

2 https://my.clevelandclinic.org/health/diseases/9357-crohns-disease.

3 Meyer, Antoine, Catherine Dong, Corinne Casagrande et al. "Food Processing and Risk of Crohn's Disease and Ulcerative Colitis: A European Prospective Cohort Study." *Clinical Gastroenterology and Hepatology* 21 (2023): 1607–1616.

4 Serrano Fernandez, Victor, Marta Seldas Palomino, José Alberto Laredo-Aguilera et al. "High-Fiber Diet and Crohn's Disease: Systematic Review and Meta-Analysis." *Nutrients* 15 (2023): 3114.

5 Jones, Patricia D., Michael D. Kappelman, Christopher F. Martin et al. "Exercise Decreases Risk of Future Active Disease in Patients with Inflammatory Bowel Disease in Remission." *Inflammatory Bowel Diseases* 2, no. 5 (May 2015): 1063–1071.

6 Albenberg, Lindsey, Colleen M. Brensinger, Qufei Wu et al. "A Diet Low in Red and Processed Meat Does Not Reduce Rate of Crohn's Disease Flares." *Gastroenterology* 157 (2019): 128–136.

7 Sadeghian, Mehdi, Parvane Saneei, Fereydoun Siassi, Ahmad Esmaillzadeh. "Vitamin D Status in Relationship To Crohn's Disease: Meta-Analysis of Observational Studies." *Nutrition* 32 (2016): 505–514.

8 Colombel, Jean-Frédéric, Tadakazu Hisamatsu, Raja Atreya et al. "Upadacitinib Reduces Crohn's Disease Symptoms Within the First Week of Induction Therapy." *Clinical Gastroenterology and Hepatology* 22, no. 8 (August 2024): 1668–1677.

9 Traboulsi, Cindy, Fares Ayoub, Alexa Silfen et al. "Upadacitinib is Safe and Effective for Crohn's Disease: Real-World Data from a Tertiary Center." *Digestive Diseases and Sciences* 68 (2023): 385–388.

10 Espi-López, Gemma V., Marta Inglés, Isabel Soliva-Cazabán, and Pilar Serra-Añó. "Effect of the Soft-Tissue Techniques in the Quality of Life in Patients in Crohn's Disease." *Medicine* 97, no. 51 (2018): e13811.

11 Naftali, Timna, Lihi Bar-Lev Schleider, Iris Dotan et al. "Cannabis Induces a Clinical Response in Patients with Crohn's Disease: A Prospective Placebo-Controlled Study." *Clinical Gastroenterology and Hepatology* 11, no. 10 (October 2013): 1276–1280.

12 Storr, Martin, Shane Devlin, Gilaad G. Kaplan et al. "Cannabis Use Provides Symptoms Relief in Patients with Inflammatory Bowel Disease but Is Associated with Worse Disease Prognosis in Patients with Crohn's Disease." *Inflammatory Bowel Diseases* 20, no. 3 (March 2014): 472–480.

13 Bae, Joon Hyun, Seo Young Kang, Si Eun You et al. "The Effects of Acupuncture on Crohn's Disease: A Systematic Review and Meta-Analysis." *Journal of Pharmacopuncture* 26, no. 3 (2023): 211–226.

14 Kitchen, Helen, Mallory Farrar, Tamara Al-zubeidi et al. "Patient's Perspective on Disease Burden, Remission Definition, and Symptoms Associated with Treatment Seeking: A Qualitative Study in Adult and Adolescent Patients with Crohn's Disease." *Crohn's and Colitis 360* 2, no. 2 (April 2020): otaa033.

15 Costa, Camila Ortiz Prospero Cavalcante, Flair José Carrilho et al. "A Snapshot of the Nutritional Status of Crohn's Disease Among Adolescents in Brazil: A Prospective Cross-Sectional Study." *BMC Gastroenterology* 15 (2015): 172.

DIVERTICULITIS

1 Matrana, Marc R. and David A. Margolin. "Epidemiology and Pathophysiology of Diverticular Disease." *Clinics in Colon and Rectal Surgery* 22, no. 3 (2009): 141–146.

2 Chabok, A., L. Påhlman, F. Hjern et al. "Randomized Clinical Trial of Antibiotics in Active Uncomplicated Diverticulitis." *British Journal of Surgery* 99, no. 4 (April 2012): 532–539.

3 de Korte, N., J. P. Kuyvenhoven, D. L. van der Peet et al. "Mild Colonic Diverticulitis Can Be Treated Without Antibiotics: A Case-Control Study." *Colorectal Disease* 14, no. 3 (March 2012): 325–330.

4 Jaung, Rebekah, Sherry Nisbet, Martijn Pieter Gosselink et al. "Antibiotics Do Not Reduce Length of Hospital Stay for Uncomplicated Diverticulitis in a Pragmatic Double-Blind Randomized Trial." *Clinical Gastroenterology and Hepatology* 19 (2021): 503–510.

5 Ogawa, Keiko, Koji Nishijima, Funio Futagami et al. "Effectiveness of Traditional Japanese Herbal (Kampo) Medicine, Daiobotanpito, in Combination with Antibiotic Therapy in the

Treatment of Acute Diverticulitis: A Preliminary Study." *Evidence-Based Complementary and Alternative Medicine* 2013 (2013): 305414.

6 Carabotti, Marilia, Francesca Falangone, Rosario Cuomo, and Bruno Annibale. "Role of Dietary Habits in the Prevention of Diverticular Disease Complications: A Systematic Review." *Nutrients* 13 (2021): 1288.

7 Crowe, Francesca, Angela Balkwill, Benjamin J. Cairns et al. "Source of Dietary Fibre and Diverticular Disease Incidence: A Prospective Study of UK Women." *Gut* 63 (2014): 1450–1456.

8 Mahmood, Mahmood W., Mirna Abraham-Nordling, Niclas Håkansson et al. "High Intake of Dietary Fibre from Fruit and Vegetables Reduces the Risk of Hospitalisation for Diverticular Disease." *European Journal of Nutrition* 58 (2019): 2393–2400.

9 Perry, Anne F., Robert S. Sandler, Dennis J. Ahnen et al. "Constipation and a Low-Fiber Diet Are Not Associated with Diverticulosis." *Clinical Gastroenterology and Hepatology* 11 (2013): 1622–1627.

10 Strate, Lisa L., Yan L. Liu, Sapna Syngal et al. "Nut, Corn and Popcorn Consumption and the Incidence of Diverticular Disease." *JAMA: Journal of the American Medical Association* 300, no. 8 (August 27, 2008): 907–914.

11 Maguire, Lillias H., Mingyang Song, Lisa E. Strate et al. "Higher Serum Levels of Vitamin D are Associated with Reduced Risk of Diverticulitis." *Clinical Gastroenterology and Hepatology* 11, no. 12 (December 2013): 1631–1635.

12 Wu, Z., J. Broad, J. Sluyter et al. "Effect of Monthly Vitamin D on Diverticular Disease Hospitalization: Post-Hoc Analysis of a Randomized Controlled Trial." *Clinical Nutrition* 40, no. 3 (March 2021): 839–843.

13 Papagrigoriadis, S., L. Macey, N. Bourantas, and J. A. Rennie. "Smoking May Be Associated with Complications in Diverticular Disease." *British Journal of Surgery* 86 (1999): 923–926.

14 Aune, Dagfinn, Abhijit Sen, Michael F. Leitzmann et al. "Body Mass Index and Physical Activity and the Risk of Diverticular Disease: A Systematic Review and Meta-Analysis of Prospective." *European Journal of Nutrition* 56 (2017): 2423–2438.

15 Song, B. K., J. M. Saavedra, E. C. Lefferts et al. "Associations Between Cardiorespiratory Fitness and Diverticulitis in Older Adults." *PLoS One* 17, no. 9 (2022): e0275433.

DYSPEPSIA

1 Baron, Jeremy Hugh and Amnon Sonnenberg. "Early History of Dyspepsia and Peptic Ulcer in the United States." *American Journal of Gastroenterology* 104, no. 12 (December 2009): 2893–2896.

2 Fujiwara, Yasuhiro and Tetsuo Arakawa. "Overlap in Patients with Dyspepsia/Functional Dyspepsia." *Journal of Neurogastroenterology and Motility* 20, no. 4 (October 2014): 447–457.

3 Azizz, I., O. S. Palsson, H. Törnblom et al. "Epidemiology, Clinical Characteristics, and Associations for Symptom-Based Rome IV Functional Dyspepsia in Adults in the USA< Canada, and the UK: A Cross-Sectional Population-Based Study." *Lancet Gastroenterology & Hepatology* 3, no. 4 (2018): 252–262.

4 Fujiwara and Arakawa. "Overlap in Patients with Dyspepsia/Functional Dyspepsia."

5 Wang, Wei Hong, Jia Qing Huang, Ge Fan Zheng et al. "Effects of Proton-Pump Inhibitors on Functional Dyspepsia: A Meta-Analysis of Randomized Placebo-Controlled Trials." *Clinical Gastroenterology and Hepatology* 5, no. 2 (February 2007): 178–185.

6 Pittayanon, R., Y. Yuan, N. P. Bollegala et al. "Prokinetics for Functional Dyspepsia: A Systematic Review and Meta-Analysis of Randomized Controlled Trials." *American Journal of Gastroenterology* 114, no. 2 (2019): 233–243.

7 Ford, Alexander C., Pavit Luthra, Jan Tack et al. "Efficacy of Psychotropic Drugs in Functional Dyspepsia: Systematic Review and Meta-Analysis." *Gut* 66 (2017): 411–420.

8 Kaji, Makiko, Yasuhiro Fujiwara, Masatsugu Shiba et al. "Prevalence of Overlaps Between GERD, FD and IBS and Impact on Health-Related Quality of Life." *Journal of Gastroenterology and Hepatology* 25, no. 6 (June 2010): 1151–1156.

9 Wei, Z., X. Yang, X. Xing et al. "Risk Factors Associated with Functional Dyspepsia in Chinese Children: A Cross-sectional Study." *BMC Gastroenterology* 21 (2021): 218.

10 Matsuzaki, J., H. Suzuki, Y. Fukushima et al. "High Frequency of Overlap Between Functional Dyspepsia and Overactive Bladder." *Neurogastroenterology & Motility* 24, no. 9 (September 2012): 8221–8227.

11 Yang, Jing-Wen, Li-Qiong Wang, Xuan Zou et al. "Effect of Acupuncture for Postprandial Distress Syndrome: A Randomized Clinical Trial." *Annals of Internal Medicine* 172, no. 12 (June 16, 2020): 777–785.

12 Tack, Jan, Peter Janssen, Tatsuhiro Masaoka et al. "efficacy of Buspirone, A Fundus-Relaxing Drug, in Patients with Functional Dyspepsia." *Clinical Gastroenterology and Hepatology* 10, no. 11 (November 2012): 1239–1245.

13 Göktas, Zeynep, Seyfettin Köklü, Derya Dikmen et al. "Nutritional Habits in Functional Dyspepsia and Its Subgroups: A Comparative Study." *Scandinavian Journal of Gastroenterology* 51, no. 8 (2016): 903–907.

14 Khodarahmi, Mahdieh and Leila Azadbakht. "Dietary Fat Intake and Functional Dyspepsia." *Advanced Biomedical Research* 5, no. 1 (2016): 76.

15 Das, D. S., G. K. Saharia, M. K. Pnigrahi, and D. Sahoo. "Association of Vitamin D and Functional Dyspepsia: A Case-Control Study." *Annals of Medicine & Surgery* 85 (2023): 4667–4673.

16 Ford, Alexander C., David Forman, Alastair G. Bailey et al. "Effect of Dyspepsia on Survival: A Longitudinal 10-Year Follow-Up Study." *American Journal of Gastroenterology* 107, no. 6 (June 2012): 912–921.

17 Esterita, T., S. Dewi, F. G. Suryatenggara, and G. Glenardi. "Association of Functional Dyspepsia with Depression and Anxiety: A Systematic Review." *Journal of Gastrointestinal and Liver Diseases* 30, no. 2 (June 18, 2021): 259–266.

18 Wei, Z., X. Xing, X. Tantai et al. "The Effects of Psychological Interventions on Symptoms and Psychology of Functional Dyspepsia: A Systematic Review and Meta-Analysis." *Frontiers in Psychology* 13 (April 2022): 827220.

19 Bonnert, Marianne, Ola Olen, Maria Lalouni et al. "Internet-Delivered Exposure-Based Cognitive-Behavioral Therapy for Adolescents with Functional Abdominal Pain or Functional Dyspepsia: A Feasibility Study." *Behavior Therapy* 50 (2019): 177–188.

FOOD POISONING

1 https://www.ift.org/news-and-publications/blog/2019/september/a-historical-look-at-food-safety.

2 https://www.cdc.gov/foodborneburden/index.html.

3 Yang, X. and R. Scharff. "Foodborne Illnesses from Leafy Greens in the United States: Attribution, Burden, and Cost." *Journal of Food Protection* 87 (2024): 100275.

4 Scharff, Robert I. "States Estimates for the Annual Cost of Foodborne Illness." *Journal of Food Protection* 78, no. 6 (2015): 1064–1071.

5 Bartsch, Sarah M., Lindsey Asti, Sindiso Nyathi et al. "Estimated Cost to a Restaurant of a Foodborne Illness Outbreak." *Public Health Reports* 133, no. 3 (2018): 274–286.

6 Park, Sung-Hee, Tong-Kyung, and Hye-Ja Chang. "Evaluation of the Food Safety Training for Food Handlers in Restaurant Operations." *Nutrition Research and Practice* 4, no. 1 (2010): 58–68.

7 Zyoud, S. J. Shalabi, K. Imran et al. "Knowledge, Attitude and Practices Among Parents Regarding Food Poisoning: A Cross-Sectional Study from Palestine." *BMC Public Health* 19 (2019): 586.

8 Mohd Yusof, A. M., N. A. A. Rahman, and M. Haque. "Knowledge, Attitude, and Practice Toward Food Poisoning Among Food Handlers and Dietetic Students in a Public University in Malaysia." *Journal of Pharmacy & BioAllied Sciences* 10, no. 4 (October–December 2018): 232–239.

9 Al-Mohaithef, Mohammed. "Awareness of Foodborne Pathogens Among Students: A Cross-Sectional Study in the Kingdom of Saudi Arabia." *International Journal of Food Science* 2021 (May 2021): 9971748.

10 Chehab, M. A., M. Nour, G. Bryant et al. "Knowledge and Practice of Emergency Physicians Regarding Food-borne Disease Surveillance at Hamad General Hospital in Qatar." *Cureus* 11, no. 6 (2019): e4934.

11 Islam, S., N. Tanjia, A. K. Mitra et al. "Inadequate Food Safety Knowledge and Hygiene Practices Among Street Food Vendors in Dhaka, Bangladesh." *Scientific Reports* 14 (2024): 17349.

12 Thaivalappil, A., I. Young, C. Paco et al. "Food Safety and the Older Consumer: A Systematic Review and Meta-Analysis of Their Knowledge and Practices at Home." *Food Control* 107 (2020): 106782.

13 Menini, A. L., G. Mascarello, M. Giarette et al. "The Critical Role of Consumers in the Prevention of Foodborne Diseases: An Ethnographic Study of Italian Families." *Foods* 11 (2022): 1006.

14 Steinberg, Ellen B., Alden Henderson, Adam Karpati et al. "Mysterious Outbreaks of Gastrointestinal Illness Associated with Burritos Supplied through School Lunch Programs." *Journal of Food Protection* 69, no. 7 (July 2006): 1690–1698.

15 Almansour, F. D., S. J. Sweitzer, A. A. Magness et al. "Temperature of Foods Sent by Parents of Preschool-Aged Children." *Pediatrics* 128, no. 3 (2011): 519–523.

GALLSTONES

1 Cárdenas-Arroyo, Felipe and Maria Cristina Martina. "Two Findings of Gallstones in Archeological Mummies from Colombia." *International Journal of Paleopathology* 24 (2019): 53–59.

2 Cárdenas-Arroyo and Martina. "Two Findings of Gallstones in Archeological Mummies from Colombia."

3 Naseri, Kaveh, Saeede Saadati, Hamid Asadzadeh-Aghdaei et al. "Healthy Dietary Pattern Reduces Risk of Gallstones: Results of a Case-Control Study in Iran." *International Journal of Preventive Medicine* 13 (2022): 66.

4 Tehrani, A. N., S. Saadati, Z. Yari et al. "Dietary Fiber Intake and Risk of Gallstone: A Case-Control Study." *BMC Gastroenterology* 23 (2023): 119.

5 Banim, Paul J. R., Robert N. Luben, Nicolas J. Wareham et al. "Physical Activity Reduces the Risk of Symptomatic Gallstones: A Prospective Cohort Study." *European Journal of Gastroenterology* 22, no. 8 (August 2010): 983–988.

6 Zhang, Yan-Peng, Ya-Lei Zhao, Yu-Ling Sun et al. "Physical Activity and the Risk of Gallstone Disease: A Systematic Review and Meta-Analysis." *Journal of Clinical Gastroenterology* 51 (2017): 857–868.

7 Misciagna, G., S. Centonze, C. Leoci et al. "Diet, Physical Activity, and Gallstones—A Population-Based, Case-Control Study in Southern Italy." *American Journal of Clinical Nutrition* 69 (1999): 120–126.

8 Wang, Siqi, Yuqiong Wang, Jinming Xu, and Yuxin Chen. "Is The Oral Contraception or Hormone Replacement Therapy a Risk Factor for Cholelithiasis." *Medicine* 96, no. 14 (2017): e6556.

9 Dai, Yu, Bujiangcun Luo, and Weizheng Li. "Incidence and Risk Factors for Cholelithiasis After Bariatric Surgery: A Systematic Review and Meta-Analysis." *Lipids in Health and Disease* 22 (2023): 5.

10 Nordenvall, Caroline, Viktor Oskarsson, and Alicja Wolk. "Inverse Association Between Coffee Consumption and Risk of Cholecystectomy in Women But Not Men." *Clinical Gastroenterology and Hepatology* 13 (2015): 1096–1102.

11 Leitzmann, Michael F., Meir J. Stampfer, Walter C. Willett et al. "Coffee Intake is Associated with Lower Risk of Symptomatic Gallstone Disease in Women." *Gastroenterology* 123 (2002): 1823–1830.

12 Wang, J., X. Duan, B. Li, and X. Jiang. "Alcohol Consumption and Risk of Gallstone Disease: A Meta-Analysis." *European Journal of Gastroenterology* 29, no. 4 (2017): e19–e28.

13 Chang, Yu, Hong-Min Lin, Kuan-Yu Chi et al. "Association Between Statin Use and Risk of Gallstone Disease and Cholecystectomy: A Meta-Analysis of 590,086 Patients." *PeerJ* 11 (April 2023): e15149.

14 Kwon, Mi Jung, Jung Woo Lee, Ho Suk Kang et al. "Association Between Gallstones Disease and Statin Use: A Nested Case-Control Study in Korea." *Pharmaceuticals* 16 (2023): 536.

15 Zhang, Junlu, Liangli Chen, Keqing Shen et al. "Association Between Metabolically Healthy Overweight/Obesity and Gallstones in Chinese." *Nutrition & Metabolism* 20, no. 1 (March 2023): 20.

16 Ratheesh, Rani, Michael T. Ulrich, Sherief Ghazy et al. "The Association Between Diabetes and Gallstones: A Nationwide Population-Based Cohort Study." *Gastroenterology Review* 18, no. 3 (2023): 292–299.

17 Zhang, Yalan, Li Sun, Xin Wang, and Zongtao Chen. "The Association Between Hypertension and the Risk of Gallstone Disease: A Cross-Sectional Study." *BMC Gastroenterology* 22 (2022): 138.

GASTRITIS

1 Sipponen, Pentti and Heidi-Ingrid Maaroos. "Chronic Gastritis." *Scandinavian Journal of Gastroenterology* 50, no. 6 (June 2015): 657–667.

2 https://www.ncbi.nlm.nih.gov/books/NBK544250/.

3 Li, Yuan, Zeqi Su, Ping Li et al. "Association of Symptoms with Eating Habits and Food Preferences in Chronic Gastritis Patients: A Cross-Sectional Study." *Evidence-Based Complementary and Alternative Medicine* 2020 (2020): Article 5197201.

4 Yang, Guo-Tao, Hong-Ying Zhao, Yu Kong et al. "Correlation Between Serum Vitamin B12 Level and Peripheral Neuropathy in Atrophic Gastritis." *World Journal of Gastroenterology* 24, no. 12 (March 28, 2018): 1343–1352.

5 Wood, I. J., M. Ralston, B. Ungar, and D. C. Cowling. "Vitamin B12 Deficiency in Chronic Gastritis." *Gut* 5 (1964): 27.

6 Woodford, Amanda M., Rabbea Chaudhry, Gabriella A. Conte et al. "Chronic Atrophic Gastritis Presenting as Hemolytic Anemia Due to Severe Vitamin B12 Deficiency." *Case Reports in Hematology* 2021 (2021): 9571072.

7 Massironi, Sara, Federica Cavalcoli, Alessandra Zilli et al. "Relevance of Vitamin D Deficiency in Patients with Chronic Autoimmune Atopic Gastritis: A Prospective Study." *BMC Gastroenterology* 18 (2018): 172

8 Zilli, Alessandra, Federica Cavalcoli, Clorinda Ciafardini, and Sara Massironi. "Deficiency of Micronutrients in Patients Affected by Chronic Atrophic Autoimmune Gastritis: A Single-Institution Observational Study." *Digestive and Liver Disease* 51 (2019): 505–509.

9 Lei, Jing, Fugang Ren, Wenyuan Li et al. "Use of Folic Acid Supplementation to Halt and Even Reverse the Progression of Gastric Precancerous Conditions: A Meta-Analysis." *BMC Gastroenterology* 22 (2022): 370.

10 Shao-hua, Zhang, Ren Lin-lin, Su Shen et al. "Atrophic Gastritis Rather Than Helicobacter Pylori Infection Can be An Independent Risk Factor of Colorectal Polyps: A Retrospective Study in China." *BMC Gastroenterology* 23 (2023): 213.

11 Sreeja, Sundara Raj, Trong-Dat Le, Bang Wool Eom et al. "Association Between the Dietary Inflammation Index and Gastric Disease Risk: Findings from a Korean Population-Based Cohort Study." *Nutrients* 14 (2022): 2662.

12 Shibata, Kazunori, Masaki Moriyama, Tetsuhito Fukushima et al. "Green Tea Consumption and Chronic Atrophic Gastritis: A Cross-Sectional Study in a Green Tea Production Village." *Journal of Epidemiology* 10, no. 5 (2000): 310–316.

13 Gebru, Demisew. "Factors Associated with Gastric Disease Among Students of Hawassa University: The Case of College of Agriculture Students." *American Journal of Theoretical and Applied Statistics* 7, no. 6 (2018): 207–214.

14 Choi, Mi-Kyeong, Myung-Hwa Kang, and Mi-Hyun Kim. "Dietary Intake Assessment and Biochemical Characteristics of Blood and Urine in Patients with Chronic Gastritis." *Clinical Nutrition Research* 4 (2015): 90–96.

15 Gao, Lei, Melanie N. Weck, Christa Stegmaier et al. "Alcohol Consumption and Chronic Atrophic Gastritis: Population-Based Study Among 9,444 Older Adults from Germany." *International Journal of Cancer* 125, no. 12 (December 2009): 2918–2922.

16 Kalkan, Çagdas and Irfan Soykan. "Differences Between Older and Young Patients with Autoimmune Gastritis." *Geriatrics & Gerontology* 17, no. 7 (July 2017): 1090–1095.

17 Lee, Sangyoon, Chang Ho Chae, Chulyong Park et al. "Relationship of Shift Work with Endoscopic Gastritis Among Workers of an Electronics Company." *Scandinavian Journal of Work, Environment & Health* 46, no. 2 (March 1, 2020): 161–167.

18 Kim, H. W., Y-H Kim, K. Han et al. "Atrophic Gastritis: A Related Factor for Osteoporosis in Elderly Women." *PLoS One* 9, no. 7 (2014): e101852.

19 Laiyemo, Adeyinka O., Farin Kamangar, Pamela M. Marcus et al. "Atrophic Gastritis and the Risk of Incidental Colorectal Cancer." *Cancer Causes & Control* 21 (2010): 163–170.

20 Nakamura, Masaru, Ken Haruma, Tomoari Kamada et al. "Cigarette Smoking Promotes Atrophic Gastritis in Helicobacter Pylori-Positive Subjects." *Digestive Diseases and Sciences* 47, no. 3 (March 2002): 675–681.

GASTROENTERITIS

1 Mitakakis, T. Z., R. Wolfe, M. I. Sinclair et al. "Dietary Intake and Domestic Food Preparation and Handling as Risk Factors for Gastroenteritis: A Case-Control Study." *Epidemiology & Infection* 132, no. 4 (August 2004): 601–606.

2 Guo, Z., J. Huang, G. Shi et al. "A Food-Borne Outbreak of Gastroenteritis Caused by Norovirus GII in a University Located in Xiamen City, China." *International Journal of Infectious Diseases* 28 (2014): 101–106.

3 Evans, Meirion R., C. Donald Ribeiro, and Roland L. Salmon. "Hazards of Healthy Living: Bottled Water and Salad Vegetables as Risk Factors for Campylobacter Infection." *Emerging Infectious Diseases* 9, no. 10 (October 2003): 1219–1225.

4 Orysbayeva, M., B. Zhuman, D. Turegeldiyeva et al. "Outbreak of Acute Gastroenteritis Associated with Drinking Water in Rural Kazakhstan: A Matched Case-Control Study." *PLOS Global Public Health* 2, no. 12 (2022): e0001075.

5 Chen, Y., Y. Wen, J. Song et al. "The Correlation Between Family Food Handling Behaviors and Foodborne Acute Gastroenteritis: A Community-Oriented, Population-Based Survey in Anhui, China." *BMC Public Health* 18 (2018): 1290.

6 Güzel, Mustafa, Orhan Akpmar, and Muhammet Burak Kılıç. "Prevalence of Rotavirus-Associated Acute Gastroenteritis Cases in Early Childhood in Turkey: Meta-Analysis." *Children* 7, no. 10 (October 2020): 159.

7 Gao, J., L. Xue, Y. Li et al. "A Systematic Review and Meta-Analysis Indicates a High Risk of Human Noroviruses Contamination in Vegetable Worldwide, with GI Being the Predominant Genogroup." *International Journal of Food Microbiology* 413 (March 2, 2024): 110603.

8 Rodrigo, Shelly, Martha Sinclair, Andrew Forbes et al. "Drinking Rainwater: A Double-Blinded, Randomized Controlled Study of Water Treatment Filters and Gastroenteritis Incidence." *American Society of Public Health* 101, no. 5 (Mary 2011): 842–847.

9 Hikita, T., T. Phan, S. Okitsu et al. "A Comparative Study of Acute Gastroenteritis Symptoms in Single-verses-Multiple-Virus Infections." *International Journal of Molecular Sciences* 24 (2023): 8364.

10 Weghorst, Anouk A. H., Irma J. Bonvanie, Gea A. Holtman et al. "Course of Uncomplicated Acute Gastroenteritis in Children Presenting to Out-of-Hours Primary Care." *BMC Primary Care* 23 (2022): 125.

11 Derakhshanfar, Hojjat, Arash Hadian Amree, Hossein Alimohammadi et al. "Results of Double-Blind Placebo Controlled Trial to Assess the Effect of Vitamin B6 on Managing of Nausea and Vomiting in Pediatrics with Acute Gastroenteritis." *Global Journal of Health Science* 5, no. 6 (2013): 197–201.

GASTROESOPHAGEAL REFLUX DISEASE (GERD)

1 https://www.researchgate.net/figure/Asher-Winkelstein-1893-1972-bottom-left-as-the-Chief-of-Gastroenterology-at-Mount_fig2_8603279.

2 El-Serag, Hashem B., Stephen Sweet, Christopher C. Winchester, and John Dent. "Update on the Epidemiology of Gastro-Oesophageal Reflux Disease: A Systematic Review." *Gut* 63, no. 6 (2014): 871–880.

3 Murao, Tetsuya, Kouici Sakurai, Syuuichi et al. "Lifestyle Change Influences on GERD in Japan: A Study of Participants in a Health Examination Program." *Digestive Diseases and Sciences* 56 (2011): 2857–2864.

4 Gong, Yan, Qiang Zeng, Yi Yan et al. "Association Between Lifestyle and Gastroesophageal Reflux Disease Questionnaire Scores: A Cross-Sectional Study of 37,442 Chinese Adults." *Gastroenterology Research and Practice* 2019 (2019): 5753813.

5 Friedenberg, Frank K., Jitha Rai, Vishwas Vanar et al. "Prevalence and Risk Factors for Gastroesophageal Reflux Disease in an Impoverished Minority Population." *Obesity Research & Clinical Practice* 4, no. 4 (2010): e261–e269.

6 Mone, I., B. Kraja, A. Bregu et al. "Adherence to a Predominantly Mediterranean Diet Decreases the Risk of Gastroesophageal Reflux Disease: A Cross-Sectional Study in a South Eastern European Population." *Diseases of the Esophagus* 29 (2016): 794–800.

7 Choi, Ji Min, Jong In Yang, Seung Joo Kang et al. "Association Between Anxiety and Depression and Gastroesophageal Reflux Disease: Results from a Large Cross-Sectional Study." *Journal of Neurogastroenterology and Motility* 24, no. 4 (2018): 593–602.

8 Fujiwara, Y., A. Machida, Y. Watanabe et al. "Association Between Dinner-to-Bed Time and Gastro-Esophageal Reflux Disease." *American Journal of Gastroenterology* 100 (2005): 2633–2636.

9 Li, Shujie, Shengying Shi, Feng Chen, and Jingming Lin. "The Effects of Baclofen for the Treatment of Gastroesophageal Reflux Disease: A Meta-Analysis of Randomized Controlled Trials." *Gastroenterology Research and Practice* 2014(2014): 307805.

10 Zhang, Chao-xian, Yong-mei Qin, and Bao-rui Guo. "Clinical Study on the Treatment of Gastroesophageal Reflux by Acupuncture." *Chinese Journal of Integrative Medicine* 16, no. 4 (August 2010): 298–303.

11 Trinh, Dieu-Thuong Thi, An Hoa Tran, Minh-Man Pham Bui, and Nguyen Lam Vuong. "Thread-Embedding Acupuncture May Improve Symptom Resolution in Patients with Gastroesophageal Reflux Disease: A Randomized Controlled Trial." *Integrative Medicine Research* 12 (2021): 100971.

12 Targownik, Laura E., Lisa M. Lix, Colleen J. Metge et al. "Use of Proton Pump Inhibitors and Risk of Osteoporosis-Related Fractures." *CMAJ* 179, no. 4 (August 12, 2008): 319–326.

13 Wang, Yun-Han, Viktor Wintzell, Jonas F. Ludvigsson et al. "Association Between Proton Pump Inhibitor Use and Risk of Fracture in Children." *JAMA Pediatrics* 174, no. 6 (2020): 543–551.

14 Hoff, M., E. Skovlund, S. Skurtveit et al. "Proton Pump Inhibitors and Fracture Risk. The HUNT Study, Norway." *Osteoporosis International* 31 (2020): 109–118.

15 den Elzen, W. P. J., Y. Groeneveld, W. de Ruijter et al. "Long-Term Use of Proton Pump Inhibitors and Vitamin B12 Status in Elderly Individuals." *Alimentary Pharmacology and Therapeutics* 27, no. 6 (March 2008): 491–497.

16 Dharmarajan, T. S., M. K. Kanagala, P. Murakonda et al. "Do Acid-Lowering Agents Affect Vitamin B1 Status in Older Adults?" *Journal of the American Medical Directors Association* 9, no. 3 (March 2008): 162–167.

17 Kandil, T. S., A. A. Mousa, A. A. El-Gendy, and A. M. Abbas. "The Potential Therapeutic Effects of Melatonin in Gastro-Esophageal Reflux Disease." *BMC Gastroenterology* 10, no. 1 (2010): 7.

18 Pereira, Ricardo de Souza. "Regression of Gastroesophageal Reflux Disease Symptoms Using Dietary Supplementation with Melatonin, Vitamins and Aminoacids: Comparison with Omeprazole." *Journal of Pineal Research* 41, no. 3 (October 2006): 195–200.

GASTROPARESIS

1 Kassander, Paul. "Asymptomatic Gastric Retention in Diabetics (Gastroparesis Diabeticorum)." *Annals of Internal Medicine* 48, no. 4 (April 1, 1958): 797–812.

2 Syed, Aslam R., Michael M. Wolfe, and Jorge Calles-Escandon. "Epidemiology and Diagnosis of Gastroparesis in the United States: A Population-Based Study." *Journal of Clinical Gastroenterology* 54, no. 1 (January 2020): 50–53.

3 Rey, Enrique, Rok Seon Choung, Cathy D. Schleck et al. "Prevalence of Hidden Gastroparesis in the Community: The Gastroparesis 'Iceberg.'" *Journal of Neurogastroenterology and Motility* 18, no. 1 (January 2012): 34–42.

4 https://www.niddk.nih.gov/health-information/digestive-diseases/gastroparesis/definition-facts.

5 Erbas, Tomris, Eerhan Varoglu, Belkis Erbas et al. "Comparison of Metoclopramide and Erythromycin in the Treatment of Diabetic Gastroparesis." *Diabetes Care* 16, no. 11 (November 1993): 1511–1514.

6 McCallum, Richard W., Dominick A. Ricci, Hebert Rakatansky et al. "A Multicenter Placebo-Controlled Clinical Trial of Oral Metoclopramide in Diabetic Gastroparesis." *Diabetes Care* 6, no. 5 (September–October 1983): 463–467.

7 Tsai, Shin-Chia, Shiow-Yunn Sheu, Li-Nien Chien et al. "High Exposure Compared with Standard Exposure to Metoclopramide Associated with a Higher Risk of Parkinsonism: A Nationwide Population-Based Cohort Study." *British Journal of Clinical Pharmacology* 84 (2018): 2000–2009.

8 Al-Saffar, Ahmad, Hans Lennernäs, and Per M. Hellström. "Gastroparesis, Metoclopramide, and Tardive Dyskinesia: Risk Revisited." *Neurogastroenterology & Motility* 31, no. 11 (November 2019): e13617.

9 Janssens, J., T. L. Peeters, G. Vantrappen et al. "Improvement of Gastric Emptying in Diabetic Gastroparesis by Erythromycin—Preliminary Studies." *New England Journal of Medicine* 322 (1990): 1028–1031.

10 Maganti, Kalyani, Kingsley Onyemere, and Michael P. Jones. "Oral Erythromycin and Symptomatic Relief of Gastroparesis: A Systematic Review." *American Journal of Gastroenterology* 98, no. 2 (2003): 259–263.

11 Larson, Jean M., Anna Tavakkoli, Walter E. Drane et al. "Advantages of Azithromycin Over Erythromycin in Improving the Gastric Emptying Half-Time in Adult Patients with Gastroparesis." *Journal of Neurogastroenterology and Motility* 16, no. 4 (October 2010): 407–413.

12 Lewis, Kim, Zuhoor Alqahtani, Lauralyn McIntyre et al. "The Efficacy and Safety of Prokinetic Agents in Critically Ill Patients Receiving Enteral Nutrition: A Systematic Review and Meta-Analysis of Randomized Trials." *Critical Care* 20, no. 1 (August 2016): 259.

13 Carbone, Florencia, Karenn Van den Houte, Egbert Clevers et al. "Prucalopride in Gastroparesis: A Randomized Placebo-Controlled Crossover Study." *American Journal of Gastroenterology* 114, no. 8 (August 2019): 1265–1274.

14 Olausson, Eva A., Stine Störsrud, Håkan Grundin et al. "A Small Particle Diet Reduces Upper Gastrointestinal Symptoms in Patients with Diabetic Gastroparesis: A Randomized Controlled Diet." *American Journal of Gastroenterology* 109 (2014): 375–385.

15 Wytiaz, Victoria, Carol Homka, Frank Duffy et al. "Food Provoking and Alleviating Symptoms in Gastroparesis: Patient Experiences." *Digestive Diseases and Sciences* 60 (2015): 1052–1058.

16 Homko, C. J., F. Duffy, F. K. Friedenberg et al. "Effect of Dietary Fat and Food Consistency on Gastroparesis Symptoms in Patients with Gastroparesis." *Neurogastroenterology & Motility* 27, no. 4 (April 2015): 501–508.

17 Ahmed, Sally S., Hala A. Abd El-Hafez, Mohammed Mohsen et al. "Is Vitamin B12 Deficiency a Risk Factor for Gastroparesis in Patients with Type 2 Diabetes?" *Diabetology & Metabolic Syndrome* 15 (2023): 33.

18 Ogorek, Carrie P., Laura Davidson, Robert S. Fisher, and Benjamin Krevsky. "Idiopathic Gastroparesis is Associated with a Multiplicity of Severe Dietary Deficiencies." *American Journal of Gastroenterology* 86, no. 4 (1991): 423–428.

19 Parkman, Henry P., Katherine P. Yates, William L. Hasler et al. "Dietary Intake and Nutritional Deficiencies in Patients with Diabetic or Idiopathic Gastroparesis." *Gastroenterology* 141 (2011): 486–498.

20 Wang, Chung-Pang, Chia-Hung Kao, Wei-Kung Chen et al. "A Single-Blinded, Randomized Pilot Study Evaluating Effects of Electroacupuncture in Diabetic Patients with Symptoms Suggestive of Gastroparesis." *Journal of Alternative and Complementary Medicine* 14, no. 7 (2008): 833–839.

HEMORRHOIDS AND FISSURES

1 https://lacolon.com/hemorrhoids/ancient-remedies-hemorrhoids-historical-perspective.

2 Beaty, Jennifer Sam and M. Shashidharan. "Anal Fissure." *Clinics in Colon and Rectal Surgery* 29 (2016): 30–37.

3 Sugarman, D. T. "Hemorrhoids." *JAMA* 312, no. 24 (December 24/31, 2014): 2698.

4 Sun, Zhifei and John Migaly. "Review of Hemorrhoid Disease: Presentation and Management." *Clinics in Colon and Rectal Surgery* 29 (2016): 22–29.

5 Sandler, Robert S. and Anne F. Peery. "Rethinking What We Know About Hemorrhoids." *Clinical Gastroenterology and Hepatology* 17 (2019): 8–15.

6 Madalinski, M. "Identifying the Best Therapy for Chronic Anal Fissure." *World Journal of Gastrointestinal Pharmacology and Therapeutics* 2, no. 2 (April 2011): 9–16.

7 Perez-Miranda, Manuel, Ana Gomez-Cedenilla, Teresa León-Colombo et al. "Effect of Fiber Supplements on Internal Bleeding Hemorrhoids." *Hepato-Gastroenterology* 43, no. 12 (1996): 1504–1507.

8 Alonso-Coello, Pablo, Ed Mills, Diane Heels-Ansdell et al. "Fiber for the Treatment of Hemorrhoids Complications: A Systematic Review and Meta-Analysis." *American Journal of Gastroenterology* 101, no. 1 (2006): 181–188.

9 Broader, J. H., I. F. Gunn, and J. Alexander-Williams. "Evaluation of a Bulk-Forming Evacuant in the Management of Haemorrhoids." *British Journal of Surgery* 61 (1974): 142–144.

10 Peery, Anne F., Robert S. Sandler, Joseph A. Galanko et al. "Risk Factors for Hemorrhoids on Screening Colonoscopy." *PLoS One* 10, no. 9 (2015): e0139100.

11 Johannsson, Helgri Örn, Wilhelm Graf, and Lars Påhlman. "Bowel Habits in Hemorrhoid Patients and Normal Subjects." *American Journal of Gastroenterology* 100 (2005): 401–406.

12 Hsu, Sheng-Pang, Hsin-Hung Chen, Tzu-Yuan Wang et al. "Association of Hemorrhoids with Hashimoto's Thyroiditis and Associated Comorbidities: A Nationwide Population-Based Cohort Study." *Frontiers in Endocrinology* 11 (October 2020): 577767.

13 Aram, Fahmi Omer. "Rubber Band Ligation for Hemorrhoids: An Office Experience." *Indian Journal of Surgery* 78, no. 4 (August 2016): 271–274.

14 Shirah, Bader Hamza, Hamza Assad Shirah, Abdelelah Hussein Fallata et al. "Hemorrhoids During Pregnancy: Sitz Baths vs. Ano-Rectal Cream: A Comparative Prospective Study of Two Conservative Treatment Protocols." *Women and Birth* 31 (2018): e272–e277.

15 Brown, Carl J., Daniel Dubreuil, Laura Santoro et al. "Lateral Internal Sphincterotomy Is Superior to Topical Nitroglycerin for Healing Chronic Anal Fissure and Does Not

Compromise Long-Term Fecal Continence: Six-Year Follow-Up of a Multicenter, Randomized, Controlled Trial." *Diseases of the Colon & Rectum* 50 (2007): 442–448.

16 Ram, Edward, Yaniv Zager, Raanan Meyer et al. "Management of Chronic Anal Fissure with a Novel Topical Hemp-Herbal-Based Ointment: A Pilot Study." *Medical Cannabis and Cannabinoids* 6 (2023): 15–20.

17 Kaushal, Manish, Arvind Shukla, P. Kovarthanan, and Yogesh Heremat Shivaprasad. "Zinc Oxide, Lidocaine, and Lateral Internal Sphincterotomy for Fissure-in-Ano: A Comparative Study." *International Surgery Journal* 9, no. 6 (June 2022): 1146–1150.

18 Sahebally, Shaheel M., Khalid Ahmed, Raminta Cerneveciute et al. "Oral Versus Topical Channel Blockers for Chronic Anal Fissures—A Systematic Review and Meta-Analysis of Randomized Controlled Trials." *International Journal of Surgery* 44 (2017): 87–93.

19 Setareh Soltany, Hamid Reza Hemmati, Jafar Alavy Toussy et al. "Therapeutic Properties of Botulinum Toxin on Chronic Anal Fissure Treatment and the Patient Factors Role." *Journal of Family Medicine and Primary Care* 9 (2020): 1562–1566.

20 Gupta, Pravin J. "Randomized, Controlled Study Comparing Sitz-Bath and Non-Sitz-Bath Treatments in Patients with Acute Anal Fissures." *ANZ Journal of Surgery* 76, no. 8 (August 2008): 718–721.

21 Tejirian, Talar and Maher A. Abbas. "Sitz Bath: Where Is the Evidence? Scientific Basis of a Common Practice." *Diseases of the Colon and Rectum* 48 (2005): 2336–2340.

HEPATITIS A, HEPATITIS B, AND HEPATITIS C

1 Feinstone, Stephen M. "History of the Discovery of Hepatitis A Virus." *Cold Spring Harbor Perspectives in Medicine* 9, no. 5 (May 2019): a031740.

2 Ogunnaike, M., S. Das, S. S. Raut et al. "Chronic Hepatitis B Infection: New Approaches Towards Cure." *Biomolecules* 13, no. 8 (August 2023): 1208.

3 Bukh, Jens. "The History of Hepatitis C Virus (HCV): Basic Research Reveals Unique Features in Phylogeny, Evolution and the Viral Life Cycle with New Perspectives for Epidemic Control." *Journal of Hepatology* 65, no. 1 Supplement (October 2016): S2–S21.

4 https://www.hhs.gov/hepatitis/learn-about-viral-hepatitis/hepatitis-b-basics/index.html.

5 Hennessey, Karen A., David R. Bangsberg, Cindi Weinbaum, and Judith A. Hahn. "Hepatitis A Seroprevalence and Risk Factors Among Homeless Adults in San Francisco: Should Homelessness Be Included in the Risk-Based Strategy for Vaccination?" *Public Health Reports* 124, no. 6 (November–December 2009): 813–817.

6 Baloch, L., G. Patel, R. Collins-Cronkright et al. "Who Really Receives Hepatitis A Vaccinations?" *American Journal of Gastroenterology* 116 (October 2021): S548.

7 Kaigh, Caroline, Andrea Blome, Kraftin E. Schreyer, and Megan Healey. "Emergency Department-Based Hepatitis A Vaccination Program in Response to an Outbreak." *Western Journal of Emergency Medicine* 21, no. 4 (July 2020): 906–908.

8 Murlidharan, S., A. L. Sangle, M. Engade, and A. B. Kale. "The Clinical Profile of Children with Hepatitis A Infection: An Observational Hospital-Based Study." *Cureus* 14, no. 8 (August 2022): e28290.

9 Hofmeister, Megan G., Shaoman Yin, Maria V. Aslam et al. "Hepatitis A Hospitalization Costs, United States, 2017." *Emerging Infectious Diseases* 26, no. 5 (May 2020): 1040–1041.

10 Rahmani, A., A. Montecucco, B. K. Vitturi et al. "Long-Term Effectiveness of Hepatitis B Vaccination in the Protection of Healthcare Students in Highly Developed Countries: A Systematic Review and Meta-Analysis." *Vaccines* 10 (2022): 1841.

11 Magri, Mariana Cavalheiro, Arielle Karen da Silva Nunes, Bianca Peixoto Dantas et al. "Meta-Analysis of the Prevalence of HBV Infection Among Alcohol Users Worldwide." *Alcohol and Alcoholism* 55, no. 2 (2020): 136–143.

12 Riyahi, Nasrin, Masood Ziaee, and Reza Dastjerdi. "The Effects of Cognitive Behavioral Therapy on Quality of Life Among Patients with Hepatitis B." *Modern Care Journal* 15, no. 3 (August 2018): e82748.

13 Huang, Wei, Xiaoli Wu, Zhenzhen Yao et al. "Investigating the Relationship Between Hepatitis B Virus Infection and Postpartum Depression in Chinese Women: A Retrospective Cohort Study." *Frontiers in Public Health* 11 (2023): 1214151

14 Zhang, Mengdi, Meijuan Wan, Wen Wang et al. "Effect of Interferon Therapy on Quality of Life in Patients with Chronic Hepatitis B." *Scientific Reports* 14 (2024): 2461.

15 Valizadeh, L., V. Zamanzadeh, R. Negarandeh et al. "Psychological Reactions Among Patients with Chronic Hepatitis B: A Qualitative Study." *Journal of Caring Sciences* 5, no. 1 (2016): 57–66.

16 Tu, An, Xiaoning Zhu, Paniz Zarghami Dastjerdi et al. "Evaluate the Clinical Efficacy of Traditional Chinese Medicine as the Neoadjuvant Treatment in Reducing the Incidence of Hepatocellular Carcinoma in Patients with Hepatitis B-Related Cirrhosis: A Systematic Review and Meta-Analysis." *Heliyon* 10, no. 3 (February 15, 2024): e24437.

17 Hu, Ye-Chao, Wei-Wei Wang, Wei-Yun Jiang et al. "Low Vitamin D Levels are Associated with High Viral Loads in Patients with Chronic Hepatitis B: A Systematic Review and Meta-Analysis." *BMC Gastroenterology* 19 (2019): 84.

18 Andreone, Pietro, Sirio Fiorino, Carmela Cursaro et al. "Vitamin E as Treatment for Chronic Hepatitis B: Results of a Randomized Controlled Pilot Trial." *Antiviral Research* 49 (2001): 75–81.

19 Rusu, Emilia, Mariana Jinga, Georgiana Enache et al. "Effects of Lifestyle Changes Including Specific Dietary Intervention and Physical Activity in the Management of Patients with Chronic Hepatitis C—A Randomized Trial." *Nutrition Journal* 12, no. 1 (2013): 119.

20 Villar, Livia Melo, Jose Antonio Del Campo, Isodora Ranchal et al. "Association Between Vitamin D and Hepatitis C Virus Infection: A Meta-Analysis." *World Journal of Gastroenterology* 19, no. 35 (September 21, 2013): 5917–5924.

21 Hyunb, Myung Han, Ji Hoon Kim, Jeong Won Jang et al. "Risk of Hepatitis C Virus Transmission Through Acupuncture: A Systematic Review and Meta-Analysis." *Korean Journal of Gastroenterology* 82, no. 3 (September 2023): 127–136.

22 Golden, Sara E., Diane Miller, Lissi Hansen et al. "The Experience of Veterans with Hepatitis C and Acupuncture: A Mixed Methods Pilot Study." *European Journal of Integrative Medicine* 10 (February 2017): 8–18.

23 Golden, Jeannette, Anne Marie O'Dwyer, and Ronan M. Conroy. "Depression and Anxiety in Patients with Hepatitis C: Prevalence, Detection Rates and Risk Factors." *General Hospital Psychiatry* 27 (2005): 431–438.

24 Egmond, Elfi, Zoe Marino, Ricard Navines et al. "Incidence of Depression in Patients with Hepatitis C Treated with Direct-Acting Antivirals." *Brazilian Journal of Psychiatry* 42, no. 1 (January–February 2020): 72–76.

25 Hallsworth, Kate, Shion Gosrani, Sarah Hogg et al. "Association of Exercise Participation Levels with Cardiometabolic Health and Quality of Life in Individuals with Hepatitis C." *BMJ Open Gastroenterology* 8 (2021): e000591.

INGUINAL HERNIA

1 Hori, Tomohide and Daiki Yasukawa. "Fascinating History of Groin Hernias: Comprehensive Recognition of Anatomy, Classic Considerations for Herniorrhaphy, and Current Controversies in Hernioplasty." *World Journal of Methodology* 11, no. 4 (July 20, 2021): 160–186.

2 https://www.ncbi.nlm.nih.gov/books/NBK513332/#:~:text=An%20inguinal%20hernia%20will%20affect,of%20women%20over%20their%20lifetime.

3 Lau, Hung, Christian Fang, Wai K. Yuen, and Nivritti G. Patil. "Risk Factors for Inguinal Hernia in Adult Males: A Case-Control Study." *Surgery* 141 (2007): 262–266.

4 Jansen, P. L., U. Klinge, M. Jansen, and K. Junge. "Risk Factors for Early Recurrence After Inguinal Hernia Repair." *BMC Surgery* 9 (2009): 18.

5 Cowan, B., M. Kvale, J. Yin et al. "Risk Factors for Inguinal Hernia Repair Among US Adults." *Hernia* 27 (2023): 1507–1514.

6 Ruhl, Constance E. and James E. Everhart. "Risk Factors for Inguinal Hernia Among Adults in the US Population." *American Journal of Epidemiology* 165 (2007): 1154–1161.

7 Hoffmann, Henry, Daniela Walther, Reinhard Bittner et al. "Small Inguinal Hernias are Independent Risk Factors for Developing Chronic Postoperative Inguinal Pain (CPIP)." *Annals of Surgery* 271, no. 4 (April 2020): 756–764.

8 Tolver, M. A., P. Strandfelt, G. Forsberg et al. "Determinants of a Short Convalescence After Laparoscopic Transabdominal Preperitoneal Inguinal Hernia Repair." *Surgery* 151, no. 4 (2012): 556–563.

9 Taghavi, Rahim, Kamyar Tavakoli Tabasi, Nasser Mogharabian et al. "The Effect of Acupuncture on Relieving Pain After Inguinal Surgery." *Korean Journal of Pain* 26 (2013): 46–50.

10 Chiu, Hon Yu, Tsz Ting Law, Lily Ng, Kin Yuen Wong. "Hernia in Pregnancy—Does It Matter?" *Surgical Practice* 26, no. 4 (November 2022): 257–261.

11 Buch, Kerri E., Parissa Tabrizian, and Celia M. Divino. "Management of Hernias in Pregnancy." *Journal of the American College of Surgeons* 207, no. 4 (2008): 539–542.

12 Lechner, M., R. Fortelny, D. Öfner, and F. Mayer. "Suspected Inguinal Hernias in Pregnancy—Handle With Care!" *Hernia* 18 (2014): 375–379.

13 Kuijer, P. P. F. M., D. Hondebrink, C. T. J. Hulshof, and H. F. Van der Molen. "Work-Relatedness of Inguinal Hernia: A Systematic Review Including Meta-Analysis and GRADE." *Hernia* 24 (2020): 943–950.

14 van Veen, R. N., A. R. Wijsmuller, W. W. Vrijland et al. "Long-Term Follow-Up of a Randomized Clinical Trial of a Non-Mesh *versus* Mesh Repair of Primary Inguinal Hernia." *British Journal of Surgery* 94 (2007): 506–510.

15 Hentati, Hassen, Wajih Dougaz, and Chadli Dziri. "Mesh Repair Versus Non-Mesh Repair for Strangulated Inguinal Hernia: Systematic Review with Meta-Analysis." *World Journal of Surgery* 38 (2014): 2784–2790.

16 Perez, Arielle J. and Shannelle Campbell. "Inguinal Hernia Repair in Older Persons." *Journal of the American Directors Association* 23 (2022): 563–567.

INTESTINAL OBSTRUCTION

1 Fevang, Bjørg-Tilde Svanes, Jonas Svanes, Stein Atle Lie et al. "Long-Term Prognosis After Operation for Adhesive Small Bowel Obstruction." *Annals of Surgery* 240, no. 2 (August 2004): 193–201.

2 Allan, Lindsey, Naomi Hatchett, Simon S. Skene et al. "Management of Inoperable Malignant Bowel Obstruction Using 4-Step BOUNCED Diet." *Journal of Human Nutrition and Dietetics* 38 (2025): e13388.

3 Sheyn, David, C. Emi Bretschneider, Sangeeta T. Mahajan et al. "Incidence and Risk Factors of Early Postoperative Small Bowel Obstruction in Patients Undergoing Hysterectomy for Benign Indications." *American Journal of Obstetrics & Gynecology* 220, no. 3 (March 2019): 251.e1–251.e9.

4 Ahmad, Bilal, Mohd Fazl Ul Haq, Mubashir Ah Shah et al. "Early Postoperative Small Bowel Obstruction After Colorectal Surgery: Incidence and Exploratory Analysis of Potential Risk Factors." *Euroasian Journal of Hepato-Gastroenterology* 14, no. 1 (2024): 70–74.

5 Mohd Suan, Mohd Azri, Wei Leong Tan, Shahrul Aiman Soelar et al. "Intestinal Obstruction: Predictor of Poor Prognosis in Colorectal Carcinoma?" *Epidemiology and Health* 37 (March 2015): e2015017.

6 Peacock, O., M. G. Bassett, A. Kuryba et al. "Thirty-Day Mortality in Patients Undergoing Laparotomy for Small Bowel Obstruction." *British Journal of Surgery* 105 (2018): 1006–1013.

7 Akrami, Majid and Mohammad Reza Sasani. "Dietary Habits Affect Quality of Life: Bowel Obstruction Caused by Phytobezoar." *Iranian Journal of Public Health* 45, no. 8 (August 2016): 1080–1082.

8 Sealey, Andrew J. and Ngee-Soon Lau. "Peanut Phytobezoar: An Unusual Cause for Small Bowel Obstruction." *Journal of Surgical Case Reports* 8 (2024): rjae564.

9 Wei, Kuang-Yu, Chih-Chien Sung, and Shih-Hua Lin. "Phytobezoar-Induced Small Bowel Obstruction in an Elderly Patient Undergoing Dialysis: A Case Report." *Journal of International Medical Research* 48, no. 10 (October 2020): 0300060520962942.

10 Rice, Amanda D., Kimberly Patterson, Evette D. Reed et al. "Decreasing Recurrent Bowel Obstructions, Improving Quality of Life with Physiotherapy: Controlled Study." *World Journal of Gastroenterology* 24, no. 19 (May 21, 2018): 2108–2119.

IRRITABLE BOWEL SYNDROME (IBS)

1 Jones, Roger. "Irritable Bowel Syndrome: Management of Expectations and Disease." *British Journal of General Practice* 54, no. 504 (July 1, 2004): 490–491.

2 Matsueda, K., S. Fukudo, M. Ogishima et al. "Efficacy and Safety of Peppermint Oil for the Treatment in Japanese Patients with Irritable Bowel Syndrome: A Prospective, Open-Label, and Single-Arm Study." *BioPsychoSocial Medicine* 18 (2024): 3.

3 Khanna, Reena, John K. MacDonald, and Barrett G. Levesque. "Peppermint Oil for the Treatment of Irritable Bowel Syndrome: A Systematic Review and Meta-Analysis." *Journal of Clinical Gastroenterology* 48 (2014): 505–512.

4 Qi, Ling-Yu, Jing-Wen Yang, Shi-Yan Yan et al. "Acupuncture for the Treatment of Diarrhea-Predominant Irritable Bowel Syndrome: A Pilot Randomized Clinical Trial." *JAMA Network Open* 5, no. 12 (2022): e2248817.

5 Bensoussan, Alan, John E. Kellow, Suzannah J. Bourchier et al. "Efficacy of a Chinese Herbal Medicine in Providing Adequate Relief of Constipation-Predominant Irritable Bowel Syndrome: A Randomized Controlled Trial." *Clinical Gastroenterology and Hepatology* 13 (2015): 1946–1954.

6 Mezzasalma, V., E. Manfrini, E. Ferri et al. "A Randomized, Double-Blind, Placebo-Controlled Trial: The Efficacy of Multispecies Probiotic Supplementation in Alleviating Symptoms of

Irritable Bowel Syndrome Associated with Constipation." *BioMed Research International* 2016 (2016): 4740907.

7 Lembo, Anthony, Mark Pimentel, Satish S. Rao et al. "Repeat Treatment with Rifaximin Is Safe and Effective in Patients with Diarrhea-Predominant Irritable Bowel Syndrome." *Gastroenterology* 151 (2016): 1113–1121.

8 Pohl, Daniel, Michael Fried, Dominic Lawrence et al. "Multicentre, Non-Interventional Study of the Efficacy and Tolerability of Linaclotide in the Treatment of Irritable Bowel Syndrome with Constipation in Primary, Secondary and Tertiary Centres: The Alpine Study." *BMJ Open* 9 (2019): e025627.

9 Chey, William D., Anthony J. Lembo, Bernard J. Lavins et al. "Linaclotide for Irritable Bowel Syndrome with Constipation: A 26-Week, Randomized, Double-Blind, Placebo-Controlled Trial to Evaluate Efficacy and Safety." *American Journal of Gastroenterology* 107 (2012): 1702–1712.

10 Brenner, Darren M., Spencer D. Dorn, Ronald P. Fogel et al. "Plecanatide Improves Symptoms of Irritable Bowel Syndrome with Constipation: Results of an Integrated Efficacy and Safety Analysis of Two Phase 3 Trials." *International Journal of General Medicine* 16 (2023): 3769–3777.

11 Abdul-Baki, Heitham, Ihab I. El Hajj, Lara ElZahabi et al. "A Randomized Controlled Trial of Imipramine in Patients with Irritable Bowel Syndrome." *World Journal of Gastroenterology* 15, no. 29 (2009): 3636–3642.

12 Ducrotte, P., J. C. Grimaud, M. Dapoigny et al. "On-Demand Treatment with Alverine Citrate/Simeticone Compared with Standard Treatments for Irritable Bowel Syndrome: Results of a Randomised, Pragmatic Study." *International Journal of Clinical Practice* 68, no. 2 (February 2014): 245–254.

13 Mitchell, S. A., A. S. Mee, G. D. Smith et al. "Alverine Citrate Fails to Relieve the Symptoms of Irritable Bowel Syndrome: Results of a Double-Blind, Randomized, Placebo-Controlled Trial." *Alimentary Pharmacology and Therapeutics* 16, no. 6 (June 2002): 1187–1195.

14 Ford, Alexander C., Alexandra Wright-Hughes, Sarah L. Alderson et al. "Amitriptyline at Low-Dose and Titrated for Irritable Bowel Syndrome as Second-Line Treatment in Primary Care (ATLANTIS): A Randomised, Double-Blind, Placebo-Controlled, Phase 3 Trial." *Lancet* 402 (2023): 1773–1785.

15 Halmos, Emma P., Victoria A. Power, Susan J. Shepherd et al. "A Diet Low in FODMAPs Reduces Symptoms of Irritable Bowel Syndrome." *Gastroenterology* 146 (2014): 67–75.

16 Staudacher, H. M., K. Whelan, P. M. Irving, and M. C. E. Lomer. "Comparison of Symptoms Response Following Advice for a Diet Low in Fermentable Carbohydrates (FODMAPS) Versus Standard Dietary Advice in Patients with Irritable Bowel Syndrome." *Journal of Human Nutrition and Dietetics* 24, no. 5 (October 2011): 487–495.

LACTOSE INTOLERANCE

1 Robles, Luelle and Ronny Priefer. "Lactose Intolerance: What Your Breath Can Tell You." *Diagnostics* 10 (2020): 412.

2 https://www.alliedmarketresearch.com/lactose-free-dairy-market-A18453#:~:text=Lactose%2DFree%20Dairy%20Market%20Research,made%20from%20lactose%2Dfree%20milk.

3 Luelle and Priefer. "Lactose Intolerance: What Your Breath Can Tell You."

4 https://www.ncbi.nlm.nih.gov/books/NBK534631/

5 Dekker, P., D. Koenders, and M. Bruins. "Lactose-Free Dairy Products: Market Developments, Production, Nutrition and Health Benefits." *Nutrients* 11 (2019): 551.

6 Barr, Susan I. "Perceived Lactose Intolerance in Adult Canadians: A National Survey." *Applied Physiology, Nutrition, and Metabolism* 38 (2013): 830–835.

7 Cassellas, F., A. Aparici, M. J. Pérez, and P. Rodríguez. "Perception of Lactose Intolerance Impairs Health-Related Quality of Life." *European Journal of Clinical Nutrition* 70 (2016): 1068–1072.

8 Baijal, Rajiv and Rakesh K. Tandon. "Effect of Lactase on Symptoms and Hydrogen Breath Levels in Lactose Intolerance: A Crossover Placebo-Controlled Study." *JGH Open* 5 (2021): 143–148.

9 Levri, Kara M., Kari Ketvertis, Mark Deramo et al. "Do Probiotics Reduce Adult Lactose Intolerance? A Systematic Review." *Journal of Family Practice* 54, no. 7 (July 2005): 613–620.

10 Tanpowpong, P., W. Aekplakorn, S. Chariyalertsak et al. "Higher Milk Consumption Is Associated with a Lower Risk of Diabetes Mellitus: A Case-Control Study." *PLoS ONE* 18, no. 8 (2023): e0289762

11 Mansouri, M., N. Pahlavani, F. Sharifi et al. "Dairy Consumption in Relation to Hypertension Among a Large Population of University Students: The MEPHASOUS Study." *Diabetes, Metabolic Syndrome and Obesity: Targets and Therapy* 13 (2020): 1633–1642.

12 Nicklas, Theresa A., Haiyan Qu, Sheryl O. Hughes et al. "Self-Perceived Lactose Intolerance Results in Lower Intakes of Calcium and Dairy Foods and Is Associated with Hypertension and Diabetes." *American Journal of Clinical Nutrition* 94 (2011): 191–198.

13 Buchowski, M. S., J. Semenya, and A. O. Johnson. "Dietary Calcium Intake in Lactose Maldigesting Intolerant and Tolerant African-American Women." *Journal of the American College of Nutrition* 21, no. 1 (2002): 47–54.

14 Morency, Marie-Elssa, Catherine S. Birken, Gerald Lebovic et al. "Association Between Noncow Milk Beverage Consumption and Childhood Height." *American Journal of Clinical Nutrition* 106, no. 2 (August 2017): 597–602.

15 Gui, J.-C., J. R. Brašić, X.-D. Liu et al. "Bone Mineral Density in Postmenopausal Chinese Women Treated with Calcium Fortification in Soymilk and Cow's Milk." *Osteoporosis International* 23 (2012): 1563–1570.

16 Black, Ruth E., Sheila M. Williams, Ianthe E. Jones, and Ailsa Goulding. "Children Who Avoid Drinking Cow Milk Have Low Dietary Calcium Intakes and Poor Bone Health." *American Journal of Clinical Nutrition* 76 (2002): 675–680.

17 Schuster, Margaret J., Xinyue Wang, Tiffany Hawkins, and James E. Painter. "Comparison of the Nutrient Content of Cow's Milk and Nondairy Milk Alternatives: What's the Difference?" *Nutrition Today* 53, no. 4 (July/August 2018): 153–159.

18 Singhal, Sarita, Robert D. Baker, and Susan S. Baker. "A Comparison of the Nutritional Value of Cow's Milk and Nondairy Beverages." *Journal of Pediatric Gastroenterology and Nutrition* 64, no. 5 (May 2017): 799–805.

METABOLIC DYSFUNCTION-ASSOCIATED STEATOTIC LIVER DISEASE

1 Oh, Sechang, Takashi Shida, Kazumasa Yamagishi et al. "Moderate to Vigorous Physical Activity Volume is An Important Factor for Managing Nonalcoholic Fatty Liver Disease: A Retrospective Study." *Hepatology* 61, no. 4 (April 2015): 1205–1215.

2 Deshpande, K., J. Olynyk, O. Ayonrinde, and K. Nosaka. "Barriers to Exercise in Patients with Metabolic Dysfunction-Associated Steatotic Liver Disease: A Patient Survey." *Journal of Clinical Medicine Research* 16, no. 2–3 (2024): 94–105.

3 Ryan, Marno C., Catherine Itsiopoulos, Tania Thodis et al. "The Mediterranean Diet Improves Hepatic Steatosis and Insulin Sensitivity in Individuals with Non-Alcoholic Fatty Liver Disease." *Journal of Hepatology* 59, no. 1 (July 2013): 138–143.

4 Deshmukh, Aniket, Vikrant Sood, Bikrant Bihari Lal et al. "Effect of Indo-Mediterranean Diet Versus Calorie-Restricted Diet in Children with Non-Alcoholic Fatty Liver Disease: A Pilot Randomized Control Trial." *Pediatric Obesity* 19, no. 11 (November 2024): e13163.

5 Akhavan Rezayat, Arash, Malihe Dadgar Moghadam, Mohammad Ghasemi Nour et al. "Association Between Smoking and Non-Alcoholic Fatty Liver Disease: A Systematic Review and Meta-Analysis." *SAGE Open Medicine* 6 (January 2018): 205031211745223.

6 Zelber-Sagi, Shira, Dana Ivancovsky-Wajcman, Naomi Fliss Isakov et al. "High Red and Processed Meat Consumption is Associated with Non-Alcoholic Fatty Liver Disease and Insulin Resistance." *Journal of Hepatology* 68 (2018): 1239–1246.

7 Raj, S. V., M. Ismail, W. K. Chan, and H. A. Majid. "A Systematic Review on Factors Associated with Non-Alcoholic Fatty Liver Disease (NAFLD) Among Adolescents." *Clinical Nutrition ESPEN* 57 (2023): 131–137.

8 Promrat, K., D. E. Kleiner, H. M. Niemeier et al. "Randomized Controlled Trial Testing the Effects of Weight Loss on Nonalcoholic Steatohepatitis (NASH)." *Hepatology* 51, no. 1 (January 2010): 121–129.

9 Xue, Yaqi, Yang Peng, Litian Zhang et al. "Effect of Different Exercise Modalities on Nonalcoholic Fatty Liver Disease: A Systematic Review and Network Meta-Analysis." *Scientific Reports* 14 (2024): 6212.

10 Hallworth, Kate, Gulnar Fattakhova, Kieren G. Hollingsworth et al. "Resistance Exercise Reduces Liver Fat and Its Mediators in Non-Alcoholic Fatty Liver Disease Independent of Weight Loss." *Gut* 60 (2011): 1278–1283.

11 Benjaminov, O., N. Beglaibter, L. Gindy et al. "The Effect of a Low-Carbohydrate Diet on the Nonalcoholic Fatty Liver in Morbidly Obese Patients Before Bariatric Surgery." *Surgical Endoscopy* 21 (2007): 1423–1427.

12 Kaewdech, A., S. Assawasuwannakit, C. Churuangsuk et al. "Effect of Smartphone-Assisted Lifestyle Intervention in MASLD Patients: A Randomized Controlled Trial." *Scientific Reports* 14 (2024): 13961.

13 Basu, Patrick P., Niraj J. Shah, Mark M. Aloysius, and Robert S. Brown Jr. "Effects of Vitamin E and Alpha Lipoic Acid in Nonalcoholic Fatty Liver Disease: A Randomized, Placebo-Controlled, Open-Label, Prospective Clinical Trial (VAIN Trial)." *Open Journal of Gastroenterology* 4, no. 5 (2014): 199–207.

14 Lavine, Joel E., Jeffrey B. Schwimmer, Mark L. Van Natta et al. "Effect of Vitamin E or Metformin for Treatment of Nonalcoholic Fatty Liver Disease in Children and Adolescents." *JAMA* 305, no. 16 (April 27, 2011): 1659–1668.

MICROSCOPIC COLITIS

1 Madisch, Ahmed, Peter Heymer, Claudia Voss et al. "Oral Budesonide Therapy Improves Quality of Life in Patients with Collagenous Colitis." *International Journal of Colorectal Disease* 20 (2005): 312–316.

2 Baert, Filip, Alain Schmit, Geert D'Haens et al. "Budesonide in Collagenous Colitis: A Double-Blind Placebo-Controlled Trial with Histologic Follow-Up." *Gastroenterology* 122 (2002): 20–25.

3 Mehlke, Stephan, Ahmed Madisch, Birgit Bethke et al. "Oral Budesonide for Maintenance Treatment of Collagenous Colitis: A Randomized, Double-Blind, Placebo-Controlled Trial." *Gastroenterology* 135 (2008): 1510–1516.

4 Nimri, Faisal M., Adel Muhanna, Zain Almonani et al. "The Association Between Microscopic Colitis and Celiac Disease: A Systematic Review and Meta-Analysis." *Annals of Gastroenterology* 35 (2022): 281–289.

5 Sandler, Robert S., Shan Sun, Temitope O. Keku et al. "Dietary Calcium and Risk of Microscopic Colitis." *Clinical and Translational Gastroenterology* 16, no. 6 (February 24, 2023): e00569.

6 Lorinczy, Katalin, Gábor Lakatos, Katalin Müllnner et al. "Low Bone Mass in Microscopic Colitis." *BMC Gastroenterology* 11 (2011): 58.

7 Rancz, Anett, Brigitta Teutsch, Marie Anne Engh et al. "Microscopic Colitis is a Risk Factor for Low Bone Density: A Systematic Review and Meta-Analysis." *Therapeutic Advances in Gastroenterology* 16 (June 15, 2023): NA.

8 Wildt, Signe, Lars K. Munck, Sabine Becker et al. "Risk of Osteoporosis in Microscopic Colitis." *Postgraduate Medicine* 130, no. 3 (2018): 348–354.

9 Forss, Anders, David Bergman, Bjorn Roelstraete et al. "Patients with Microscopic Colitis Are at High Risk of Major Adverse Cardiovascular Events: A Matched Cohort Study." *Clinical Gastroenterology and Hepatology* 21 (2023): 3356–3364.

10 Kane, John S., Andrew J. Irvine, Yannick Derwa et al. "High Prevalence of Irritable Bowel Syndrome-Type Symptoms in Microscopic Colitis: Implications for Treatment." *Therapeutic Advances in Gastroenterology* 11 (January 2018): 1756284818783600.

11 Bergman, David, Bjorn Roelstraete, Jiangwei Sun et al. "Psychiatric Disorders Among 5,800 Patients with Microscopic Colitis: A Nationwide Population-Based Matched Cohort Study." *American Journal of Gastroenterology* 119, no. 12 (December 2024): 2516-2525.

12 Bergman, David, Bjorn Roelstraete, Jiangwei Sun et al. "Microscopic Colitis and Risk of Incident Psoriasis: A Nationwide Population-Based Matched Cohort Study." *Clinical Epidemiology* 16 (2024a): 213–225.

13 Kane, John S., Andrew J. Irvine, Yannick Derwa, and Alexander C. Ford. "Fatigue and Its Associated Factors in Microscopic Colitis." *Therapeutic Advances in Gastroenterology* 11 (September 13, 2018): NA.

14 Sjöberg, Klas, Lina Vigren, Bodil Roth et al. "Vitamin D Levels in Microscopic Colitis." *Scandinavian Journal of Gastroenterology* 48 (2013): 987–988.

15 Larsson, J. K., E. Sonestedt, B. Ohlsson et al. "The Association Between the Intake of Specific Dietary Components and Lifestyle Factors and Microscopic Colitis." *European Journal of Clinical Nutrition* 70 (2016): 1309–1317.

16 Bonderup, Ole K., Gunnar L. Nielsen, Michael Dall et al. "Significant Association Between the Use of Different Proton Pump Inhibitors and Microscopic Colitis: A Nationwide Danish

Case-Control Study." *Alimentary Pharmacology & Therapeutics* 48, no. 6 (September 2018): 618–625.

17 Fine, Kenneth D. and Edward L. Lee. "Efficacy of Open-Label Bismuth Subsalicylate for the Treatment of Microscopic Colitis." *Gastroenterology* 114 (1998): 29–36.

PANCREATITIS

1 https://www.aafp.org/pubs/afp/issues/2007/0515/p1513.html#:~:text=Mild%20acute%20pancreatitis%20has%20a%20very%20low%20mortality%20rate%20(less,of%20sterile%20versus%20infected%20necrosis.

2 https://www.facs.org/media-center/press-releases/2023/largest-study-on-long-term-follow-up-of-chronic-pancreatitis-patients-highlights-need-for-closer-monitoring-after-surgery/.

3 Pannala, Rahul, Mark Kidd, and Irvin M. Modin. "Acute Pancreatitis: A Historical Perspective." *Pancreas* 38, no. 4 (May 2009): 355–366.

4 Navarro, Salvador. "Chronic Pancreatitis. Some Important Historical Aspects." *Gastroenterología y Hepatología* 41, no. 7 (August 2018): 474.e1–474.e8.

5 https://www.ncbi.nlm.nih.gov/books/NBK538337/.

6 Jøker-Jensen, Henriette, Anne Sofie Mathiasen, Marianne Køhler et al. "Micronutrient Deficits in Patients with Chronic Pancreatitis: Prevalence, Risk Factors and Pitfalls." *European Journal of Gastroenterology & Hepatology* 32 (2020): 1328–1334.

7 Martínez-Moneo, Emma, Serena Stigliano, Aleksandra Hedström et al. "Deficiency of Fat-Soluble Vitamins in Chronic Pancreatitis: A Systematic Review and Meta-Analysis." *Pancreatology* 16 (2016): 988–994.

8 Oskarsson, V., N. Orsini, O. Sadr-Azodi, and A. Wolk. "Fish Consumption and Risk of Non-Gallstone-Related Acute Pancreatitis: A Prospective Cohort Study." *American Journal of Clinical Nutrition* 101 (2015): 72–78.

9 Setiawan, Veronica Wendy, Stephen J. Pandol, Jacqueline Porcel et al. "Dietary Factors Reduce Risk of Acute Pancreatitis in a Large Multiethnic Cohort." *Clinical Gastroenterology and Hepatology* 15 (February 2017): 257–265.

10 Jang, Dong Kee, Jun Kyu Lee, Chan Yung Jung et al. "Electroacupuncture for Abdominal Pain Relief in Patients with Acute Pancreatitis: A Three-Arm Randomized Controlled Trial." *Journal of Integrative Medicine* 21, no. 6 (November 2023): 537–542.

11 Monaghan, Brenda, Ann Monaghan, Qurat Ul Ain et al. "Significantly Lower Physical Activity Participation in Individuals with Chronic Pancreatitis Compared to Controls: An Exploratory Study of Objectively Assessed Physical Activity Levels." *Digestive Surgery* 40 (2023): 69–75.

12 Parhiala, Mikael, Mika Ukkonen, Juhani Sand, and Johanna Laukkarinen. "Osteoporosis and Sarcopenia Are Common and Insufficiently Diagnosed Among Chronic Pancreatitis Patients." *BMC Gastroenterology* 23 (2023): 124.

13 Koh, Amanda, Olamide Oyende, David J. Humes, and Dileep N. Lobo. "Risk of Osteopenia, Osteoporosis and Osteoporotic Fractures in Patients with Chronic Pancreatitis: A Systematic Review and Meta-Analysis." *Clinical Nutrition* 42 (2023): 1086–1094.

14 Wiese, Mats, Simone Gärtner, Nele von Essen et al. "Malnutrition is Highly Prevalent in Patients with Chronic Pancreatitis and Characterized by Loss of Skeletal Muscle Mass but Absence of Impaired Physical Function." *Frontiers in Nutrition* 9 (June 2022): 889489.

15 Singh, S., S. Midha, N. Singh et al. "Dietary Counseling Versus Dietary Supplements for Malnutrition in Chronic Pancreatitis: A Randomized Controlled Trial." *Clinical Gastroenterology and Hepatology* 6 (2008): 353–359.

16 Du, Wei-Dong, Zu-Rong Yuan, Jian Sun et al. "Therapeutic Efficacy of High-Dose Vitamin C on Acute Pancreatitis and Its Potential Mechanisms." *World Journal of Gastroenterology* 9, no. 11 (2003): 2565–2569.

17 Siriwardena, Ajith K., James M. Mason, Srinivasan Balachandra et al. "Randomised, Double Blind, Placebo Controlled Trial of Intravenous Antioxidant (N-Acetylcysteine, Selenium, Vitamin C) Therapy in Severe Acute Pancreatitis." *Gut* 56 (2007): 1439–1444.

18 Huh, Ji Hye, Jae Woo Kim, and Kyong Joo Lee. "Vitamin D Deficiency Predicts Severe Acute Pancreatitis." *United European Gastroenterology Journal* 7, no. 1 (February 2019): 90–95.

19 Ocal, Serkan, Kubra Cerci, Osman Cagin Buldukoglu et al. "Effect of Serum Vitamin D Levels on the Severity of Acute Pancreatitis: A Prospective Study." *Pancreatology* 24 (2024): 206–210.

20 Yaghoobi, M., J. McNabb-Baltar, R. Bijarchi, and P. B. Cotton. "Pancreatic Enzyme Supplements Are not Effective for Relieving Abdominal Pain in Patients with Chronic Pancreatitis: Meta-Analysis and Systematic Review of Randomized Controlled Trials." *Canadian Journal of Gastroenterology and Hepatology* 2016 (2016): 8541839.

PEPTIC ULCER DISEASE

1 Salas, Maribel, Alexandra Ward, and Jaime Caro. "Are Proton Pump Inhibitors the First Choice for Acute Treatment of Gastric Ulcers? A Meta Analysis of Randomized Clinical Trials." *BMC Gastroenterology* 2 (July 15, 2002): 17.

2 Mo, Chen, Gang Sun, Yan-Zhi Wang et al. "PPI versus Histamine H2 Preceptor Antagonists for Prevention of Upper Gastrointestinal Injury Associated with Low-Dose Aspirin: Systematic Review and Meta-Analysis." *PLoS ONE* 10, no. 7 (2015): e0131558.

3 Schöttker, Ben, Mariam A. Adamu, Melanie N. Weck, and Hermann Brenner. "Helicobacter Pylori Infection Is Strongly Associated with Gastric and Duodenal Ulcers in a Large Prospective Study." *Clinical Gastroenterology and Hepatology* 10, no. 5 (May 2012): 487–493.

4 Pyo, J. H., H. Lee, J. E. Kim et al. "Obesity and Risk of Peptic Ulcer Disease: A Large-Scale Health Check-Up Cohort Study." *Nutrients* 11 (2019): 1288.

5 Andersen Bak, Inger, Torben Jørgensen, Olaf Bonnevie et al. "Smoking and Alcohol Intake as Risk Factors for Bleeding and Perforated Peptic Ulcers: A Population-Based Cohort Study." *Epidemiology* 11, no. 4 (July 2000): 434–439.

6 Yen, Pei-Chi, Jiun-Hung Geng, Pei-Yu Wu et al. "Secondhand Smoke Is Associated with Peptic Ulcer Disease and Gastroesophageal Reflux Disease in Non-Smoker in a Large Taiwanese Population Study." *Frontiers in Public Health* 12 (2024): 1450481.

7 Levenstein, Susan, Steffan Rosenstock, Rikke Kart Jacobsen et al. "Psychological Stress Increases Risk for Peptic Ulcer, Regardless of *Helicobacter pylori* Infection of Use of Nonsteroidal Anti-Inflammatory Drugs." *Clinical Gastroenterology and Hepatology* 13 (2015): 498–506.

8 Lee, Young Bok, Jihan Yu, Hyun Ho Choi et al. "The Association Between Peptic Ulcer Diseases and Mental Health Problems." *Medicine* 96, no. 34 (August 2017): e7828.

9 Goodwin, Renee D. and Murray B. Stein. "Generalized Anxiety Disorder and Peptic Ulcer Disease Among Adults in the United States." *Psychosomatic Medicine* 64 (2002): 862–866.

10 Yim, M., Hong, Keun Ho Kim, and Bum Ju Lee. "The Number of Household Members as a Risk Factor for Peptic Ulcer Disease." *Scientific Reports* 11 (2021): 5274.

11 Svanes, C., J. A. Søreide, A. Skarstein et al. "Smoking and Ulcer Perforation." *Gut* 41 (1997): 177–180.

12 Cheng, Y., C. A. Macera, D. R. Davis, and S. N. Blair. "Physical Activity and Peptic Ulcers." *Western Journal of Medicine* 173, no. 2 (August 2000): 101–107.

13 Leone, Alessandro, Carmen De la Fuente-Arrillaga, Mariano Valdrés Mas et al. "Association Between the Consumption of Ultra-Processed Foods and the Incidence of Peptic Ulcer Disease in the SUN Project: A Spanish Prospective Cohort Study." *European Journal of Nutrition* 63 (2024): 2367–2378.

14 Loke, Song-Seng and Wen-Cheng Li. "Peptic Ulcer Disease Associated with Central Obesity." *Journal of Personalized Medicine* 12 (2022): 1968.

15 Wu, Chieh-Hsin, Yi-Ching Tung, Chee-Yin Chai et al. "Increased Risk of Osteoporosis in Patients with Peptic Ulcer Disease." *Medicine* 95, no. 16 (April 2016): e3309.

16 Segawa, Kose, Yasumasa Niwa, Tomiyasu Arisawa et al. "Incidence of Peptic Ulcer in Men Is Inversely Correlated with Blood Pressure: Study in an Apparently Healthy Japanese Population." *American Journal of Gastroenterology* 90, no. 3 (1995): 399–402.

17 Ogura, M., Y. Yamaji, Y. Hikiba et al. "Gastric Cancer Among Peptic Ulcer Patients: Retrospective, Long-Term Follow-Up." *Digestive and Liver Disease* 38 (2006): 811–814.

ULCERATIVE COLITIS

1 https://www.crohnscolitisfoundation.org/about/our-beginning#:~:text=Ulcerative%20colitis%20was%20first%20described,diseases%20caused%20by%20infectious%20agents.

2 Sands, Bruce W., Laurent Peyrin-Biroulet, Edward V. Loftus et al. "Vedolizumab versus Adalimumab for Moderate-to-Severe Ulcerative Colitis." *New England Journal of Medicine* 381 (2019): 1215–1226.

3 Berinstein, Jeffrey A., Jessica Sheehan, Michael Dias et al. "Tofacitinib for Biologic-Experienced Hospitalized Patients with Acute Severe Ulcerative Colitis: A Retrospective Case-Control Study." *Clinical Gastroenterology and Hepatology* 19, no. 10 (October 2021): 2112–2120.

4 Hanauer, Stephen, Remo Panaccione, Silvio Danese et al. "Tofacitinib Induction Therapy Reduces Symptoms Within Three Days for Patients with Ulcerative Colitis." *Clinical Gastroenterology and Hepatology* 17 (2019): 139–147.

5 Wang, Xiao, Nan-qi Zhao, Yu-xin Sun et al. "Acupuncture for Ulcerative Colitis: A Systematic Review and Meta-Analysis of Randomized Clinical Trials." *BMC Complementary Therapies and Medicine* 20 (2020): 309.

6 Gilat, T., A. Suissa, G. Leichtman et al. "A Comparative Study of Metronidazole and Sulfasalazine in Active, Not Severe, Ulcerative Colitis." *Journal of Clinical Gastroenterology* 9, no. 4 (1987): 415–417.

7 Gilat, T., G. Leichtman, G. Delpre et al. "A Comparison of Metronidazole and Sulfasalazine in the Maintenance of Remission in Patients with Ulcerative Colitis." *Journal of Clinical Gastroenterology* 11, no. 4 (1989): 392–395.

8 Panaccione, Remo, Subrata Ghosh, Stephen Middleton et al. "Combination Therapy with Infliximab and Azathioprine is Superior to Monotherapy with Either Agent in Ulcerative Colitis." *Gastroenterology* 146 (2014): 392–400.

9 Ben-Horin, Shomron, Ofir Har-Noy, Konstantinos H. Katsanos et al. "Corticosteroids and Mesalamine Versus Corticosteroids for Acute Severe Ulcerative Colitis: A Randomized Controlled Trial." *Clinical Gastroenterology and Hepatology* 20, no. 12 (December 2022): 2868–2875.

10 Hou, Jason K., Bincy Abraham, Hashem El-Serag. "Dietary Intake and Risk of Developing Inflammatory Bowel Disease: A Systematic Review of the Literature." *American Journal of Gastroenterology* 106, no. 4 (April 2011): 563–573.

11 Weisshof, Roni and Irit Chermesh. "Micronutrient Deficiencies in Inflammatory Bowel Disease." *Current Opinion in Clinical Nutrition & Metabolic Care* 18,, no. 6 (November 2015): 576–581.

12 Pan, Yun, Ya Liu, Haizhuo Guo et al. "Associations Between Folate and Vitamin B12 Levels and Inflammatory Bowel Disease: A Meta-Analysis." *Nutrients* 9 (2017): 382.

13 Khazdouz, Maryam, Naser Ebrahimi Daryani, Makan Cheraghpour et al. "The Effect of Selenium Supplementation on Disease Activity and Immune-Inflammatory Biomarkers in Patients with Mild-to-Moderate Ulcerative Colitis: A Randomized, Double-Blind, Placebo-Controlled Clinical Trial." *European Journal of Nutrition* 62, no. 8 (December 2023): 3125–3134.

14 Fritsch, Julia, Luis Garces, Maria A. Quintero et al. "Low-Fat, High-Fiber Diet Reduces Markers of Inflammation and Dysbiosis and Improves Quality of Life in Patients with Ulcerative Colitis." *Clinical Gastroenterology and Hepatology* 19 (2021): 1189–1199.

15 Tarar, Zahid Ijaz, Umer Farooq, Muhammad Usman Zafar et al. "A National Study of Pregnancy-Related Maternal and Fetal Outcomes in Women with Inflammatory Bowel Disease." *International Journal of Colorectal Disease* 37 (2022): 1535–1543.

INDEX

ABOUT THE AUTHORS

Myrna Chandler Goldstein, MA, has been a freelance writer and independent scholar for more than thirty-five years. She is the author of Bloomsbury's *Treatments for Anxiety: Fact versus Fiction* and *Pain Management: Fact versus Fiction* and other Bloomsbury books.

Mark A. Goldstein, MD, is the founding chief emeritus of the Division of Adolescent and Young Adult Medicine at Massachusetts General Hospital and Associate Professor of Pediatrics at Harvard Medical School. He is co-author of *Treatments for Anxiety: Fact versus Fiction* and *Pain Management: Fact versus Fiction.*